Advanced Electroencephalography Analytical Methods

Advanced Electroencephalography Analytical Methods: Fundamentals, Acquisition, and Applications presents the theoretical basis and applications of electroencephalography (EEG) signals in neuroscience, involving signal analysis, processing, signal acquisition, representation, and applications of EEG signal analysis using nonlinear approaches and machine learning. It explains the principles of neurophysiology, linear signal processing, computational intelligence, and the nature of signals including machine learning. Applications involve computer-aided diagnosis, brain-computer interfaces, rehabilitation engineering, and applied neuroscience.

This book:

- Includes a comprehensive review of biomedical signals nature and acquisition aspects.
- Focuses on selected applications of neuroscience/cardiovascular/muscle-related biomedical areas.
- Provides a machine learning update to a classical biomedical signal processing approach.
- Explains deep learning and its application to biomedical signal processing and analysis.
- Explores relevant biomedical engineering and neuroscience state-of-the-art applications.

This book is intended for researchers and graduate students in biomedical signal processing, electrical engineering, neuroscience, and computer science.

Biomedical Signal and Image Processing

Series Editor: Ganesh Naik, *MARCS Institute for Brain, Behaviour, and Development, Western Sydney University, Sydney, Australia*

Biomedical signal and image processing involves the analysis of physiological measurements to provide useful information upon which clinicians can make decisions. Working with traditional bio-measurement tools, the signals and images can be computed by software to provide physicians with real-time data and greater insights to aid in clinical assessments. These challenges motivate the further study of biomedical signal and image analysis, and this book series intends to report the new results of these efforts. Topic coverage aims to include neurological signal processing, pathological speech signal analysis, electromyography (EMG) signal processing, electroencephalography (EEG), electrocardiography (ECG), brain-computer interface (BCI), and all associated analytical techniques. This book series is intended for both biomedical engineers and clinicians (researchers and graduate students) who wish to get novel research ideas and some training in theory and recent advances in clinical, neural engineering and biomedical signal/image processing applications.

Biomedical Signal Processing

A Modern Approach

Edited by Ganesh Naik and Wellington Pinheiro dos Santos

Advanced Electroencephalography Analytical Methods

Fundamentals, Acquisition, and Applications

Edited by Ganesh Naik, Wellington Pinheiro dos Santos, and Gaetano Gargiulo

For more information about this series, please visit www.routledge.com/Biomedical-Signal-and-Image-Processing/book-series/BSIP

Advanced Electroencephalography Analytical Methods

Fundamentals, Acquisition, and Applications

Edited by
Ganesh Naik, Wellington Pinheiro dos Santos,
and Gaetano Gargiulo

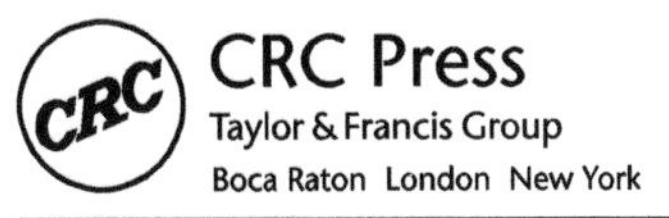

CRC Press
Taylor & Francis Group
Boca Raton London New York

CRC Press is an imprint of the
Taylor & Francis Group, an **informa** business

Designed cover image: Shutterstock

MATLAB® is a trademark of The MathWorks, Inc., and is used with permission. The MathWorks does not warrant the accuracy of the text or exercises in this book. This book's use or discussion of MATLAB® software or related products does not constitute endorsement or sponsorship by The MathWorks of a particular pedagogical approach or particular use of the MATLAB® software.

First edition published 2025
by CRC Press
2385 NW Executive Center Drive, Suite 320, Boca Raton FL 33431

and by CRC Press
4 Park Square, Milton Park, Abingdon, Oxon, OX14 4RN

CRC Press is an imprint of Taylor & Francis Group, LLC

Library of Congress Cataloging-in-Publication Data
Names: Naik, Ganesh R., editor. | Santos, Wellington Pinheiro dos, editor.
| Gargiulo, Gaetano, editor.
Title: Advanced electroencephalography analytical methods : fundamentals,
acquisition, and applications / edited by Ganesh Naik, Wellington
Pinheiro dos Santos, and Gaetano Gargiulo.
Description: First edition. | Boca Raton FL : CRC Press, 2025. | Includes
bibliographical references and index. Identifiers: LCCN 2024026279 (print) | LCCN 2024026280 (ebook) |
ISBN 9781032171708 (hardback) | ISBN 9781032171715 (paperback) | ISBN
9781003252092 (ebook)
Subjects: MESH: Electroencephalography | Signal Processing,
Computer-Assisted | Image Interpretation, Computer-Assisted—methods |
Brain-Computer Interfaces | Brain Diseases—diagnosis
Classification: LCC RC386.6.E43 (print) | LCC RC386.6.E43 (ebook) | NLM
WL 150 | DDC 616.8/047547—dc23/eng/20241010
LC record available at https://lccn.loc.gov/2024026279
LC ebook record available at https://lccn.loc.gov/2024026280

ISBN: 978-1-032-17170-8 (hbk)
ISBN: 978-1-032-17171-5 (pbk)
ISBN: 978-1-003-25209-2 (ebk)

DOI: 10.1201/9781003252092

Typeset in Times
by codeMantra

Contents

SECTION I   EEG Applications and Challenges

SECTION II   EEG – Signal Processing

SECTION III   EEG – Signal Classification

About the Editors

Ganesh Naik ranked in the top 2% of researchers in biomedical engineering (Stanford University Research), is a leading expert in biomedical engineering and signal processing. He received his Ph.D. degree in electronics engineering, specializing in biomedical engineering and signal processing, from Royal Melbourne Institute of Technology (RMIT) University, Melbourne, Australia, in December 2009. Currently, he is an academic and research theme co-lead at Flinders University, Adelaide, Australia. He held a Postdoctoral Research Fellow position at the MARCS Institute, Western Sydney University (WSU), between July 2017 and July 2020 and worked on a Cooperative Research Centres (CRC) project for sleep. During his tenure at WSU, he has developed several novel algorithms for wearables related to sleep projects. Before that, he held a Chancellor's Post-Doctoral Research Fellowship position in the Centre for Health Technologies, University of Technology Sydney (UTS), between February 2013 and June 2017. As a mid-career researcher, he has edited 12 books and authored around 150 papers in peer-reviewed journals and conferences. He serves as an associate editor for *IEEE Access, Frontiers in Neurorobotics*, and two Springer journals (*Circuits, Systems, and Signal Processing* and *Australasian Physical & Engineering Sciences in Medicine*). He is a Baden–Württemberg Scholarship recipient from Berufsakademie, Stuttgart, Germany (2006–2007). In 2010, he was awarded an ISSI overseas fellowship from Skilled Institute Victoria, Australia.

Wellington Pinheiro dos Santos holds a degree in electrical and electronic engineering (2001) and a master's degree in electrical engineering (2003) from the Federal University of Pernambuco and a Ph.D. degree in electrical engineering from the Federal University of Campina Grande (2009). He is currently an associate professor (exclusive dedication) at the Department of Biomedical Engineering at the Center for Technology and Geosciences/School of Engineering of Pernambuco, Federal University of Pernambuco, working in the undergraduate program in biomedical engineering and the graduate program in biomedical engineering. He has also been a member of the graduate program in computer engineering at Escola Politécnica de Pernambuco, Universidade de Pernambuco, since 2009. He has experience in the field of computer science, with an emphasis on graphics processing, working mainly in the following areas: digital image processing, pattern recognition, computer vision, evolutionary computing, numerical optimization methods, computational intelligence, image formation techniques, virtual reality, game design, and applications of computing and engineering in medicine and biology. He is a member of the Brazilian Society of Biomedical Engineering (SBEB), the Brazilian Society of Computational Intelligence (SBIC, ex-SBRN), and the International Federation of Medical and Biological Engineering (IFMBE).

Gaetano Gargiulo received his Ph.D. degree in biomedical engineering from the University of Bologna, Bologna, Italy, in 2010. Currently, he is a research professor at the School of Engineering, Design and Built Environment, Western Sydney University. He is also a research affiliate at the "Federico II" University of Naples, Naples, Italy. His research interests include medical instrumentation/devices, telemedicine, human-computer interfaces, and bio-inspired systems. He is a coauthor of more than 100 papers in these research areas and has edited four scholarly books in applied biomedical engineering; he is an inventor on 10 patents and has contributed to spin out four commercial companies all in the field of biomedical engineering.

Contributors

Sheikh Farhana Binte Ahmed
Department of Electrical and Electronic
  Engineering
Islamic University of Technology
Gazipur, Bangladesh

Jarina Akter
Department of Electrical and Electronic
  Engineering
Independent University
Dhaka, Bangladesh

Shafiq Alam
School of Management
Massey University
Auckland, New Zealand

Maisha Anjum
Department of Electrical and Electronic
  Engineering
Independent University
Dhaka, Bangladesh

Anusha A N
Department of ECE
BNM Institute of Technology
Bengaluru, India

M Krishna Chaitanya
School of Electronics Engineering
VIT-AP University
Amaravati, India

Yi-Hsuan Cheng
Department of Electrical and Electronic
  Engineering
School of Engineering
RMIT University
Melbourne, Australia

**Belmira Lara da Silveira
Andrade da Costa**
Department of Physiology and
  Pharmacology
Universidade Federal de Pernambuco
Recife, Brazil

Júlio César Sousa Dantas
Neurobots Research and Development
  Ltd
Recife, Brazil

**Jeniffer Emídio de Almeida
Albuquerque**
Department of Physiology and
  Pharmacology
Universidade Federal de Pernambuco
Recife, Brazil

Vitor de Carvalho Hazin
Neurobots Research and Development
  Ltd
Recife, Brazil

Marília Marinho de Lucena
Department of Physiology and
  Pharmacology
Universidade Federal de Pernambuco
Recife, Brazil

José Antonio Alves de Menezes
University of Pernambuco
Recife, Brazil

Igor Tchaikovsky Mello de Oliveirab
Department of Physiology and
  Pharmacology
Universidade Federal de Pernambuco
Recife, Brazil

Kusumika Krora Dutta
Electrical & Electronics Engineering
M. S. Ramaiah Institute of Technology
Bengaluru, India

Tasnuva Faruk
Department of Electrical and Electronic
    Engineering
Independent University
Dhaka, Bangladesh

Juliana Carneiro Gomes
Department of Biomedical Engineering
Universidade Federal de Pernambuco
Recife, Brazil

Mehedi Hasan
Department of Electrical and Electronic
    Engineering
Independent University
Dhaka, Bangladesh

Md. Kafiul Islam
Department of Electrical and Electronic
    Engineering
Independent University
Dhaka, Bangladesh

Margaret Lech
Department of Electrical and Electronic
    Engineering
School of Engineering
RMIT University
Melbourne, Australia

Saiful Islam Leon
Department of Electrical and Electronic
    Engineering
Independent University
Dhaka, Bangladesh

Sourav Maity
Department of Instrumentation &
    Control Engineering
Dr. BR Ambedkar National Institute of
    Technology
Jalandhar, India

Chetan S Mukundan
Axxonet System Technologies Pvt Ltd
Bengaluru, India

Jyoti R Munavalli
Department of ECE
BNM Institute of Technology
Bengaluru, India

Shafaq Mushtaq
Pakistan Institute of Medical Sciences
Islamabad, Pakistan

Abida Nazir
Department of Biomedical Engineering
    and Sciences
School of Mechanical and
    Manufacturing Engineering
National University of Sciences and
    Technology
Islamabad, Pakistan

Rabia Nazir
Electrical Engineering Department
National University of Sciences and
    Technology
Islamabad, Pakistan

Imran Khan Niazi
Center of Chiropractic Research
New Zealand College of Chiropractic
Auckland, New Zealand
Center for Sensory-Motor Interaction
Department of Health Science and
  Technology
Aalborg University
Aalborg, Denmark
Department of Clinical Sciences
Auckland University of Technology
Auckland, New Zealand

Pedro Luís Gurgel Nogueir
Federal University of Pernambuco
Recife, Brazil

Md. Tawhid Islam Opu
Department of Electrical and Electronic
  Engineering
Independent University
Dhaka, Bangladesh

Pooja
IIT Mandi iHub and HCi
  Foundation
Indian Institute of Technology
Himachal Pradesh, India

Marcelo Cairrão Araújo Rodrigues
Department of Physiology and
  Pharmacology
Universidade Federal de Pernambuco
Recife, Brazil

Nazmus Sakib
Department of Electrical and Electronic
  Engineering
Independent University
Dhaka, Bangladesh

Priya R Sankpal
Department of ECE
BNM Institute of Technology
Bengaluru, India

Arun Sasidharan
Scientist-C (Neurosciences)
Center for Consciousness Studies
Neurophysiology, NIMHANS
Bengaluru, India

Faisal Bin Shahin
Department of Electrical and Electronic
  Engineering
Independent University
Dhaka, Bangladesh

Lakhan Dev Sharma
School of Electronics Engineering
VIT-AP University
Amaravati, India

Sumit Sharma
Axxonet System Technologies Pvt Ltd
Bengaluru, India

Md. Ahsan-Ul Kabir Shawon
Department of Electrical and Electronic
  Engineering
Independent University
Dhaka, Bangladesh

K R Shylaja
Department of AIML
Ambedkar Institute of Technology
Bengaluru, India

Sumathi A
Department of ECE
BNM Institute of Technology
Bengaluru, India

Karan Veer
Department of Instrumentation &
    Control Engineering
Dr. BR Ambedkar National Institute of
    Technology
Jalandhar, India

Vrinda M
Axxonet Brain Research Lab
Axxonet System Technologies Pvt Ltd
Bengaluru, India
Department of Psychiatry
NIMHANS
Bengaluru, India
Center for Consciousness Studies
    Neurophysiology
NIMHANS
Bengaluru, India

Asim Waris
Department of Biomedical Engineering
    and Sciences
School of Mechanical and
    Manufacturing Engineering
National University of Sciences and
    Technology
Islamabad, Pakistan

Richardt H Wilkinson
Department of Electrical and Electronic
    Engineering
School of Engineering
RMIT University
Melbourne, Australia

Jammisetty Yedukondalu
School of Electronics Engineering
VIT-AP University
Amaravati, India

Preface

The use of electroencephalography (EEG) as a noninvasive measure of electrical brain activity to gather insight into human brain functions has seen tremendous growth across various disciplines due to the technology's increased ease of use and affordability. Recent advances in this field yield the potential to improve the accuracy and reliability of sleep staging, a plethora of brain disorder-related medical diagnoses, as well as precision medicine and therapy efficacy monitoring. This book presents recent advances in EEG applications.

Our editorial goal for this book is to bring together various scientific perspectives and research approaches related to EEG analysis that provide an integrated, cutting-edge overview of the field's current state. This edited book comprises contributions from leading researchers within various allied disciplines. This book is intended for biomedical signal processing experts, biomedical, computer science, and electronics engineers (researchers and graduate students) who wish to get novel research ideas and some training in EEG signal analysis, signal processing, and classification methods. Furthermore, the research results previously scattered in many scientific articles worldwide are collected methodically and presented in the book in a unified form.

This book is organized into three sections. The first section is devoted to *EEG Applications and Challenges*. In this section, we have collected four chapters with several novel contributions. The second section focuses on *EEG – Signal processing applications* and contains four chapters. The final section covers *EEG – Signal Classification* using novel machine learning methods and has three chapters.

We want to thank the authors for their excellent submissions (chapters) to this book, which have helped ensure this publication's high quality. With their contributions, this book could come successfully into existence.

Ganesh Naik, Wellington Pinheiro dos Santos,
and Gaetano Gargiulo

Section I

EEG Applications and Challenges

1 Diagnostic Applications of EEG Signal Patterns in Neuroscience

Arun Sasidharan, Sumit Sharma, Vrinda M, Kusumika Krora Dutta, and Chetan S Mukundan

1.1 INTRODUCTION

Electroencephalography (EEG) is the process of detecting, recording, and analysing the minute electrical activity emitted from the brain. The electrical signals could be acquired from the scalp (non-invasive), surface of the brain (invasive), and depth of the brain (invasive). EEG is an affordable medical technique that has been in clinical use for several decades. Often, its diagnostic application has been limited to visual interpretation for spike patterns in patients with epilepsy and for sleep stage determination in patients with sleep disorders. With advances in signal processing algorithms, increased computational power in portable devices, and accessibility to high-quality EEG devices, there is an opportunity to utilise the diagnostic power of EEG patterns in more areas and in a more application-friendly manner. On the contrary, neuroscience research using EEG has leaned towards acquiring high-density (>64 sensors) data and examining EEG patterns that need long and computationally intensive signal processing. Moreover, the inferences from such data are made at group level, which is not suitable for application at most clinical set-ups. In this chapter, we will introduce some approaches that could address a few of the above lacunae in the diagnostic application of EEG in neuroscience. In this chapter, we focus on three common mental health conditions, namely, epilepsy, schizophrenia, and chronic non-organic pain, to show how EEG-based methods could be used in clinical diagnosis and management, reducing the burden on clinical manpower. We then highlight the technical aspects of implementing or incorporating such research methods into practically viable software and hardware modules for clinical set-ups.

1.2 UNDERSTANDING OF EEG SIGNAL PATTERNS USED IN CLINICAL APPLICATIONS

In EEG, a series of scalp voltage values are repeatedly collected simultaneously from multiple sites from the scalp/brain, in ultrashort time intervals (usually in 1–8 ms intervals). So, an EEG signal can be interpreted in two ways – either as voltage

DOI: 10.1201/9781003252092-2

TABLE 1.1
Visually Appreciable EEG Features

Sl. No.	Visually Appreciable EEG Feature	What it Signifies
1	'Spike and wave pattern'	Epileptic episode
2	'Lambda waves'	Visual exploration
3	'Wicket waves'	Drowsy state
4	'Spindle waves'	Non-dream sleep stage
5	'Saw tooth waves'	Dreaming sleep stage
6	'Delta brush'	Encephalitis or brain inflammation
7	'Non-reactive' oscillations	Coma
8	'Generalised slowing'	Delirium or dementia
9	'Choppy activity' or irregular low amplitude fast activity	Psychosis or schizophrenia
10	Frontal intermittent rhythmic delta activity (FIRDA)	Chronic schizophrenia

waveforms from each scalp/brain site (this will look like an 'audio signal', like an electrocardiogram (ECG) recording) or as voltage maps across scalp sites and time (this will look like a 'video signal').

The 'audio signal' approach has been widely used among clinical experts and signal analysis experts alike. Clinical experts tend to describe the EEG waveforms in terms of their visually appreciable features (like shape, context, location, etc.), and there are numerous patterns identified and matched to possible brain states (see Table 1.1 and Figure 1.1) [1].

Signal analysis experts prefer to describe EEG waveforms in terms of their sinusoidal spectral features (like frequency, amplitude, phase, etc.), and several studies have identified their relation to various mental conditions (see Table 1.2 and Figure 1.2).

The 'video signal' approaches could provide important insights into the temporal dynamics of whole-brain neuronal networks as with EEG microstates (see [5] for a review). But such approaches are seldom used and will not be further discussed in this chapter.

1.3 SELECTING THE APPROPRIATE EEG SIGNAL ANALYSIS BASED ON MENTAL HEALTH CONDITION

In this section, we describe three different EEG signal analyses as examples to show how the domain knowledge on mental health conditions can help choose the appropriate analysis approach.

1.3.1 EEG Waveform Pattern Detection: For Early Detection of Epilepsy

1.3.1.1 What Is Epilepsy?

Epilepsy, commonly known in layman's term as fits, is considered a neural network disorder in current neuroscience research. It is characterised by aberrant hypersynchronous electrical discharges in neural networks and manifests as spontaneous

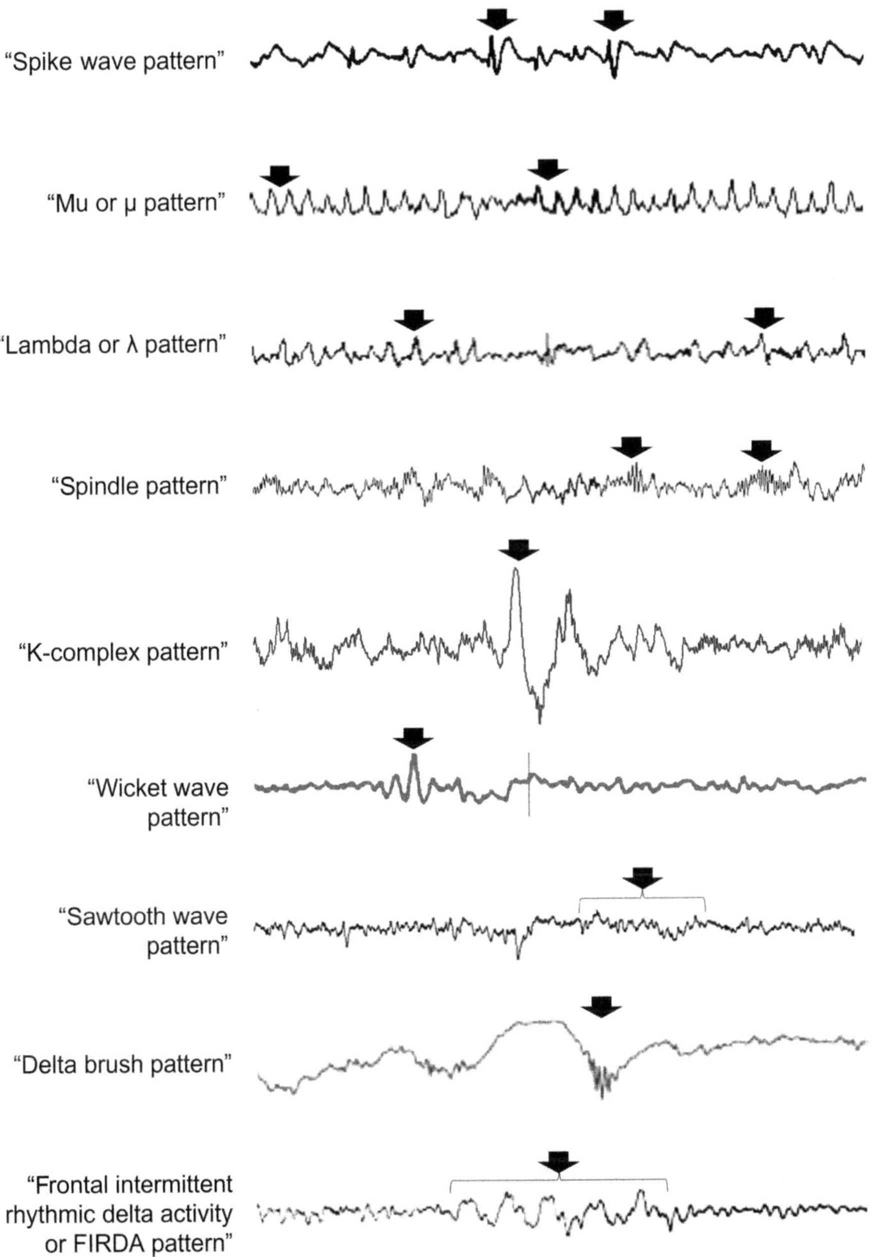

FIGURE 1.1 Examples of some visually appreciable EEG waveform patterns. The events are marked using a downward arrow.

TABLE 1.2
Sinusoidal Spectral EEG Features

Sl. No.	Sinusoidal Spectral EEG Feature	Associated Clinical Condition	Reference
1	Increase in delta absolute power	Depression, schizophrenia, ADHD, obsessive-compulsive disorder (OCD)	[2]
2	Increase in theta absolute power	Depression, schizophrenia, ADHD, OCD, alcohol addiction	[2]
3	Decrease in alpha absolute power	Schizophrenia, OCD	[2]
4	Increase in beta absolute power	Alcohol addiction, depression	[2]
5	Decrease in theta coherence in parietal region	Autism	[3]
6	Increase in delta and alpha coherence	Schizophrenia	[4]

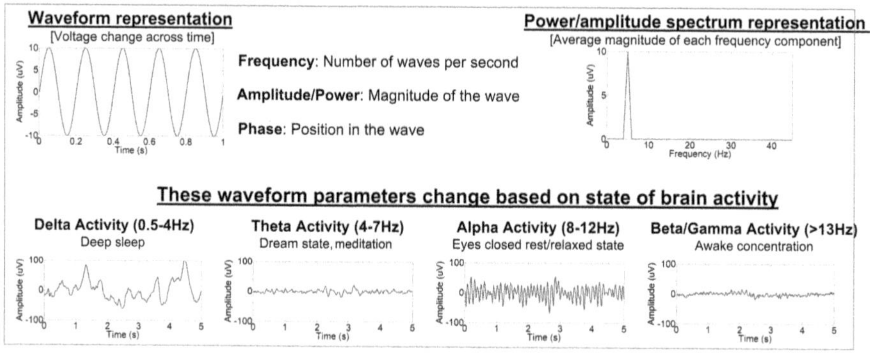

FIGURE 1.2   Sinusoidal and spectral features of EEG waveform.

recurrent behavioural and electrographic seizures. Generally, epilepsy is diagnosed after the spontaneous occurrence of two or three seizures (treatment may start even after a single seizure episode). As per the International League Against Epilepsy (ILAE; www.ilae.org), seizure types are classified into focal onset, generalised onset, and unknown onset, and epilepsy types are classified into focal, generalised, combined generalised and focal, and unknown. Generalised epilepsies may have a spectrum of seizure types, including absence, myoclonic, atonic, tonic, and tonic-clonic seizures. In addition to seizure types and epilepsy types, epilepsy can be categorised as epilepsy syndrome, which includes a cluster of features like seizure types, imaging, and EEG features occurring together. The epileptic discharges can be appreciated in the EEG recording. Figure 1.3a shows the EEG reading of a healthy person, whereas Figures 1.3b and c show the EEG recording of focal and generalised epileptic seizures, respectively. In the figure, it can be observed that focal epileptic discharges occur in localised brain regions, whereas generalised epileptic discharges occur across the entire brain. In some cases, a person may have more than one type of seizure classification, which makes the diagnosis more complicated. Therefore,

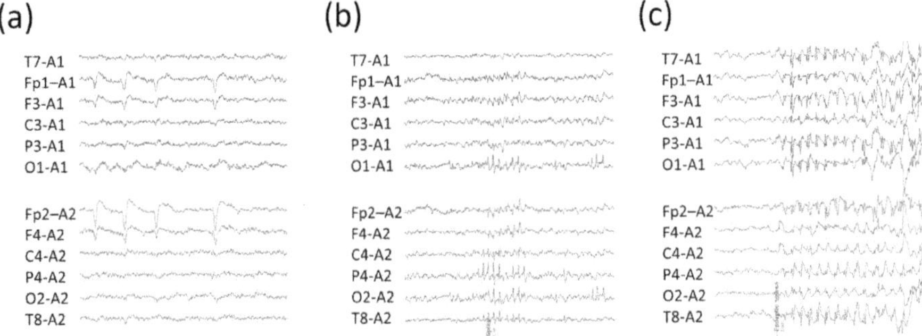

FIGURE 1.3 EEG showing (a) resting pattern in a healthy person (eye blinks are visible), (b) focal spikes in focal epilepsy, (c) widespread spikes in generalised epilepsy. Dark grey traces are from the left side of the head and light grey traces are from the right side.

regardless of the great progress made in drug treatment options for the different types of epilepsy and decades of worldwide research in this area, a major challenge lies in making correct diagnosis [6–8].

1.3.1.2 How Can EEG Waveform Pattern Detection Be Implemented for Epilepsy Diagnosis?

As discussed, EEG waveforms are random signals, but can show several complex morphological patterns. Such patterns are usually examined using template-matching algorithms. Many mathematical models, algorithms, and procedures have been applied to increase the accuracy of type detection from the EEG signals (which is the most used electrophysiological method in the clinical diagnosis of epilepsy). With the advent of deep learning, different signal analysis techniques are explored towards automated EEG pattern detection. Some of the most common deep learning techniques used to classify seizures include 1D-convolutional neural networks (CNNs); 2D-CNNs; recurrent neural networks (RNN); long short-term memory (LSTM) networks; pretrained networks like residual network (ResNet), visual geometry group (VGGNet), GoogleNet, and sparse autoencoders (SAEs) [9–25].

1.3.1.3 Deep Learning Techniques and Their Architectures

There are four major network architectures used in deep learning. Figure 1.4 shows the four main architectures along with their different varieties popularly used.

1.3.1.3.1 Unsupervised Pre-trained Networks (UPNs)

A challenge in deep learning is to train a model with many layers in deep networks using adaptive parameters. Here, the main function is an extremely non-convex function of the attributes. Because of this, many local minima are created in the parameter space of the model, and all these minima don't provide comparable errors. This requires optimisation of stochastic gradient descent (SGD), which can be better executed by starting the discriminative neural network with an unsupervised pre-trained network. This architecture is shown in Figure 1.5 with restricted Boltzmann machine (RBM) layers.

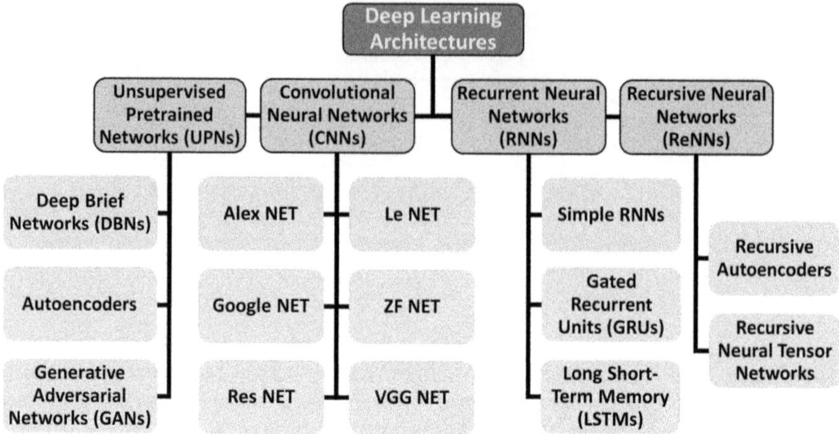

FIGURE 1.4   Different network architectures used in deep learning.

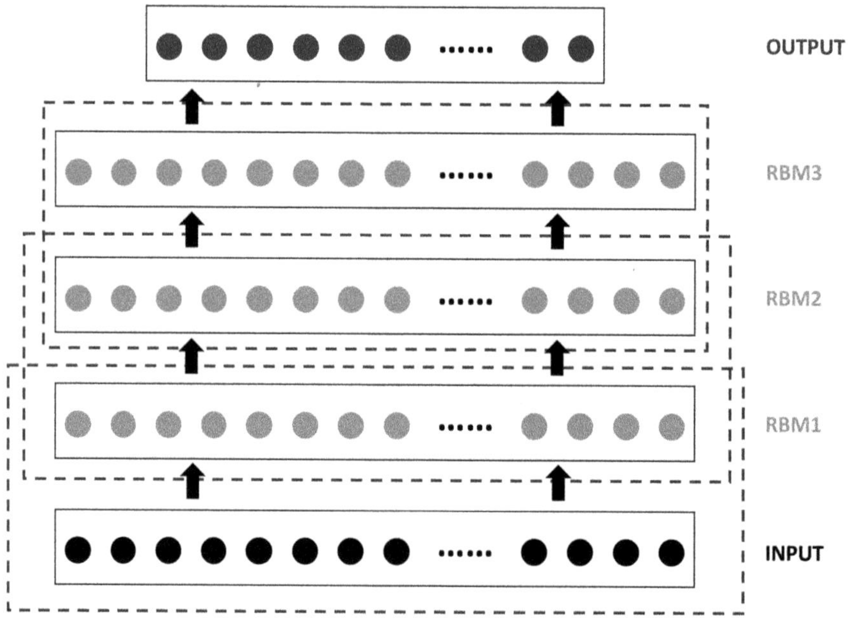

FIGURE 1.5   Unsupervised pre-trained network architecture.

This network can use three different architectures, and they are as follows:

1. Auto encoders
2. Deep belief networks
3. Generative adversarial networks

1.3.1.3.2 *Convolutional Neural Networks (CNN)*

CNN architecture basically has three types of layers, namely, input layer, convolutional layer, and output layer. In the convolutional layer, the main feature extraction step takes place through convolution, pooling, and activation. Figure 1.6 shows the architecture of deep CNNs.

1.3.1.3.3 *Recurrent Neural Networks (RNNs)*

The RNN consists of input, hidden, and output layers with a recurrent structure between the output and input layers, after completion of an epoch learning. A sequence data with finite length unfolds the self-loop of hidden neurons into a feedforward network that resembles the traditional network. The self-loop allows back propagation learning within hidden layers for weight updating in discrete steps and employs the same function for each neuron. The architecture of RNN is shown in Figure 1.7.

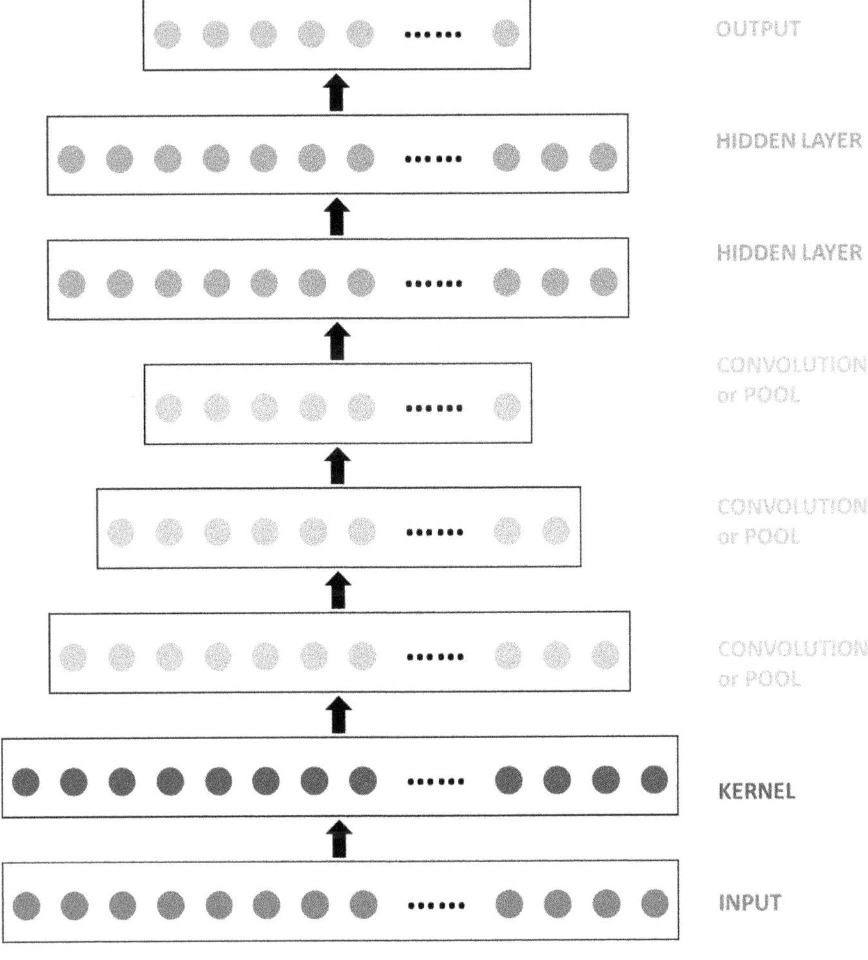

FIGURE 1.6 Deep CNN Architecture.

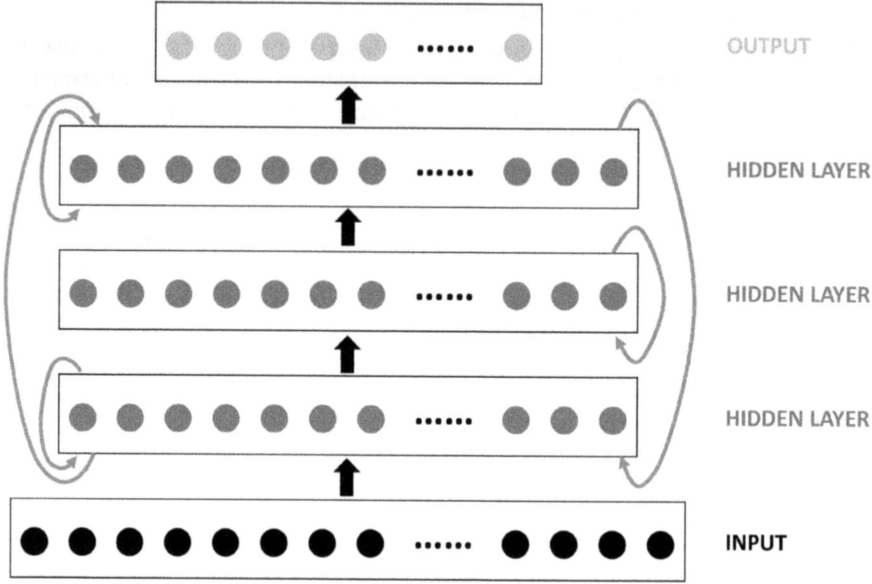

FIGURE 1.7 RNN architecture.

RNN handles both real values (time series) and symbolic values of variable length inputs. Semantic interpretation of text using time-layered RNN structure has found applications in new research areas, such as sentiment analysis, machine translation, and information analytics. RNN holds memory in the form of hidden layers. In RNN, the information is transferred among individual layers of the network and the sequence positions.

1.3.1.3.4 Long Short-Term Memory (LSTM)

LSTMs follow an artificial RNN architecture, which has both feedforward and feedback connections. They can process an entire sequence of data at a time. One of the most important advantages is that they can also work with sequences of different lengths, which makes them very popular in the field of deep learning. Figure 1.8 shows the architecture of an LSTM network describe its mathematical model.

The LSTM network takes a sequence of data as input into its network and makes predictions/classifications considering the temporal order of the data. Time-domain pre-processing is not usually required for such a network.

1.3.1.4 Implementation of Deep Learning in Automatic Seizure Type Diagnostic

The steps towards implementing deep learning techniques for seizure type detection are as follows.

1.3.1.4.1 Selecting the Right Data Set

Data sets play the most important role in the training of any network (supervised or unsupervised) for detecting seizure type. The data sets can be obtained from

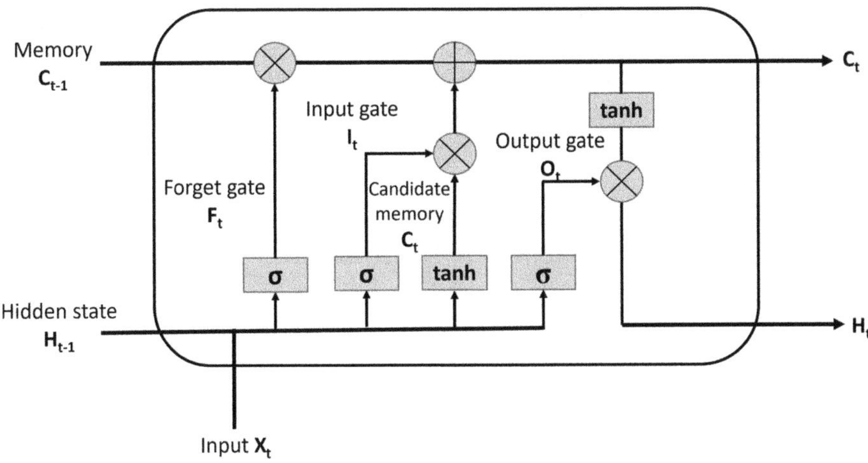

FIGURE 1.8 Architecture of LSTM networks.

various sources. Temple University EEG Corpus (TUH EEG Corpus) [26] is one such data set, which is a huge collection of clinical EEG data collected over more than a decade. The data are stored in the form of European data format (EDF) files and consists of 24–36 channels of signal data, sampled at 250 Hz, with 16-bits resolution. Selected data follows the average reference (AR) channel configuration, while the annotations follow the temporal central parasagittal (TCP) channel configuration. Each EDF file is accompanied by an anonymised report given by a neurologist, including patient's medical history like symptoms during seizure, medication details, along with that age, gender, and frequency of seizure occurrence. It also includes clinician's findings and analysis of seizure events.

Similarly, other data sets are available from many sources like GitHub, Kaggle, hospitals and research organisations. The data sets are both available in raw and pre-processed form. If it's in raw form, then the next step is to pre-process the same before exposing them to a deep learning algorithm.

1.3.1.4.2 Pre-processing of EEG Signals

In most data sets, the number of channels and the length of the signals are not the same. So, to start, we need to make these two parameters compatible. LSTM is the only algorithm which can handle different length sequences at a time, whereas other algorithms require the same length. To achieve this, several approaches can be adopted, such as resampling the data, reshaping the data or converting to frequency domain. Some of the different frequency domain approaches include Hilbert transforms, discrete cosine transforms and short-time Fourier transforms.

1.3.1.4.3 Prediction of Seizure Types Using Deep Learning Techniques

After pre-processing of the EEG signals, the analysis is carried out with various deep learning algorithms. Among all, LSTM is the most popular as it can handle multiple sequences at a time. Whereas, for feature extraction, CNNs are better, and they are also available as pre-trained networks for faster execution and better accuracy. RNNs are also gaining popularity, as their gated structures help retain information in their memory.

Most of the time, the prediction of seizure types is done using two ways: (i) binary classification (predict between presence or absence), (ii) multiclass classifications (prediction among many classes of seizures). Overall, deep learning techniques offer a huge variety in terms of usage and are quickly developing into an essential EEG analysis method for easily classifying seizure types from EEG signals and aid in clinical diagnosis.

1.3.2 EEG Connectivity Dynamics: To Measure the Brain Network Dysconnectivity in Schizophrenia

1.3.2.1 What Is Schizophrenia?

Schizophrenia is a well-known mental disorder with an inability to make valid predictions about expected sensations and experiences – a form of thought disorder. They can present with a myriad of symptoms, but most patients will only experience a subset of them at a given time. They may show an excessive tendency to perceive mental thoughts as real external voices (hallucinations) or show excessive belief in irrational ideas (delusions), which are grouped as positive symptoms. They may show abnormal reduction in communication, social interaction, and motivation, which are called negative symptoms. Additionally, they would also have several cognitive deficits and disorganisation of thought structure. So, clinical diagnosis of schizophrenia involves identifying the onset, duration, and progression of such symptoms and exclusion of other conditions that show similar symptoms.

Based on over a century of research on this elusive disorder, our best guess about the underlying brain mechanism is that there is a dynamic disconnection among the thought-generating brain regions. This means that the symptoms of schizophrenia could be produced by not one but many different permutations and combinations of brain disconnection. Even the reason for auditory hallucinations (one of the major symptoms) is thought to involve language, auditory, and memory/limbic brain networks in varying proportions [27]. Accordingly, an overinfluence of striatal regions on auditory-language regions, imbalanced fronto-temporal connections, and weak interhemispheric auditory pathway all play significant roles in the generation of this symptom. A similar hybrid picture could be responsible for other symptoms. Therefore, brain connectivity patterns should be the main criterion for the diagnosis of schizophrenia.

1.3.2.2 What Is the Basis for EEG Brain Connectivity?

EEG, due to its inherent property of being generated from synchronised activity of large patches of brain neural networks, has many signal patterns that reflect brain connectivity. For instance, the increase in amplitude or power of different frequency bands of the EEG signal could be an indirect indication of increased brain connectivity. However, a more reliable indicator of brain connectivity would be to see EEG signals from different brain regions being in sync at a particular frequency band. Hence, this is the common approach to study EEG-based brain connectivity. The synchrony could be in terms of the simultaneous increase or decrease in amplitude/magnitude of a specific frequency band, which has been a popular approach used in literature. This can be easily computed using fast Fourier transform (FFT) or by taking the root mean square (RMS) of band-passed filtered data. But the oscillatory activities between two brain regions could also be in sync, in terms of their phase relations (i.e. relative position of peaks and troughs between signals across time). This latter aspect could occur independent of magnitude changes and hence be missed in magnitude-based connectivity measures. Therefore, a combination of both magnitude-based and phase-based spectral connectivity would be required to get a better picture of inter-brain region synchrony. There are several FFT-based methods that capture either magnitude- or phase-based connectivity and are usually termed magnitude coherence and imaginary coherence, respectively. The same could be achieved with higher temporal resolution using time–frequency analysis methods like complex wavelet transform and Hilbert transform. For the magnitude-based connectivity using the above techniques, the instantaneous amplitude of specific frequencies of signal pairs could be extracted and then a direct correlation is performed to determine the extent of synchrony or connectivity. On the contrary, the instantaneous phase time series extracted for specific frequencies of signal pairs could be examined for phase difference consistencies (e.g. phase lag index), as a measure of connectivity. Connectivity measures could also ignore the spectral structure of EEG signals and look for a plain statistical correlation of voltage values between signal pairs.

To understand the possibility of other approaches to estimate connectivity, we need to know more formal definitions of connectivity. One, being functional connectivity, is defined as "the statistical dependence or mutual information between two neuronal systems" [28]. All the measures mentioned above satisfy this description. Another definition, that is more related to the goal of this approach, is to understand "the casual relationship among neural entities" [29]. To satisfy this latter description, more complex relations been signal pairs need to be examined. One such relation is the concept of causality introduced by Ganger [30], wherein if the prediction of the future of a signal can be improved by the knowledge of the past of another signal, then that latter signal could be considered causally influencing or connected to the former signal. This method is called Granger causality and has started to become popular in EEG connectivity studies. Transfer entropy builds on this concept by incorporating principles of information theory (specifically conditional probabilities) to estimate connectivity between signal pairs [31]. Most of such connectivity measures are done between each signal pair independently as bivariate analysis. However, there are multivariate data-driven variants too. Mapping between channel pairs based on such connectivity measures could then be subjected to various network analysis techniques to find patterns of groupings in brain networks (see Figure 1.9). A popular method is called graph theory, which uses mathematical concepts on graph metrics (considers electrodes as nodes and their connectivity measures as edges) (see [32] for a review).

Similarly, another factor to consider is the temporal aspect of the measured connectivity indices. Most studies explore an average measure of functional connectivity across a rest or an experimental session. Such static connectivity measures assume that the brain connectivity remains constant during the measurement period. Several recent studies have highlighted that the fluctuations in functional connectivity are common during rest [33–35]. Figure 1.10 shows how the connectivity measure could change every few minutes. Moreover, the measurement of such dynamic connectivity patterns could find crucial derangements that are sometimes missed by static connectivity measures, as in studies on schizophrenia patients [36,37].

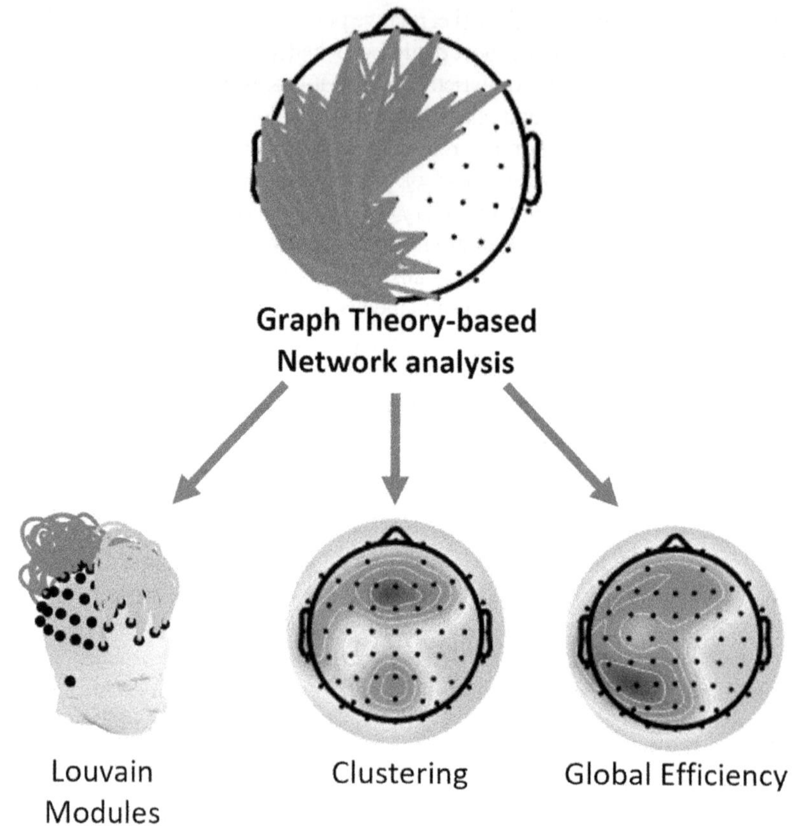

FIGURE 1.9 Graph theory-based network analysis on channel-pair connectivity data. Note that the frontal module shows higher clustering ('small-world' or local connectivity), whereas the posterior module shows higher global efficiency ('big-world' or long-range connectivity). The connectivity measure was based on the phase of 10 Hz (alpha frequency) during resting eyes closed state.

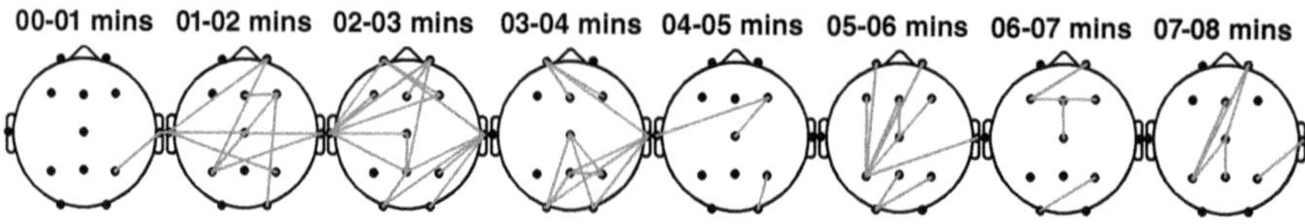

FIGURE 1.10 Connectivity dynamics across time. Eyes open resting state. Alpha phase connectivity.

1.3.2.3 How Would EEG Connectivity Be Helpful to Measuring Dysconnectivity in Schizophrenia?

EEG connectivity measures could thus aid in the objective diagnosis of schizophrenia, which otherwise relies purely on qualitative inference by trained psychiatrists/psychologists. A recent meta-analysis of multi-modal connectivity results (including EEG as well as functional magnetic resonance imaging (fMRI) results across 70 studies and >2,500 schizophrenia patients) suggested that brain hypoconnectivity could localise to auditory network, default mode network (DMN), or somatomotor network [38]. These were from studies that followed a seed-based connectivity approach, wherein key brain regions that might be involved were pre-decided and whole brain connectivity was not performed. Another recent study that used whole brain connectivity in two independent schizophrenia patients' sample (total of 100 patients) found significant hypoconnectivity within the cingulo-opercular network in one sample but hyperconnectivity within the temporal-thalamic network in the other sample [39]. Therefore, interpreting such EEG patterns is a non-trivial task as they are non-unique and dynamic. This is the main reason many earlier studies have found inconsistent results for brain activity measures that directly or indirectly capture the strength of brain connectivity.

Hence, there is a need to search for subject-specific connectivity abnormalities that may show up in different brain networks that may be related to different perceptual or cognitive functions from a 'predictive coding framework'.

1.3.3 EEG-Derived Event-Related Potentials (ERP): To Understand the Complex Cognitive Profile in Chronic Pain

1.3.3.1 What Is Chronic Pain?

Pain is an unpleasant sensory and emotional experience associated with or resembling that associated with actual or potential tissue damage [40]. Chronic pain is a pain that persists for long periods and, in most cases, extends beyond the period of healing (more than 3 months) of the original insult or injury [41]. It can also occur in the absence of prior injury and also without any threat to the body. It is sometimes called chronic non-organic pain when the pain is without any known aetiology. Chronic pain is an agonising and major global health issue, having a severe impact on the individuals and the country's health care system and economy [42]. The worldwide prevalence rate of chronic pain is 20% [43] and 19.3% in India [44]. Chronic pain is more prevalent in women and also in the elderly population beyond the age of 65 years [44]. Some of the examples of chronic pain are fibromyalgia, back pain, somatoform pain disorder, and musculoskeletal pain.

Chronic pain is considered a disease of the central nervous system, particularly the brain. The transition from acute pain to chronic pain involves myriad changes in the brain (both structural and functional plasticity), which are maladaptive and result in aberrant top-down pain modulation. Alterations occur at many different interconnected levels, ranging from the molecular to the network level, at several anatomical avenues in the nociceptive pathway. These include aberrant structural and functional plasticity in the regions like the primary sensory and motor cortex, thalamus, medial prefrontal cortex, nucleus accumbent, hippocampus, cingulate cortex, insula, orbitofrontal cortex, dorsal pons, cerebellum, and amygdala [45,46].

The majority of these occur subconsciously and this results in altered conscious perception of pain. In addition to aberrant pain perception, chronic pain patients also suffer from other comorbidities like anxiety, depression, cognitive deficits (attention bias, memory impairment, abnormal processing speed, and executive function) [47], emotional instability [48], and aberrant sensory perception (hypervigilance, abnormal sensory gating, and somatosensory amplification) [49–51]. These are the result of alterations in the pathways and the brain regions involved in the chronic pain pathophysiology.

The comorbidities along with the pain are generally assessed by questionnaire-based subjective ratings, which are highly prone to discrepant results. Hence there is an urgent need to have an objective assessment of these comorbidities and pain and to create a specific profile out of them.

1.3.3.2   What Is Event-Related Potential?

ERPs are minute changes seen in EEG signals, time-locked to stimuli or events. They aid in the assessment of brain processes at millisecond resolution [52]. They are usually derived from EEG signals by averaging several EEG segments time-locked to specific stimulus/event repetitions (see Figure 1.11a and b). ERPs are informative about the exact timing of the cognitive process (high temporal resolution). Though EEG-based measures have lower spatial resolution in comparison to many imaging techniques, this can often be improved for ERPs by increasing the number of electrodes or sensors (using high-density EEG). Additionally, the signal-to-noise ratios of many ERP components are much higher than regular EEG measures, making their source estimation more accurate. It gives a direct measure of the brain activity with no measurable conduction delay between the electrical activity generated by the

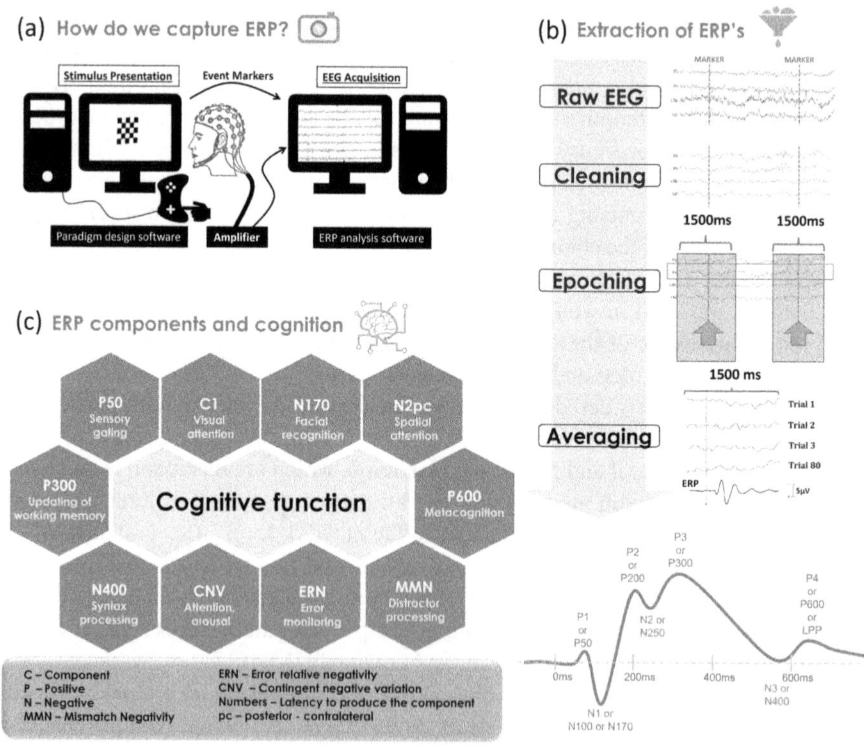

FIGURE 1.11   Details of ERP acquisition, analysis, and the different components.

brain and ERPs acquired from the scalp [53]. ERP components are usually named based on their polarity ('N' & 'P' for negative- and positive-going wave, respectively) and ordinal (1 for first, 2 for the second, etc.). Researchers often choose to use temporal labelling after the indication of polarity (for example P300 in place of P3, occurring around 300 ms after stimulus onset). ERPs are measured in terms of latency (time from stimulus to reach the peak) and amplitude (peak of the wave).

ERPs can be elicited using somato-sensory/touch/laser/vibration/electrical (intensity, duration, and frequency), auditory (loudness, duration, auditory frequency, and complexity), and visual (luminance, size, duration, colour, and visual frequency). In most of the diagnostic studies, auditory and visual ERPs are studied. ERPs can be classified based on the latency as short-latency-evoked potentials, mid-latency-evoked potentials, and long-latency-evoked potentials. Short-latency-evoked potential peaks within 10 ms post stimulus elicited by peripheral auditory nerve and brainstem. They are not affected by attention, psychological salience, and level of sleep but they are affected by physical aspects of the stimulus. Mid-latency-evoked potential peaks between 10 and 200 ms. It reflects processing in the thalamus and primary auditory or visual cortex. Long-latency-evoked potentials peak above 200 ms and reflect higher cortical functions. Both mid- and long-latency-evoked potentials are affected by attention, psychological salience, and level of sleep. Short- and mid-latency-evoked potentials are elicited by the bottom-up process, whereas long latency components are majorly elicited by the top-down process.

Mid- and long-latency ERP components facilitate the understanding of the cognitive process. These ERP components and their functions are mentioned in the Figure 1.11c.

1.3.3.3   How Can ERPs Be Implemented for Understanding Cognitive Deficits in Chronic Non-Organic Pain?

Aberrant functional plasticity with a greater temporal resolution can be assessed using ERP [54,55]. However, the spatial resolution of EEG/ERP methods can be further improved by increasing the number of EEG/ERP sensors [56]. Chronic pain is known to be associated with cognitive deficits and many of the cognitive deficits can be measured using ERP.

The study has shown increased P3 latency in chronic back pain because of delayed cognitive processing [57]. Chronic back pain also showed altered implicit pain memories and selective attention to the pain-related materials by showing enhanced N100 and N200 amplitudes to the pain-related words in comparison to the healthy controls [58]. Similarly, fibromyalgia patients have also shown enhanced N100 amplitude because of preconscious allocation of attention to pain and anger faces reflecting the development of implicit memory for pain (that is attentional bias towards pain) [59]. Additionally, chronic back pain has also shown a decreased speed of pre-attentive cognitive processing by exhibiting increased latency in the mismatch negativity (MMN) component [60]. This reflects insufficient recall time due to decreased cognitive processing speed rather than an actual memory problem. Somatosensory gating is not seen in fibromyalgia (no changes in the amplitude of P50 component between two paired stimuli) as a result of impaired habituation because of a lack of inhibitory control to repetitive somatosensory stimuli [61].

Previously mentioned studies have tried to conduct the ERP measurement of cognition in chronic pain conditions in isolation. As different types of chronic pain have varied functional abnormalities, the development of an ERP profile would give a broad overview of the abnormality of each patient (Figure 1.12). This would help

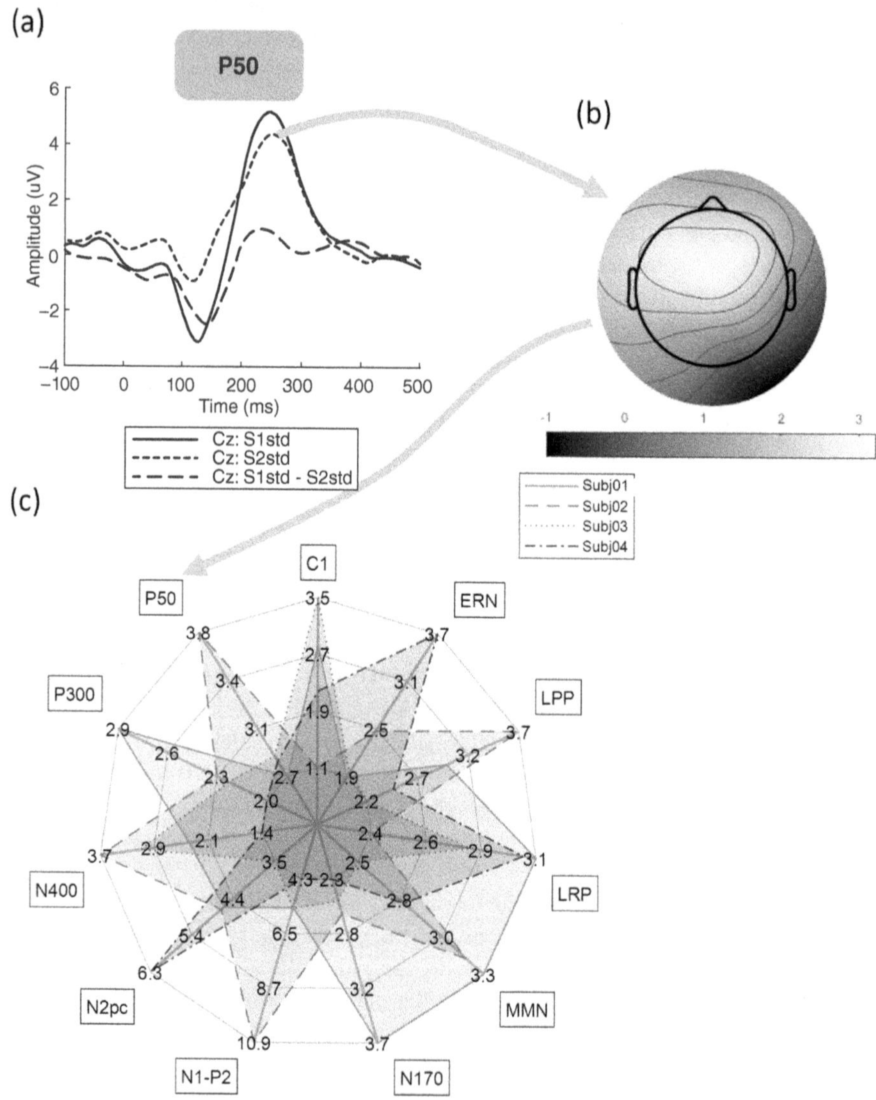

FIGURE 1.12 Figure showing the generation of ERP profiles for each subject. For P50 (sensory gating) condition (a) the ERP waveforms from Cz electrode and (b) the scalp distribution of the averaged difference P50 waveform is shown from a single subject. The ERPs were generated by regression approach and are beta values. (c) The spider plot shows the distribution of such ERP values extracted across multiple subjects and conditions. This helps in understanding and comparing the cognitive profiles of different subjects. This ERP profile is obtained from a single audio–visual ERP paradigm.

clinicians design a comprehensive treatment model for chronic pain, which would address the co-morbidities in addition to pain. The objective measure of pain and comorbidities can be obtained using EEG measures, one such measure being ERP.

Current treatment strategies fail to give any sort of relief to the pain patients. That mandates the development of better diagnostic tools, such as the ERP profile of the patient and novel tailor-made treatment strategies. So, apart from conventional diagnostic tools, brain electrophysiological patterns can be used in both screenings as well as treating chronic pain subjects.

ERPs give a better picture of the pain experience. Using the ERP paradigm, we can extract ERP components related to perception, cognition, and emotion in chronic pain subjects. Both bottom-up and top-down regulation of the brain can be elaborately understood. So, the development of a cognitive ERP model with a wider framework is imperative in treating pain. This model should encompass objective assessment of perceptual (sensory gating, self-monitoring, image perception, auditory perception, motor readiness), emotional (valence and arousal), and cognitive (congruence detection, attention, memory, error monitoring, and spatial attention). This comprehensive investigation facilitates both the diagnosis and development of a non-pharmacological treatment strategy (alongside conventional approaches) which would help in addressing the issue at multiple levels and thereby restoration of normal perception in chronic pain conditions.

1.4 CHALLENGES IN USING EEG-BASED DIAGNOSTIC SOLUTIONS

To become a diagnostic application, the approaches and algorithms mentioned above need to be translated into viable software and hardware tools that can be used reliably in various clinical set-ups or by patients themselves. There can be multiple roadblocks that need to be negotiated during such a transition.

1.4.1 SOFTWARE CHALLENGES

Research-level signal processing solutions are often implemented in high-level programming languages (like MATLAB and Python) and work on top of several existing open-source libraries. So, this could require rewriting many of the codes in lower-level languages (like C, C++, C# or Java, etc.) and shifting to software libraries with appropriate licences that allow commercial use. Medical devices and the software that are part of it are highly regulated by law. This implies that each and every component of the software will need to be verified and validated before it can be released for use. This also means that normal third party libraries cannot be used off the shelf for medical device applications directly unless the libraries come with all the documentations and testing results as required for medical device software. These third party libraries get termed as software of unknown province (SOUP), and unless these libraries were designed and maintained specially for medical device application by following the IEC 62304 guidelines, it becomes a major challenge to integrate them.

1.4.1.1   Medical Device Software Safety Classification

Medical device software can be classified into three categories based on severity of harm it can cause the patient or the user operating the medical device. Depending on the class of the software, the records in the development and maintenance can change. The three categories of medical device software are

Class A – No injury or damage to health is possible,
Class B – Non-serious injury is possible, and
Class C – Death or serious Injury is possible.

1.4.1.2   IEC 62304 and FDA Guideline Documents for Medical Device Software

FDA provides many guidelines for the development of software and mobile applications that are used in medical devices [62]. The software functions are generally categorised into either software as a medical device (SaMD) or software in a medical device (SiMD). The software, including the firmware, user interface, software modules, etc., that are deployed inside a medical device and are required for its operation is known as the SiMD. The term SaMD is defined by International Medical Device Regulator Forum (IMDRA) which specifies it as the part of the software which is intended to be used for medical purposes and performs these functions without being part of the hardware of the medical device. These devices were earlier referred to by names, such as medical device software or health software, etc.

The development and maintenance of the medical device software is defined in the ANSI/AAMI/IEC 62304 standards [63]. The standard identifies the various stages and phases that are essential for the development and maintenance of the medical device software where the software itself is the medical device (SaMD) and also where the software is embedded or is an integral part of the medical device (SiMD). The development and maintenance process for medical device software has to be guided by the risk analysis guidelines using IEC 14971. The development also has to be guided by usability engineering which is defined by the guidelines provided by FDA under the heading of human factors and IEC 62366 guidelines.

The various phases for the development of medical device software are listed below (also see Figure 1.13) and there has to be a documented record for each of the processes listed. For simplicity, the various record requirements according to software class have not been made here.

1. Software Development Planning
   - Includes planning for development, verification, risk management, configuration management, integration & integration testing, development standards, etc.
2. Software Requirement Analysis
   - Must define and document the requirements of the system, including requirement documents, risk analysis, risk control measures, etc.
3. Software Architectural Design
   - Architecture of software items, SOUPS, hardware & software requirement of SOUPS, software segregation that are necessary, etc.

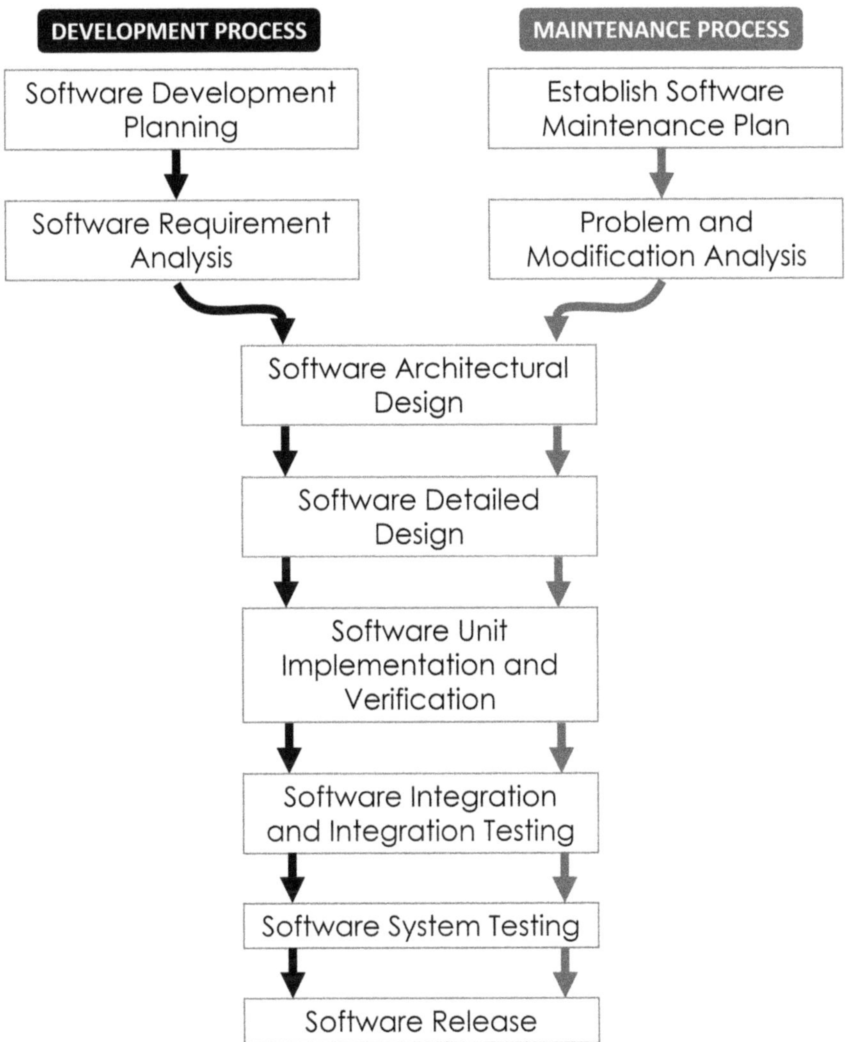

FIGURE 1.13 Visual representation of the software development and maintenance process.

4. Software Detailed Design
   - Software units based on architecture, detailed design and interfaces for each unit, verification of detailed design, etc.
5. Software Unit Implementation and Verification
   - Development of each unit, verification testing of each unit with records, etc.
6. Software Integration and Integration Testing
   - Integration of all units, verification of integration of units, testing of integrated software, regression test, software problem resolution process, etc.

7. Software System Testing
   - Testing of each requirement defined in SRS, use of problem resolution process, retesting after changes, risk management activities, etc.
8. Software Release
   - Release of the medical device to end user, versioning and backing up of the software with release tag, document residual anomalies, etc.

The various phase of the maintenance of medical device software are listed below (also see Figure 1.13) and there has to be a documented record for each of the processes listed.

1. Establish Software Maintenance Plan
   - Includes planning for maintenance process of medical device software, verification, risk management, etc.,
   - Procedures for documentation, evaluation, resolving, and tracking, and
   - Criteria for determining feedback as a problem.

2. Problem and Modification Analysis
   - Document and evaluate feedback from users, market, safety aspects, etc.,
   - Software resolution process,
   - Change request and approval process, and
   - Communication with users and regulators.

3. The modification implementation will follow the process of points 3–8 that are listed in the medical device development process. After the process is completed, a re-release of the modified software is followed.

1.4.1.3 Usability Engineering and Human Factor for Medical Device Software

Human factor/usability engineering is an important part of the medical device design because it deals with the people's interaction with the device for its intended purpose. The process is a very important component in order to minimise use-related hazards and reduce risks thereby allowing a safe use of the medical device. The aim of this engineering process is to increase effectiveness, efficiency, ease of learning for a user and to give a user satisfaction during usage. The human factor should be applied during the process of design input, design verification, and design validation. FDA provides many guidelines for human factor engineering [64]. Another guideline that is available is the IEC 62366 – 'Medical devices – Application of usability engineering to medical devices'.

The human factor needs to consider the following points – the type of user, the environment it will be used in, and the device/interface to the user (see Figure 1.14) [65]. The outcome should be to produce a safe and effective device and also identify the unsafe and ineffective usage types.

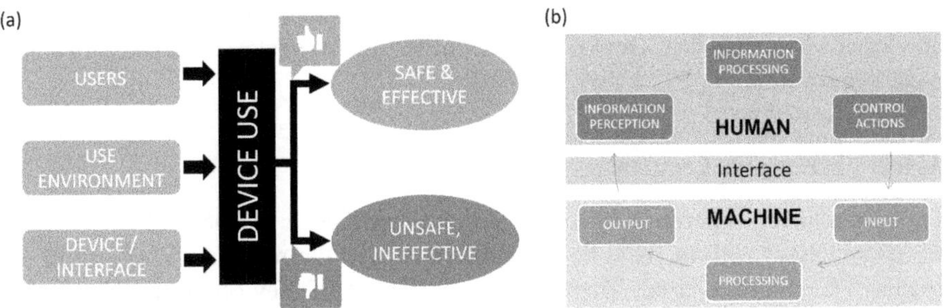

FIGURE 1.14   Human factors of (a) device and (b) the device–user interface.

1.4.1.4   FDA Guidelines for ML System

FDA has a good guideline for the usage of ML systems in medical devices [66]. It is known as the good machine learning practises (GMLP) and has 10 guiding principles that will effectively promote safe, effective and a high-quality medical device that uses artificial intelligence (AI) and machine learning (ML). This guidance document and its guidance principles have been jointly identified by FDA, Health Canada, and United Kingdom's medicines and healthcare product regulatory agency (MHRA).

The guiding principles are

1. Multi-disciplinary expertise involvement for the total product life cycle,
2. Implementation of good engineering and security practises,
3. Clinical study participants are representative of the intended patient population,
4. Training data sets are independent of test sets,
5. Selected reference data set are based on best available methods,
6. Model design should reflect the intended use of the device,
7. Focus is placed on the performance of the human–AI team,
8. Demonstrates device performance during clinically relevant conditions,
9. Users are provided clear and essential information, and
10. Deployed models are monitored for performance, and retraining risks are managed.

1.4.1.5   FDA Guidelines for Cyber Security

The international medical device regulators forum (IMDRF) with FDA as a part came up with the global medical device cyber security guidelines. The importance of cyber security has become even more important with the medical devices increasingly being connected to network-connected devices wirelessly or via internet. The availability of the device without disruption should be ensured and that the possibility of resource takeover by other malicious programs or devices should be prevented. This will allow the patient to get timely information and diagnosis or therapy, as intended from the medical device's software. The IMDRF guideline document – 'Principles and Practises for Medical Device Cybersecurity' that was released in March 2020 is a useful resource.

1.4.2 Hardware Challenges

Even the real-time operating system (OS) that is used inside the medical device needs to be compliant with medical device guidelines, and the regular OS we use in our regular PC cannot be used. There are few portable EEG devices in the market, but the design of portable ERP and specialised neurofeedback devices can become challenging because of the need to synchronise the stimulus with the recording and to run some pre-processing and further analysis on the EEG signals. Such algorithms would also

- Need to work on multiple platforms,
- Need to work on varying medical devices,
- Conform to several hospital and legal standards,
- Need a dedicated support and maintenance team, and
- Need to provide regular training.

All these above points need a specialised and experienced team and various resources, including human resources (HR), document management tools, design tools, development tools, testing tools, and regulatory certified labs tests.

The various analysis steps for clinical analysis, algorithms for detection, and other new ideas discussed earlier can lead to changes in the scope of the medical device. For example, the device may make a claim to be able to either detect a condition or to be used as therapeutic option for the patient. This could lead to additional requirements, including additional documentation, pre-market approval process, non-predicate device process, clinical evaluation, and clinical trials.

1.4.3 Clinical Evaluation - Regulatory Challenges

As mentioned above, any change in the scope or used case or intended purpose, could lead to the requirement of a clinical trial of the medical device with the regulatory bodies. The clinical evaluation/clinical trial would need to evaluate the effectiveness of the intended purpose and safety of the device according to the various regulations. The trial would require additional resources, time, and budget to conduct.

IMDRF in association with FDA has released a guideline document – 'Software as a Medical Device: Clinical Evaluation', which covers this topic extensively [67].

The SaMD utilises an algorithm that may be based on models, logic, or set of rules in order to produce an intended clinical output from one or more clinical inputs (see Figure 1.15). The output should be relevant clinically by way of providing or assisting in the area of inform, drive, diagnose, or treat.

Clinical evaluation is an ongoing life cycle process for SaMD, and it starts from pre-market period where the evidence of accuracy, reliability, sensitivity, sensitivity, scope of usage, based on the intended purpose need to be demonstrated (see Table 1.3).

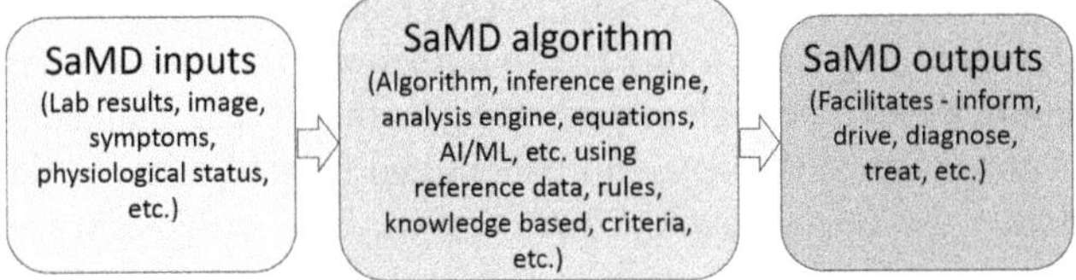

FIGURE 1.15   SaMD algorithm (https://www.fda.gov/regulatory-information/search-fda-guidance-documents/software-medical-device-samd-clinical-evaluation).

TABLE 1.3

Diagram Comparing Clinical Validation Types: Analytical, Clinical, and Regulatory

	Clinical Evaluation	
(1) Valid Clinical Association	**(2) Analytical Association**	**(1) Clinical Validation**
Dose the SaMD output and the targeted clinical condition have a valid clinical association?	Dose the SaMD process and generate accurate, reliable and precise output data for the input data?	Dose the SaMD output data achieve the intended purpose for the traget population in the context of the clinical care?

Source: https://www.fda.gov/regulatory-information/search-fda-guidance-documents/softwaremedical-device-samd-clinical-evaluation.

Once the SaMD is in the market, post-market process of collecting real-time data of usage, customer complaints, safety data, customer needs to be analysed and will serve as inputs for further improvement of the medical device software.

1.5 CONCLUSION

EEG signal processing constitutes a dynamic field with immense potential for diagnostic and brain monitoring applications, provided comprehensive attention is directed towards continuous research and development efforts. Despite the challenges in utilising EEG signal processing for the various diagnostic or therapeutic applications, its notable attributes, such as high temporal resolution, non-invasiveness, affordability, and user-friendliness, render it a valuable diagnostic biomarker in both clinical and research settings. There are several tools, analysis, and application frameworks available in the open-source community for evaluating and prototyping algorithms before using them as standalone diagnostic products, thus streamlining the process which can save months of effort. EEG has found extensive use in the healthcare system, with neurologists using EEG for the diagnosis and classification of epilepsy, audiologists using evoked potential and ERP to diagnose auditory system issues, and psychologists using quantitative EEG for the diagnosis of attention deficit hyperactivity disorder (ADHD) and EEG neurofeedback for therapy. The widespread application of EEG in numerous diagnostic contexts signifies its substantial untapped potential, necessitating further research and development in the realms of diagnostics, therapy, and patient and normal user monitoring. These imperative drives the further exploration of novel EEG-based software and hardware tools.

REFERENCES

1. Chandra SR, Asheeb A, Dash S, et al. Role of electroencephalography in the diagnosis and treatment of neuropsychiatric border zone syndromes. *Indian Journal of Psychological Medicine* 2017; 39:243–249. DOI: 10.4103/0253-7176.207336

2. Newson JJ, Thiagarajan TC. EEG frequency bands in psychiatric disorders: a review of resting state studies. *Frontiers in Human Neuroscience* 2019; 12:521. DOI: 10.3389/fnhum.2018.00521

3. Markovska-Simoska S, Pop-Jordanova N, Pop-Jordanov J. Inter- and intra-hemispheric EEG coherence study in adults with neuropsychiatric disorders. *PRILOZI* 2018; 39:5–19. DOI: 10.2478/prilozi-2018–0037

4. Kam JWY, Bolbecker AR, O'Donnell BF, et al. Resting state EEG power and coherence abnormalities in bipolar disorder and schizophrenia. *Journal of Psychiatric Research* 2013; 47:1893. DOI: 10.1016/j.jpsychires.2013.09.009

5. Michel CM, Koenig T. EEG microstates as a tool for studying the temporal dynamics of whole-brain neuronal networks: a review. *NeuroImage* 2018; 180:577–593. DOI: 10.1016/j.neuroimage.2017.11.062

6. Dutta KK. Epilepsy is a curse: myth or reality. *InnoHEALTH Magazine.* 2020. Available from: https://innohealthmagazine.com/2020/issues/epilepsy-is-a-curse-myth-or-reality/

7. Xue-Ping W, Hai-Jiao W, Li-Na Z, et al. Risk factors for drug-resistant epilepsy: a systematic review and meta-analysis. *Medicine* 2019; 98(30):e16402. DOI: 10.1097/MD.0000000000016402

8. Kaculini CM, Tate-Looney AJ, Seifi A. The history of epilepsy: from ancient mystery to modern misconception. *Cureus* 2021; 13:e13953. Available from: https://www.cureus.com/articles/53579-the-history-of-epilepsy-from-ancient-mystery-to-modern-misconception. DOI: 10.7759/cureus.13953

9. Costa RP, Oliveira P, Rodrigues G, et al. Epileptic seizure classification using neural networks with 14 features. In: Lovrek I, Howlett RJ, Jain LC, editors. *Knowledge-Based Intelligent Information and Engineering Systems.* Berlin, Heidelberg: Springer; 2008, pp. 281–288. (Lecture Notes in Computer Science; vol. 5178). Available from: https://link.springer.com/10.1007/978-3-540-85565-1_35. DOI: 10.1007/978-3-540-85565-1_35

10. Altman NS. An introduction to Kernel and nearest-neighbor nonparametric regression. *The American Statistician* 1992; 46:175–185.

11. Park Y, Luo L, Parhi KK, et al. Seizure prediction with spectral power of EEG using cost-sensitive support vector machines. *Epilepsia* 2011; 52(10):1761–1770. DOI: 10.1111/j.1528-1167.2011.03138.x

12. LeCun Y, Bengio Y, Hinton G. Deep learning. *Nature* 2015; 521(7553):436–444. DOI: 10.1038/nature14539

13. Dutta KK, Venugopal K, Swamy SA. Removal of muscle artifacts from EEG based on ensemble empirical mode decomposition and classification of seizure using machine learning techniques. In: *2017 International Conference on Inventive Computing and Informatics (ICICI).* Coimbatore: IEEE; 2017, pp. 861–866. Available from: https://ieeexplore.ieee.org/document/8365259/. DOI: 10.1109/ICICI.2017.8365259

14. Wong S, Simmons A, Rivera-Villicana J, et al. EEG datasets for seizure detection and prediction: a review. *Epilepsia Open* 2023; 8(2):252–267. DOI: 10.1002/epi4.12704.

15. Dutta KK. Multi-class time series classification of EEG signals with recurrent neural networks. In: *2019 9th International Conference on Cloud Computing, Data Science & Engineering (Confluence)*. Noida, India: IEEE; 2019, pp. 337–341. Available from: https://ieeexplore.ieee.org/document/8776889/. DOI: 10.1109/CONFLUENCE.2019.8776889

16. Halabi N, Daou RAZ, Achkar R, et al. Monitoring system for prediction and detection of epilepsy seizure. In: *2019 Fourth International Conference on Advances in Computational Tools for Engineering Applications (ACTEA)*. Beirut, Lebanon: IEEE; 2019, pp. 1–7. Available from: https://ieeexplore.ieee.org/document/8851094/. DOI: 10.1109/ACTEA.2019.8851094

17. Dutta KK, Manohar PKI, Naaz F, et al. Seven epileptic seizure type classification in pre-Ictal, Ictal and inter-Ictal stages using machine learning techniques. *Research Square* 2022. Available from: https://www.researchsquare.com/article/rs-2100432/v1. DOI: 10.21203/rs.3.rs-2100432/v1

18. Dutta KK, Manohar P, Naaz F, et al. Epileptic seizure classification based on energy compaction of different transformation technique and machine learning classifiers. *International Journal of Mechanical Engineering (IJME)* 2022; 7(1):484. Available from: https://kalaharijournals.com/resources/IJME_Vol7.1_484.pdf

19. Wang L, Xue W, Li Y, et al. Automatic epileptic seizure detection in EEG signals using multi-domain feature extraction and nonlinear analysis. *Entropy* 2017; 19(6):222. DOI: 10.3390/e19060222

20. Hu X, Yuan S, Xu F, et al. Scalp EEG classification using deep Bi-LSTM network for seizure detection. *Computers in Biology and Medicine* 2020; 124:103919. DOI: 10.1016/j.compbiomed.2020.103919

21. Takahashi H, Emami A, Shinozaki T, et al. Convolutional neural network with auto-encoder-assisted multiclass labelling for seizure detection based on scalp electroencephalography. *Computers in Biology and Medicine* 2020; 125:104016. DOI: 10.1016/j.compbiomed.2020.104016

22. Emami A, Kunii N, Matsuo T, et al. Seizure detection by convolutional neural network-based analysis of scalp electroencephalography plot images. *NeuroImage: Clinical* 2019; 22:101684. DOI: 10.1016/j.nicl.2019.101684

23. Birjandtalab J, Heydarzadeh M, Nourani M. Automated EEG-based epileptic seizure detection using deep neural networks. In: *2017 IEEE International Conference on Healthcare Informatics (ICHI)*. Park City, UT: IEEE, pp. 552–555. Available from: https://ieeexplore.ieee.org/document/8031211/. DOI: 10.1109/ICHI.2017.55

24. Raghu S, Sriraam N, Temel Y, et al. EEG based multi-class seizure type classification using convolutional neural network and transfer learning. *Neural Networks* 2020; 124:202–212. DOI: 10.1016/j.neunet.2020.01.017

25. Sasidharan A, Dutta KK. Application of machine learning techniques in electroencephalography signals. In: Sahu M, Sinha GR, editors. *Brain and Behaviour Computing*. 1st ed. Boca Raton, FL: CRC Press; 2021, pp. 61–84.

26. Shah V, von Weltin E, Lopez S, et al. The temple university hospital seizure detection corpus. *Frontiers in Neuroinformatics* 2018; 12:83. DOI: 10.3389/fninf.2018.00083

27. Ćurčić-Blake B, Ford JM, Hubl D, et al. Interaction of language, auditory and memory brain networks in auditory verbal hallucinations. *Progress in Neurobiology* 2017; 148:1–20. DOI: 10.1016/j.pneurobio.2016.11.002

28. Friston K, Moran R, Seth AK. Analysing connectivity with Granger causality and dynamic causal modelling. *Current Opinion in Neurobiology* 2013; 23:172–178. DOI: 10.1016/j.conb.2012.11.010

29. Reid AT, Headley DB, Mill RD, Sanchez-Romero R, Uddin LQ, Marinazzo D, et al. Advancing functional connectivity research from association to causation. *Nature Neuroscience* 2019; 22(11):1751–1760. DOI: 10.1038/s41593-019-0510-4

30. Indira K, Dutta KK, Poornima S, et al. Deep learning methods for data science. In: Mire A, Malik S, Tyagi AK, editors. *Advanced Analytics and Deep Learning Models.* 1st ed. New York: Wiley; 2022, pp. 149–179. Available from: https://onlinelibrary.wiley. com/doi/10.1002/9781119792437.ch7. DOI: 10.1002/9781119792437.ch7

31. Vicente R, Wibral M, Lindner M, et al. Transfer entropy—a model-free measure of effective connectivity for the neurosciences. *Journal of Computational Neuroscience* 2011 Feb; 30(1):45–67. DOI: 10.1007/s10827-010-0262-3

32. Fallani FDV, Richiardi J, Chavez M, et al. Graph analysis of functional brain networks: practical issues in translational neuroscience. *Philosophical Transactions of the Royal Society B: Biological Sciences* 2014; 369:0521. DOI: 10.1098/rstb.2013.0521

33. Allen EA, Damaraju E, Plis SM, et al. Tracking whole-brain connectivity dynamics in the resting state. *Cerebral Cortex* 2014; 24:663–676. DOI: 10.1093/cercor/bhs352

34. Hutchison RM, Womelsdorf T, Gati JS, et al. Resting-state networks show dynamic functional connectivity in awake humans and anesthetized macaques: dynamic functional connectivity. *Human Brain Mapping* 2013; 34:2154–2177. DOI: 10.1002/ hbm.22058

35. Chang C, Glover GH. Time–frequency dynamics of resting-state brain connectivity measured with fMRI. *NeuroImage* 2010; 50:81–98. DOI: 10.1016/j.neuroimage.2009.12.011

36. Ma S, Calhoun VD, Phlypo R, et al. Dynamic changes of spatial functional network connectivity in healthy individuals and schizophrenia patients using independent vector analysis. *NeuroImage* 2014; 90:196–206. DOI: 10.1016/j.neuroimage.2013.12.063

37. Damaraju E, Allen EA, Belger A, et al. Dynamic functional connectivity analysis reveals transient states of dysconnectivity in schizophrenia. *NeuroImage: Clinical* 2014; 5:298–308. DOI: 10.1016/j.nicl.2014.07.003

38. Li S, Hu N, Zhang W, et al. Dysconnectivity of multiple brain networks in schizophrenia: a meta-analysis of resting-state functional connectivity. *Frontiers in Psychiatry* 2019; 10:482. DOI: 10.3389/fpsyt.2019.00482

39. Culbreth AJ, Wu Q, Chen S, et al. Temporal-thalamic and cingulo-opercular connectivity in people with schizophrenia. *NeuroImage: Clinical* 2021; 29:102531. DOI: 10.1016/j.nicl.2020.102531

40. Raja SN, Carr DB, Cohen M, et al. The revised international association for the study of pain definition of pain: concepts, challenges, and compromises. *Pain* 2020; 161:1976–1982. DOI: 10.1097/j.pain.0000000000001939

41. Kuner R, Flor H. Structural plasticity and reorganisation in chronic pain. *Nature Reviews Neuroscience* 2017; 18:20–30. DOI: 10.1038/nrn.2016.162

42. Mills SEE, Nicolson KP, Smith BH. Chronic pain: a review of its epidemiology and associated factors in population-based studies. *British Journal of Anaesthesia* 2019; 123:e273–e283. DOI: 10.1016/j.bja.2019.03.023

43. Goldberg DS, McGee SJ. Pain as a global public health priority. *BMC Public Health* 2011; 11:770. DOI: 10.1186/1471-2458-11-770

44. Saxena AK, Jain PN, Bhatnagar S. The prevalence of chronic pain among adults in India. *Indian Journal of Palliative Care* 2018; 24:472–477. DOI: 10.4103/IJPC.IJPC_141_18

45. Borsook D, Sava S, Becerra L. The pain imaging revolution – advancing pain into the 21st century. *Neuroscientist* 2010; 16:171–185. DOI: 10.1177/1073858409349902

46. May A. Chronic pain may change the structure of the brain. *Pain* 2008; 137:7–15. DOI: 10.1016/j.pain.2008.02.034

47. Nadar MS, Jasem Z, Manee FS. The cognitive functions in adults with chronic pain: a comparative study. *Pain Research & Management* 2016; 2016:5719380. DOI: 10.1155/2016/5719380

48. Lumley MA, Cohen JL, Borszcz GS, et al. Pain and emotion: a biopsychosocial review of recent research. *Journal of Clinical Psychology* 2011; 67:942–968. DOI: 10.1002/jclp.20816

49. Ceko M, Bushnell MC, Gracely RH. Neurobiology underlying fibromyalgia symptoms pain research and treatment. *Hindawi* 2011; 2012:e585419. DOI: 10.1155/2012/585419

50. McDermid AJ, Rollman GB, McCain GA. Generalized hypervigilance in fibromyalgia: evidence of perceptual amplification. *Pain* 1996; 66:133–144. DOI: 10.1016/0304-3959(96)03059-x

51. Raphael KG, Marbach JJ, Gallagher RM. Somatosensory amplification and affective inhibition are elevated in myofascial face pain. *Pain Medicationes* 2000; 1:247–253. DOI: 10.1046/j.1526–4637.2000.00034.x

52. Woodman GF. A brief introduction to the use of event-related potentials (ERPs) in studies of perception and attention. *Attention, Perception, & Psychophysics* 2010; 2031:72. DOI: 10.3758/APP.72.8.2031

53. Nunez PL, Srinivasan R. *Electric Fields of the Brain.* Oxford: Oxford University Press; 2006. https://doi.org/10.1093/acprof:oso/9780195050387.001.0001

54. Miltner WHR, Weiss T. Brain electrical correlates of pain processing. *Zeitschrift für Rheumatologie* 1998; 57:S14–S18. DOI: 10.1007/s003930050227

55. Sator-Katzenschlager S. Pain and neuroplasticity. *Revista Médica Clínica Las Condes* 2014; 25:699–706. DOI: 10.1097/ACO.0b013e32834a1079

56. Song J, Davey C, Poulsen C, et al. EEG source localization: sensor density and head surface coverage. *Journal of Neuroscience Methods* 2015; 256:9–21. DOI: 10.1016/j.jneumeth.2015.08.015

57. Tandon OP, Kumar S. Contingent negative variation response in chronic pain patients. *Indian Journal of Physiology and Pharmacology* 1996; 40(3):257–261.

58. Flor H, Knost B, Birbaumer N. Processing of pain- and body-related verbal material in chronic pain patients: central and peripheral correlates. *Pain* 1997; 73:413–421. DOI: 10.1111/j.1365–2842.2005.01450.x

59. González-Roldán AM, Munoz MA, Cifre I, et al. Altered psychophysiological responses to the view of others' pain and anger faces in fibromyalgia patients. *The Journal of Pain* 2013; 14:709–719. DOI: 10.1016/S0304–3959(97)00137-1

60. Yao S, Liu X, Yang W, et al. Preattentive processing abnormalities in chronic pain: neurophysiological evidence from mismatch negativity. *Pain Medications* 2011; 12:773–781. DOI: 10.1111/j.1526–4637.2011.01097.x

61. Montoya P, Sitges C, García-Herrera M, et al. Reduced brain habituation to somatosensory stimulation in patients with fibromyalgia. *Arthritis & Rheumatology* 2006; 54:1995–2003. DOI: 10.1002/art.21910

62. Policy for Device Software Functions and Mobile Medical Applications/FDA. U.S. Food and Drug Administration, 2019. Available from: https://www.fda.gov/regulatory-information/search-fda-guidance-documents/policy-device-software-functions-and-mobile-medical-applications.

63. IEC 62304:2006(en), Medical device software: Software life cycle processes, 2006. Available from: https://www.iso.org/obp/ui/#iso:std:iec:62304:ed-1:v1:en.

64. Applying Human Factors and Usability Engineering to Medical Devices/FDA U.S. Food and Drug Administration, 2019. Available from: https://www.fda.gov/regulatory-information/search-fda-guidance-documents/applying-human-factors-and-usability-engineering-medical-devices.

65. Human Factors and Medical Devices/FDA, 2019. Available from: https://www.fda.gov/medical-devices/device-advice-comprehensive-regulatory-assistance/human-factors-and-medical-devices.
66. Good Machine Learning Practice for Medical Device Development: Guiding Principles/FDA, 2021. Available from: https://www.fda.gov/medical-devices/software-medical-device-samd/good-machine-learning-practice-medical-device-development-guiding-principles.
67. Software as a Medical Device (SAMD): Clinical Evaluation/FDA. U.S. Food and Drug Administration, 2017. Available from: https://www.fda.gov/regulatory-information/search-fda-guidance-documents/software-medical-device-samd-clinical-evaluation.

2 Deep Learning Techniques for Automatic Sleep Pattern Identification and Disorder Evaluation Using EEG Signals

K R Shylaja

2.1 INTRODUCTION

In recent times, a majority of road accidents worldwide are found to be related to sleep. The current lifestyle of people has a greater influence on their mental health, especially on the quality of sleep in Western countries. The study of sleep is becoming a prominent area of research to study the patterns of sleep in individuals to diagnose sleep disorders in early stages. The quality of sleep impacts the day-to-day performance of general tasks in individuals and their physical and mental health. Sleep is necessary for cells in the body to recover from damages and also to integrate and consolidate memory. Sleep disorders can lead to anxiety, depression, and other mental problems, such as imparity in decision-making in simple tasks (Acharya et al., 2020). Sleep research has been a focus of interest in medical science, biomedical engineering, and transportation, military security, aviation and aerospace.

2.1.1 SLEEP

Sleep is a natural state of mind, a psychological process with altered consciousness, inhibited sensory activity, inhibition of all voluntary muscles activities, and reduced interactions with surroundings. During sleep, the body is in an anabolic state with reduced heartbeat and breathing rates that help in restoring the immune, nervous, skeletal, and muscular systems. During sleep, the brain shows major physiological changes with reduced activity and consumes less energy. The quality of sleep directly affects the mood, memory, cognitive functions, endocrine system, and immune system of living organisms. Hence, the study of sleep to determine its quality is becoming a research focus to address the challenges of sleep-related disorders as a large population in Western countries suffers from sleep-related disorders (Krueger et al., 2015).

DOI: 10.1201/9781003252092-3

Sleep is broadly classified into two different behavioral states called random eye movement (REM) and non-REM (NREM) sleep. Non-REM sleep is also called slow-wave sleep or deep sleep, during which an individual is away from the environment and cannot be woken up. During this phase, the body temperature and heartbeat rate fall and the brain consumes less energy. REM sleep is paradoxical sleep, during which an individual generally gets dreams or nightmares. This state is characterized by fast brain waves, eye movements, loss of muscle tone, and suspension of homeostasis (a state of steady internal, physical, and chemical condition maintained by an organism).

The sleep cycle in humans is a sequence of alternating cycles of NREM and REM sleeps. The entire sleep consists of a succession of four cycles of 90–120 minutes each. Non-REM sleep consists of three stages, N1, N2, and N3. The sleep cycle starts with a slow-wave sleep of stages 1 and 2 and is followed by REM sleep, which occurs generally at the end of the cycle. There is a greater amount of deep sleep (stage N3) earlier in the night, while the proportion of REM sleep increases in two cycles just before natural awakening and one will tend to get dreams or nightmares during these two cycles of REM. During REM sleep, the body is virtually paralyzed (Krueger et al., 2015).

The study of sleep is conducted to read brain signals and various body movements by using sensors to identify abnormalities in sleep cycles. The electrical activity of the brain and other body movements are recorded using polysomnogram (PSG), which involves electroencephalography (EEG), electrooculography (EOG) for eye movements (Iber et al., 2007), electrocardiography (ECG) for cardiac activity, and electromyography (EMG) for skeletal muscle activity. The signals are decoded by experts using standard methods as specified by Rechtschaffen and Kales (R&K) (Rechtschaffen and Kales, 1968) and the American Academy of Sleep Medicine (AASM).

The human and non-human physiological systems work in a synchronized manner with an internal biological clock, called the circadian clock, which controls sleep cycles. It controls the secretion of hormones and in turn the body's activities. This biological clock is a biochemical oscillator that oscillates in cycles with a stable phase, synchronized with solar time. It enables living organisms to anticipate daily environmental changes corresponding with the day-night cycle and adjust their biology and behavior accordingly. During the night, the brain secretes a hormone called melatonin in response to darkness that puts one into sleep. The concentration of this hormone is more during sleep. The brain also restores the supply of adenosine triphosphate (ATP), a molecule used for short-term storage and transportation of energy. After adequate sleep, the body restores to a normal state with rejuvenated energy (Fuller et al., 2006; Zee and Turek, 1999; Derk-Jan and Edgar, 1999).

The AI and ML approaches have made a significant reduction in determining sleep-related decisions by automating sleep-stage identification and the duration of the stages by using trained neural networks. Researchers have been working on the variants of deep networks, such as CNNs, RNNs, and long short-term memory (LSTM) in combinations. These deep learning models are built by using multiple layers of linear and non-linear processing units to identify hierarchical features from the given sleep datasets that help recognize sleep-stage scoring. The following sections discuss the processes involved in building AI models for sleep-stage identification.

2.1.2 SLEEP DISORDERS

Sleep disorders are the most common health issues found in a majority of the population all over the world. Sleep insomnia and apnea are major disorders that are life threatening; hence, timely diagnosis and treatment become important. The disorders are mainly characterized by disturbed sleep cycles. The patterns of major disorders are discussed in the subsequent sections (Thorpy, 1999, 2000).

2.1.2.1 Insomnia

A common sleep disorder is insomnia in which people find difficulty in falling asleep or maintaining sleep. Generally, a person having insomnia experiences delayed and interrupted sleep cycles. They experience poor sleep quality as the individual does not reach stage 3 or delta sleep, which is attributed to restorative properties. The three symptoms of insomnia are increased activity of the hypothalamus-pituitary-adrenal (HPA) axis and arousal; increased utilization of glucose during NREM sleep and wakefulness; and, finally, full-body metabolism and increase in heartbeat rate. Generally, to diagnose insomnia, the actigraphy test can be conducted using non-invasive devices to study parameters, such as time to bed, sleep onset time, the number of awakenings by capturing body movements, along with medications prescribed, time of awakening, and subjective feeling after awakening.

2.1.2.2 Sleep Apnea

The common symptoms of sleep apnea are shallow breathing or pause in breathing during sleep lasting for a few seconds to a few minutes. This pause of breathing for a longer number of cycles will reduce the oxygen level in blood or increase carbon dioxide levels that can damage body cells and in turn organs. As the breathing cycles change, normal sleep cycles are affected, which disrupts normal sleep. With the lack of sleep during the night, an individual may experience sleepiness and feel tired during daytime. Sleep apnea is two types: obstructive sleep apnea (OSA) in which breathing is interrupted due to blockage of airflow, which may be due to anatomical compromises, such as narrow and collapsed upper airways, and central sleep apnea, which is a malfunctioning of neurological controls that fail to signal to inhale, leading to a sudden stoppage of breathing for a few cycles. People with sleep apnea experience slow-wave sleep and spend less time in REM sleep (Cao et al., 2020; Mostafa et al., 2019).

2.1.2.3 Circadian Rhythm Disorder

This disorder is concerned with the inability to sleep when desired, needed, or expected as per the circadian sleep clock rhythm. This results in inappropriate wake episodes at inappropriate times. These patients have delayed onset of sleep and delayed major sleep episodes involving REM and NREM cycling. Adolescents experience a delayed major sleep phase, and older adults experience an advancement in the major sleep phases, which concerns the desired sleep onset and wake-up times. A major feature of this disorder is a persistent or recurrent misalignment between the sleep patterns compared to normal sleep cycles (Abad and Guilleminault, 2003; Zee and Turek, 1999).

2.1.2.4   Hypersomnia

This disorder has symptoms of daytime sleepiness and a lack of the ability to stay alert and awake during major waking episodes during daytimes, leading to unintended sleep cycles. The term hypersomnia in diagnostic terminology refers to excessive daytime sleepiness and the daily sleep time amounts to more than nine hours. The diagnosis of hypersomnia of central origin has to be ensured that the disturbed sleep is not due to other sleep disorders (Bollu et al., 2018).

2.1.2.5   Parasomnia

This disorder is related to abnormal sleep-related movements, behaviors, dreaming emotions, and perception. It is manifested through activation of the central nervous system that initiates skeletal muscle activity, which is a predominant feature of this disorder. It is a disorder of arousal, partial arousal, and sleep-stage transition. This often occurs in conjunction with other sleep disorders, such as OSA syndrome. A typical pattern is associated with arousal from NREM sleep due to mental confusion or disordered arousal that occurs during or after arousal from sleep (Cao et al., 2020).

There are many human disorders connected with the quality of sleep and can be cured by diagnosing them at the right time. Reading brain signals during sleep and recognizing the stages of sleep is a prerequisite for identifying the disorders (Abad and Guilleminault, 2003).

The challenging part of studying sleep is reading the continuous signals and identifying the structure of the signal to classify it into the sleep stage. This phase generally requires manually scoring the signal patterns by an expert to identify the stages. It requires a lot of time and expertise otherwise leading to non-precise classification. AI in recent times mainly focuses on machine learning and deep learning for pattern recognition and classification problems (Boostani et al., 2016).

The machine learning techniques and neural network models are driven by huge and consistent datasets. The models result in good accuracy if they are trained using meaningful and consistent datasets. The flow diagram (Figure 2.1) shows the general steps adopted in building ML/deep learning models.

2.2   DATA COLLECTION OF SLEEP

Data collection on sleep was generally done in a lab environment where the subject was made to wear the sensors under the supervision of an expert and go to sleep without using any medicine. The sensors used were of two types: non-invasive and invasive. The advancement in wearable devices like Apple wristwatches, which are comfortable to wear and sleep in a home environment, can read multiple body parameters. The various methods of collecting sleep data are discussed below.

The EEG, EOG, EMG, and ECG record specific patterns during the sleep state. Sleep data used in most of the research are taken from PhysioNet's Sleep-EDF database collected in a lab environment. For sleep-stage identification, the standard adopted is as specified in R&K and AASM standards (Rechtschaffen and Kales, 1968; Iber et al., 2007). This chapter covers the literature on single-channel EEG datasets. The following section elaborates on EEG signals and brain waves.

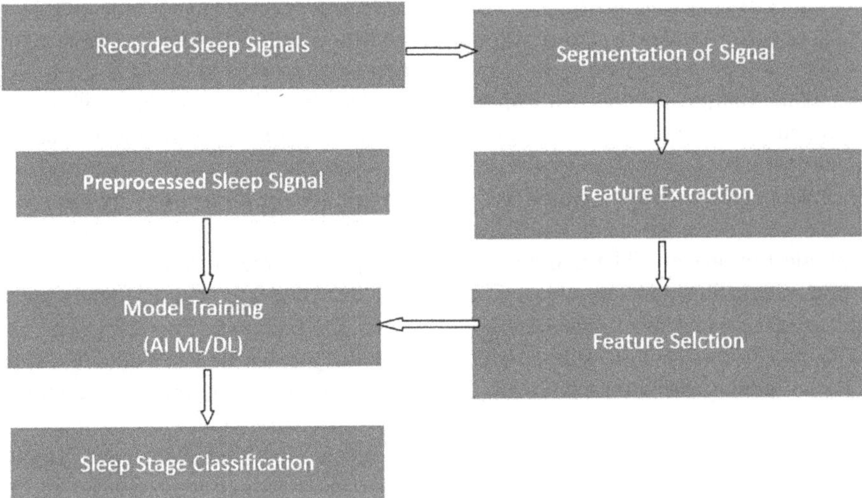

FIGURE 2.1 A diagram illustrating the design process for creating a model. It showcases the step-by-step stages involved in sleep model development.

2.2.1 EEG Signals and Brain Waves

EEG signals are read through electrodes placed on the subject's scalp to read the neural oscillations called brain waves that are read as spectral EEG signals. The summation of electric potential generated by a set of neurons involved in collective synchronous firing becomes brain waves. EEG is the most commonly used for diagnosing brain disorders, such as sleep disorders, tumor detection, stroke prediction, epilepsy, and brain death. The oscillations recorded are categorized by frequency ranges for each state of brain functioning, such as sleeping, reading, listening, and so on (Jebelli et al., 2018).

The technician identifies reference positions, such as the nasion, a point between the forehead and nose; the inion, a middle point on the back of the skull; and the preauricular on both sides of the head as indentation points. All other electrodes are placed at equal distances to cover different regions of the brain. The electric activity of brain waves is read through differential amplifiers using montages. The consecutive pair of electrodes are connected to two-channel amplifiers such that electrode input 2 of one channel is connected to input 1 of the subsequent channel to form a bipolar montage that reads the voltage difference between two consecutive electrodes, whereas referential montage is formed by connecting the input of various electrodes to input 1 of the amplifier and the input of the reference electrode (current inactive electrode) to input 2. The referential montage reads the difference between the given electrode and the referential voltage.

The following theoretical frequency bands used in brain study are also called cerebral rhythm. The rhythmic activities of humans generate oscillations in the frequency band of 8–12 Hz are called alpha waves, which are characterized by a certain distribution in the scalp region. These frequency bands are extracted using spectral methods of free software tools, such as EEGLAB. The delta band frequency that is less than 4 Hz is found when an adult is in slow-wave sleep or a constant attention state. A theta wave characterized by a frequency band of 4–7 Hz is spiked when a person is continuously trying to repress a response. The frequency band of 8–15 Hz is characterized as an alpha wave that is generally found during a relaxed state with eyes closed and trying to inhibit activities in different parts of the brain. Beta waves of 16–31 Hz are found during active thinking, focus, and high alert or anxiety. The gamma waves of frequency greater than 32 Hz are read while integrating multiple sensory inputs like watching a movie and listening to dialogues or when short-term memory is accessed to recognize an object, whereas EEG uses a frequency band less than 4 Hz as delta, greater than 4 Hz and less than 8 Hz as theta, greater than 8 Hz and less than 14 Hz as alpha, and any frequency greater than 14 Hz as beta waves.

The non-REM sleep with slow brain waves and eye movement completely stopped is observed in stage 2 with a wave pattern sleep spindles and K complexes represented by a sharp negative wave followed by a slow positive wave that lasts for 0.5 seconds. The waves of stage 2 are transient and rhythmic in the frequency band of 12–14 Hz and are characterized as sigma waves. In stage 3, the extremely slow brain waves called delta waves start appearing with a frequency range between 1 and 3 Hz with high amplitude. Stage 4 is characterized by a deep sleep stage with deeper delta waves appearing in the brain. In stage 5, which is before coming to a wakeful state, the subject shows rapid eye movements and muscular twitches with predominant theta waves. These generally follow a rhythmic wave of frequency domain identified as cerebral rhythms. Sleep cycle stages 3 and 4 are dominated by a delta rhythm of 1–4 Hz covering more than 50% of the spectrum and stages 1 and 5 are dominated by theta rhythm (Aserinsky and Kleitman, 1953; Ronzhina et al., 2012).

Experts study these signals by localizing the electrodes to particular regions of the brain to interpret the normalcy or abnormality of the signals. In a bipolar montage, phase reversal is a deflection of two channels within a chain pointing to opposite directions, which is identified to see the transitions. In a referential montage, all channels may show deflections or movements in the same direction. If the electrical activity at the active electrodes is positively compared to the activity at the reference electrode, the deflection will be downward. Electrodes, where the electrical activity is the same as at the reference electrode, do not show any deflection.

2.2.1.1 Signal Pre-processing, Feature Extraction, and Feature Selection of Sleep Signals

The stages of sleep signals are characterized by distinct frequency domains and the time of occurrence. They also differ in proportion. Sleep scoring identifies sleep stages and also the transitions from one stage to another.

The sleep signal waveform is interpreted to identify the patterns by using amplitude and frequency band filters. These patterns are described using mathematical and statistical methods to identify them as features. Feature extraction is a process of identifying the various frequency bands and time-domain variations from a continuous sleep signal. The parameters required for training the model are extracted using different techniques as discussed below.

2.2.2 Frequency-Domain Features of Sleep Signal

The frequency-domain parameters from the EEG signal of sleep data capture four different cerebral rhythms, such as delta rhythms, alpha rhythms, beta rhythms, and theta rhythms that describe sleep stages. Each of these rhythms is characterized by different frequency band waveforms. As discussed in the previous sections, the wakeful state is dominated by alpha rhythm, and theta and delta rhythms in the N3 and N4 deep sleep stages. The slow-wave sleep or deep sleep stage is generally dominated by a large amount of delta rhythm. The various frequency band filters and wavelet transform techniques are adopted to capture the features of sleep stages of an EEG signal. In Fast Fourier Transform (FFT), the time domain signal is converted into a frequency domain, which gives the ratio of the power of certain frequency activity in a particular band (Inoue et al., 2005; Alam and Sameni, 2020; Delimayanti et al., 2020).

2.2.3 Discrete Wavelet Transformation (DWT) Approach for Feature Extraction from Sleep Signal

In the current research scenarios, feature extraction and sleep-stage classification have been automated to a greater extent. One of the research papers on single-channel EEG signal quantification by da Silveira et al. (2016) demonstrated automatic scoring of sleep stages using three basic steps, such as signal pre-processing, features extraction, and ML classification. They experimented using 106,376 samples of 30-second epochs available in PhysioNet's Sleep-EDF public data. The raw signals were normalized and applied with discrete wavelet transformation (DWT) to decompose each 30-second epoch into different frequency bands using Daubechies wavelet transformation with two vanishing points and four Db2 filters to capture the variations.

The sleep-stage classification is performed by identifying the features extracted from raw sleep signals. These generally follow a rhythmic wave of frequency domain identified as cerebral rhythms. In the sleep cycle, stages 3 and 4 are dominated by a delta rhythm of 1–4 Hz covering more than 50% of the spectrum. Stages 1 and 5 are dominated by theta rhythm (Lopes et al., 2017; Ronzhina et al., 2012; Ahmed et al., 2009).

2.2.4 Non-Linear Time Series Parameters

The approximate entropy method calculates the entropy of the time series sequence to statistically quantify the regularity and complexity of the signal. This determines the unpredictable fluctuations of a time-series signal. The sample entropy helps measure the regularity of a continuous sleep signal, which is independent of the pattern length. The higher the complexity of the sequence the larger the corresponding approximate entropy. The average approximate entropy calculated will be considered as a feature (Acharya et al., 2020, 2015; Hassan et al., 2015).

2.2.5 Time-Domain Parameters

The standard statistical analysis methods, such as the average of amplitude, variance, maximum, minimum, zero-crossing numbers, skewness, and kurtosis, are used to analyze the sleep signal to extract the features.

The time-domain features are collected in three steps: pre-processing, feature extraction, and classification. In the pre-processing phase, the alpha rhythm of the awakening state is extracted as features as it becomes easier to recognize the other frequencies. The raw sleep signals are interpreted by an expert clinician by using three rules. These rules are framed as procedures to eliminate the clutter in raw EEG signals to enhance the featured rhythm for time-domain analysis of the signal. The first rule focuses on eliminating pseudo-turning points that do not change the trend of the sequence. This rule also extracts the local maxima and local minima of the signal sequence to form a new time sequence. The second rule eliminates pseudo peaks by comparing the amplitude of two adjacent peaks. The third rule eliminates a clutter that contains two peaks that are small with amplitude Max1 and Max2, and Min1 forms the trough of the sequence. If Max1−Min1 < 5 μv, the point Min1 is seen as a pseudo trough. This rule removes the pseudo trough and uses rule 1 to smooth the sequence. These three rules convert a raw sleep signal into an appropriate characteristic waveform for feature extraction 5 (Xu et al., 2020).

To extract features from the processed signal, the procedure counts the number of peaks of each frequency band in a 1-second sample signal. The frequency band of the alpha rhythm is 8–13 Hz, and in initial signal recording, these frequency band peaks are dominated. Later, the delta and theta rhythm frequency band peaks appear and are extracted as features by the procedure.

The features extracted for the sleep stage show that in the wakeful state, the alpha and beta rhythms dominate. As the sleep becomes deeper, the theta and delta waves dominate slow-wave sleep as shown in Figure 2.2 (Zhang et. al., 2017).

The feature extraction process is important in sleep staging as appropriate feature parameters can dramatically improve classification accuracy. The dimensionality reduction of EEG signal data is effectively done using feature extraction methods. The time-domain features are extracted by averaging of amplitude, variance,

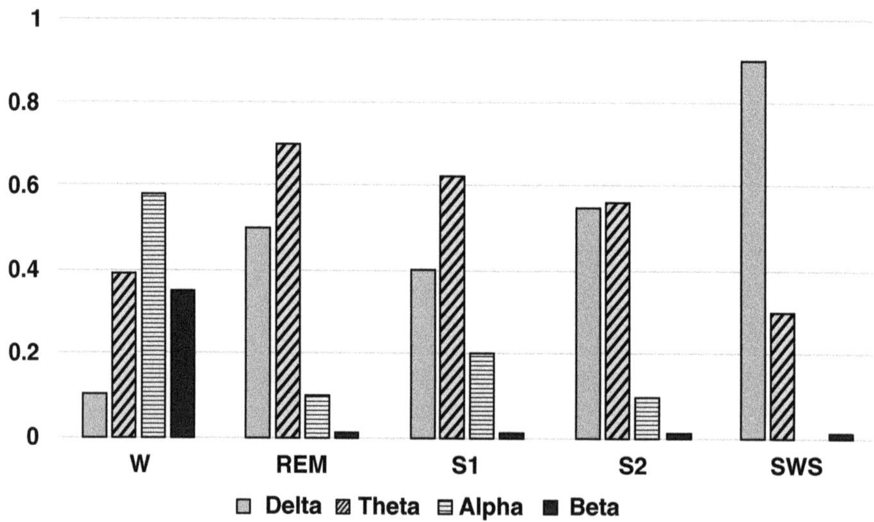

FIGURE 2.2 Brain rhythms of sleep stages (Zhang et al., 2017).

skewness, kurtosis, zero-crossing, or maximum, and minimum methods (Hjorth, 1970). Another type of parameter is derived from a transformed domain, such as the power spectral density (PSD) of the EEG signal. The theory of non-linear time series can capture brain dynamics reflected in EEG signals (Acharya et al., 2015, 2016). Methods, such as correlation, largest Lyapunov entropy, approximate entropy, data complexity, and permutation entropy, are derived from non-linear analysis. Frequency-domain features are extracted by using wavelet transformation techniques to extract peak frequency in the time series of EEG signal data (Inoue et al., 2005, 2020; Ahmed et al., 2009).

2.3 AI/ML AND DL TECHNIQUES

The automatic sleep-stage classification using sleep signals requires a trained AI model for recognizing patterns. The AI approach is required to learn the patterns existing in valid sleep signals. The ML techniques and DL models are the most general techniques of AI used in the current literature. Classification techniques, such as support vector machine (SVM) (Aboalayon et al., 2014; Evgeniou and Pontil, 2001) and K-nearest neighbor (KNN), are the most frequently used ML approach, and CNN, RNN with LSTM technique are more accurate models built for automatic sleep scoring (Yildirim et al., 2019; Supratak et al., 2017; Mohamed et al., 2019). The following section discusses the models in detail.

2.3.1 SVM AND KNN FOR CLASSIFICATION

SVMs are widely used for the classification of EEG signals for automatic sleep scoring in many papers. SVM is a good generalizer and shows good performance for high-dimensional data. The SVM finds an optimal hyperplane as a solution for a classification problem using kernel k to define the hypothesis space (Hochreiter et al., 1997; Evgeniou and Pontil, 2001).

KNN is also used for classification problems that create clusters of input data by calculating the distance between the mean of the cluster and the new instance. The KNN uses either Euclidian distance or Hamming distance to find the nearest cluster (Cunningham and Delany, 2021; Aboalayon et al., 2016).

2.3.2 DECISION TREES FOR CLASSIFICATION

Decision trees belong to a class of supervised learning methods used for both regression and classification problems. The intermediate nodes in the decision tree represent the features of the dataset, and branches signify the decision guidelines framework to reach the leaf nodes where the leaf nodes represent the labels of classification. Once the dataset is divided based on characteristics, the estimated entropy and information gain ascertain the next node to be chosen for branching. The entropy must decrease and information gain must increase as the tree grows and expect zero entropy at leaf nodes with information gain being high. The trained model is analyzed for performance by generating a confusion matrix, using the accuracy, specificity, sensitivity, precision, and F-score (Hassan and Subasi, 2017).

2.3.3 DL Techniques for Classification

DL is a subfield of ML inspired by artificial neural networks (ANNs) that can automatically learn patterns from the dataset without explicitly mentioning them. Deep learning is more accurate and performs better when the data size is too big compared to ML algorithms. More often this technique is adopted for applications involving image classification, speech recognition, natural language processing (NLP), recommendation systems, and so on. The different variations of neural networks are used for building DL models, such as CNN, RNN, and LSTM models. The following sections briefly explain the working mechanism of each of these models.

2.3.4 Convolution Neural Networks (CNN)

ANN are computing networks, such as the brain with a network of neurons, that are used in recent times for implementing learning on machines. These networks are very efficient for implementing regression and classification problems, especially on image data. The computations in nodes in ANN are the simple linear summations of weighted edge and input. Various activation functions used at each node, such as rectified linear unit (ReLU), sigmoid, Softmax, tanh, and so on, control the output of the node.

The CNNs are an extension of ANN that generally involve a combination of fully connected layers, convolution layers, and pooling layers in different order starting from the input layer. Based on the complexity of the dataset used and the level of features that need to be identified, the number of nodes in each layer and the number of hidden layers vary themselves while building the model. This decision requires domain expertise, data visualization, and the working mechanism of CNN (Figure 2.3).

The input layer in CNN is fed with features extracted from previous layers or multichannel signals. The convolution layer uses time-invariant linear filters to process

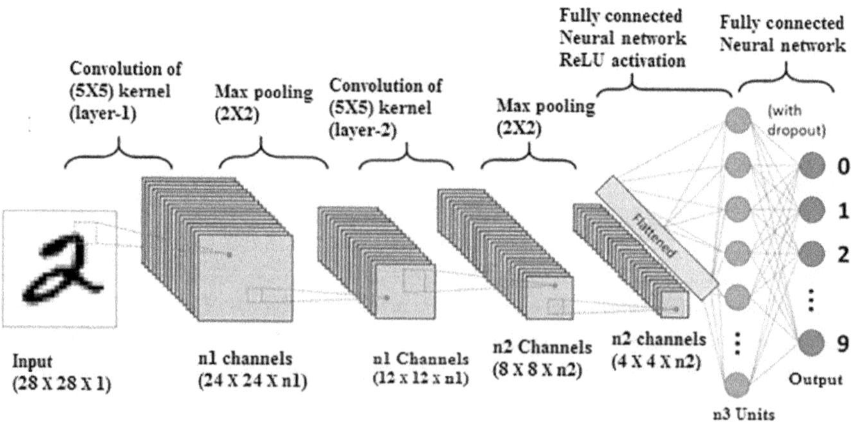

FIGURE 2.3 CNN architecture.

the features. The pooling layer controls the exponential growth of intermediate features by merging the output of the filter using pointwise summations. In this layer, local summaries of features are generated and the feature components, as a weighted average of adjacent components in the linear form or as a maximum value among adjacent components in the non-linear form, are replaced. It also conducts sub-sampling of the summarized output to reduce the dimensionality with a small loss of information as the summarization function is a low-pass operation. The output of each layer is a result of non-linear activation functions that are passed as input to the next layers. The CNN models are proved to be efficient for applications involving NLP, search query retrieval, sentence modeling, audio and video signal processing, image processing, and many unsupervised learning tasks. CNN works with better accuracy even with a certain degree of invariance of scale and deformation of the perception.

2.3.4.1   RNN and LSTM Models

The RNNs are the improved version of CNNs that are considered to be more efficient for sequence prediction problems as in sleep signals. In addition, the patterns are sequenced in some order and it is required to remember the previous patterns. RNNs consider the predictions of previous steps in making predictions for the future. They work well for simple and short contexts but fail to remember the concept behind the sequence for longer time-dependent contexts. They fail to remember the relevant information at the point where it is needed, which is their biggest drawback. Another limitation is the vanishing gradient, which results during the back-propagation of the error term.

The LSTM models are an extended and improved version of an RNN, which was introduced by Hochreiter and Schmidhuber (1997) to address the drawback of remembering the context for a longer duration. LSTM makes simple modifications to the information by using addition and multiplication to selectively remember or forget the information. They are similar to standard networks with many hidden layers along with input and output layers. The unique structure of LSTM over RNN is that the nodes in the hidden layer are replaced with memory modules. Each module consists of a memory cell, forget cell, and input and output gates. The memory cell consists of a self-connected loop edge with a fixed weight of one that takes the gradient through many time steps to overcome the vanishing gradient problem (Figure 2.4).

The cell state represented as a horizontal line at the top portion of the cell carries the information from cell to cell down the chain with a small modification of information in each cell while passing through the cell using some operations. The cell state is controlled by the sigmoid layer, also known as the "forget gate layer," which controls what information to keep or throw away. The sigmoid gate takes $ht-1$ and xt as inputs and generates a value between 0 and 1, where 0 indicates "completely get rid of the information" and 1 indicates "completely keep the information."

The next step in the LSTM memory module is to generate an updated information vector by using the tanh layer, and the other sigmoid gate determines which information must get updated. This updated information vector is combined with the output

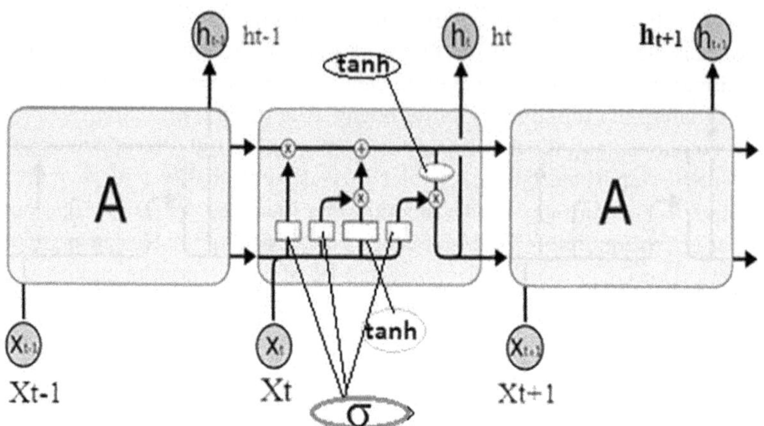

FIGURE 2.4   LSTM memory module.

of the sigmoid function to create the updated cell state. Finally, the scaled-cell state is created by using a combination of tanh and sigmoid layers.

2.4   CASE STUDIES ON TRAINED AI/ML/DL MODELS FOR INTERPRETATION OF SLEEP

This section covers the latest CNN models designed and built for sleep staging and sleep disorder identification. One of the DL models is discussed in detail in the next section as a case study. The comparative table is created to highlight the techniques adopted, parameters used, and performance obtained in each of the models.

The basic models of deep neural network (DNN) were implemented by Mohamed H. Al-Meer (Mohamed et al., 2019) for sleep-stage classification. The three-layered neural network model was a feed-forward network with 100 nodes in the first layer, and in the hidden layer, which is densely connected, the output layer consists of six nodes for classifying six stages of sleep. The activation functions used in the first two layers were ReLU, and the output layer uses the Softmax activation. Initial weights were given by using a Gaussian distribution with a mean of 0 and a variance of 2. The dataset used for the training was collected in a clinical environment with eight healthy persons and four subjects with difficulty falling asleep. The Electro Polysomnography (EPG) signal recorded is decomposed into 57,600 epochs of 30-second samples. The dataset was further split into 65% and 35% proportions for training and testing, respectively. This model obtained a training accuracy of 92%.

Yildirim et al. (2019) proposed a one-dimensional CNN by using EEG and EOG signals for the classification of sleep stages. The dataset used in this work is taken from the PhysioNet Sleep-EDF database, which consists of PSG recordings from eight healthy males and four females. The convolution layer is used for feature extraction from the input EEG signal. These feature maps are further sub-sampled by using a subsequent pooling layer. The output of this layer is fed into the final fully connected layer, which performs the classification. The number of layers and initial values of parameters are assigned using the brute force technique. The model learned to extract time and frequency domain features from raw EEG signals, which are fed as input. The model achieved an accuracy of 98% for stage 2 and the least accuracy of 89.3% for stage 6 during training.

Chambon et al. (2018) and Eldele et al. (2021) used multimodal, multivariate PSG signal readings from EEG, EMG, and EOG with 30-second sequential segments of continuous time-series signals. The DL model built into this work automatically learns the frequency bands of each sleep stage as well as valid transitions from one stage to another. This problem is treated as a multi-class predictive classification problem. The major issue in sleep scoring is its imbalanced sleep stages in the entire sleep signals collected, such as the number of N1 stages being very rare compared to N2. This imbalance in the dataset can cause the model to fail in predicting the rarest sleep stages. The other challenge is learning transition rules that determine the time of occurrence of a sleep stage. These time-domain transitions are very important to capture from the signal as they determine the performance of the model predictions, which are done as temporal sleep staging. The research work in this paper proposes a single DNN that can work on multivariate and multimodal sleep signals collected from EEG, EMG, and EOG through different channels to address the issues. The network architecture used consists of three convolution layers: each layer followed by a max-pool layer for feature extraction and a dropout layer that gives input to a fully connected Softmax classifier. The model is trained in two stages: in the first stage, the linear spatial filter is used to recognize virtual channels and convolution to recognize spectral features. In the second stage, the model is trained for a Softmax classifier. The proposed architecture shows good performance for the waking state compared to other sleep stages.

Eldele et al. (2021) propose a DNN that works on an attention model called AttnSleep. The model is built in three parts: the first part for feature extraction, the second part for temporal relations among features, and the third part for classification. For feature extraction, a multi-resolution CNN (MRCNN) and adaptive features calibration (AFC) modules are used. The MRCNN is a general convolution network that recognizes the intra-segment features, such as low- and high-frequency bands, whereas alternate frame rendering (AFR) encodes the interdependencies to learn the features more accurately. The second part of the model temporal context encoder (TCE) is a simple convolution network that captures the temporal dependencies among the features extracted. The last part uses a Softmax classifier, which is a fully connected layer. Finally, the model adopts a class-aware loss function to address the imbalance issue. In MRCNN, filters of different sizes are used in convolution layers to capture different frequency bands. The filter sizes are matched to the high- and low-frequency bands of sleep stages and sampling rates. In the AFR module, the residual squeeze and excitation (SE) block helps in exploiting the contextual information by using two convolution layers with different kernel sizes, followed by a max pool layer to capture the features and the adaptive average pooling to capture the global spatial information.

The self-attention concept is applied by giving more weightage to the region of interest in input signals and low weights for other regions. Multi-head Attention is used to improve self-attention by expanding the model's ability to encode the heads of different positions to capture the temporal contexts. Splitting the input signal into a different partition and encoding each partition head increases the representational spaces and thereby increases the performance accuracy of the classifier. The model shows an overall accuracy of 85.6% and an $F1$ score of 80.9.

Hafezi et al. (2020) proposed a DL model for estimating the severity of sleep apnea by identifying the disturbance in sleep stages. The dataset used for training the model was collected at a sleep laboratory at the Toronto Rehabilitation Institute from subjects in the age group of 18–85 years who were referred for an overnight diagnostic sleep study. The data recorded include PSG signals, chest and abdominal movements, airflow by nasal pressure, and peripheral oxyhemoglobin saturation (SpO_2) by pulse oximetry. The features extracted were average tracheal movement from inhalation to exhalation; the average duration of the breathing duty cycle; the average ratio of inspiratory duration to the breathing duration; an average of the area under the inspiratory signal; the average slope of the signal during inspiration; the average area under the whole breadth; and signal drop, which is the distance between the minimum movement value of the current window and the maximum movement value of the previous non-overlapping window.

The model consists of four convolution layers followed by one LSTM layer along with input and output layers. In the convolution layers, a filter size of 4 with a stride value of 1 is used to extract 64 features. The model uses a dropout with a probability of 0.5 to avoid over-fitting, and the layer is embedded with batch normalization to speed up the training process. Each node uses the ReLU activation function for non-linearity. The model could preserve the temporal dependencies in the input signal. The results depict the severity of the disorder for the data collected in different sleep postures of the subjects. In the following section, one of the DL models is discussed in detail.

2.4.1 DeepSleepNet

The DeepSleepNet model is proposed by Supratak et al. (2017) in their research paper used for automatic sleep-stage scoring. The dataset was used from two sources – Montreal Archive of Sleep Studies (MASS) and Sleep-EDF from PhysioNet. The EEG and EOG recordings were pre-processed with a notch filter of 60 Hz, and band-pass filters of 0.30–100 Hz (EEG) and 0.10–100 Hz (EOG). These signals were manually classified into five stages.

DeepSleepNet is a CNN model built for automated sleep-stage scoring using raw single-channel EEG signals. It uses CNN to automatically extract features by using convolution operation with different filter sizes in the beginning layers to extract time-invariant features and a bidirectional LSTM (Bi-LSTM) model to detect temporal information like the sleep-stage transition rule. Small filters were good to recognize temporal features, such as a pattern occurrence in EEG signal, and large filter sizes were good for capturing frequency domain information. The model is designed as a two-step training algorithm with a back propagation technique so that it can overcome the class imbalance. The model worked better for datasets with different scoring standards.

The Bi-LSTM neural network processes the input data in two directions through two LSTMs, computes the forward hidden layer sequence, and iteratively computes the backward hidden layer sequence. The hidden layers of the Bi-LSTM neural network are coupled with the same output layer so that the output of the model can simultaneously utilize information about the past and the future in the time series. This paper uses two layers of deep Bi-LSTM neural network structure with a time step length of 5. The Bi-LSTM neural network is constructed by stacking multiple layers of LSTM layers. Each subsequent layer receives the implicit state of the upper layer as a time series input. When the network is updated, the information is transmitted along the hierarchy and the time context information is added at each layer. The input sequence at each moment undergoes a multilayer non-linear transformation before the output to enable the Bi-LSTM neural network to learn the inputs on different time scales.

2.4.2 METHODOLOGY AND ARCHITECTURE OF TRAINING IN DEEPSLEEPNET

The authors propose an architecture that includes two stages: training to learn filter extract time-invariant features and learning transition rules. The model was built by using two CNNs with each one containing four convolution layers and two max pool layers with filter sizes of 2, 4, and 16 in both CNNs. The neurons use the ReLU activation function where the output is max$(0, x)$.

A sequence of n samples each of 30-second epochs of single-channel EEG signals represented as $\{X1, X2, X3,...Xn\}$ is fed parallel to two CNNs. To extract with attribute and convert it into a feature vector, the model adopts a function $h(Xi)$=CNN(Xi) on both CNN networks and a concatenation operation to combine the output of these two CNNs to extract the ith attribute. This indicates that by taking N samples, the CNN generates N features, one from each sample.

The second part of the training is for residual learning, which trains the filters to recognize sleep transition patterns or rules. The Bi-LSTM is trained to remember the subject in the N2 sleep stage, and the EEG signals show low amplitude and a mixed frequency EEG activity. Hence, it detects successive epochs as the N2 stage if they also show amplitude and mixed frequency. The Bi-LSTM uses forward and backward processing of the input sequence independently. This enables the model to exploit the information from the past and future. The LSTM uses a peephole mechanism to inspect the memory cell before modification. The feature vector detected in CNN is added to the output from the LSTM. These layers perform matrix multiplication of the weight matrix with batch normalization and use the ReLU activation function.

2.4.3 CASE STUDY ON ML APPROACH FOR SLEEP-STAGE SCORING

A major part of research in studying sleep is focused on automatic sleep-stage recognition using AI and ML. In this section, the ML classification algorithms used for sleep-stage scoring are discussed in detail. The main classification techniques used are K-means and SVM algorithms. Case studies of these are covered in the following section.

2.4.4 Multiclass SVM Classification of Sleep Stages

The experiment was conducted on a dataset that was collected using single-channel EEG on the A1:C3 and C4:A2 areas of the brain. The frequency bandwidth features were extracted using Butterworth band-pass filters that are designed to filter and decompose the EEG signal into five frequency sub-bands: delta wave (0–4 Hz), theta wave (4–8 Hz), alpha wave (8–12 Hz), beta wave (12–30 Hz), and gamma wave (>30 Hz). The algorithm is implemented in four steps, such as acquiring the EEG signal; filtering and decomposition of the signal; feature extraction; and, finally, the SVM classification for sleep-stage identification.

The dataset consists of 61 participants, both male and female, whose sleep data are collected for almost 24 hours, and samples at 100-Hz patterns, which are available on the PhysioNet website. Each hypnogram file is manually scored by an expert as per the R&K (1968) manual that is sampled into 60-second frames.

In the filtering and decomposition stage, the signals are classified into different bands using infinite impulse response (IIR) Butterworth band-pass filters.

The feature extraction stage analyzes each frequency band to identify and extract various statistical features, such as energy, entropy, and standard deviation, to identify the sleep stages. The energy gives the net power of a signal at a given time; the entropy indicates the uncertainty of an outcome; and the standard deviation indicates the distribution of the data to determine sleep stages (Aboalayon et al., 1999).

The sleep-stage classification is done by using the SVM as a binary classifier. The classifier locates a hyperplane by projecting the data to higher dimensions by using a linear kernel function. The one-against-all approach is used for multiclass classification by constructing k SVM models for k classes. The performance measure of the model is done by generating a confusion matrix to determine accuracy. The model gave an overall accuracy of 92% for the wake, stage 1, stage 2, stage 3, and stage 4 (Aboalayon, 2014; Xu et al., 2020).

2.4.5 Decision Support System for Automated Scoring of Sleep Stages

Hassan and Subasi (2017) propose a decision support system for automatic sleep scoring using EEG raw signals. The process involves sampling the EEG signals into epochs, and each epoch is further decomposed into sub-bands using tunable Q-wavelet transform (TQWT), extracting statistical moment features, such as mean, variance, skewness, and kurtosis, from each band. For each of these sub-bands, further statistical analysis is made to figure out the sleep stage for classification. The dataset used in this work is taken from PhysioNet's Sleep-EDF database consisting of EEG signals recorded for subjects in the age group of

21–35 years. The feature selection is done by using Kruskal–Wallis ANOVA, performed at a confidence level of 95%. Ensemble learning techniques, such as bootstrap aggregating, which is used for creating and combining multiple classification methods, are adopted.

2.4.6 COMPLEX NETWORKS APPROACH FOR EEG SIGNAL SLEEP-STAGES CLASSIFICATION

This research paper published by Mohammed Diykh and Yan Li (2016) discusses a model to recognize sleep stages automatically using classification methods. The raw EEG signal is sampled into 30-second segments and each segment is further divided into 75 sub-segments. The model extracts 12 statistical features in the form of a vector from each segment, such as the mean, min, mode, max, median, range, variation, skewness, kurtosis, first quartile, second quartile, and standard deviation. These statistical features were ranked and sorted in descending order based on the accuracy achieved, and then, the top nine features were used for experimentation.

A vector of nodes is mapped into a complex weighted undirected network. After mapping the time series data into a complex network, the network properties are determined for classification. The graph constructed includes a set of nodes for each segment of the EEG signal, and the edges are created if the space distance between the corresponding nodes is less or equal to the predetermined value. The graph properties, such as average degree and Jacquard coefficients (Anuradha and Sairam, 2011), are evaluated for classification. It shows that the network parameters vary for each sleep stage, which is identified by the least square-SVM (LS-SVM) classifier. The results obtained are compared against Naïve, k-nearest, and multiclass SVM (Table 2.1).

2.4.7 SUMMARY

The chapter discusses the significance of sleep and related disorders in detail from a neuropsychological approach. The recent technological advancements and methods adopted for reading the signals by using various non-invasive methods are covered. In studying and recognizing sleep disorders, it becomes important to extract the features from continuous signal waveforms read through wearable devices. The chapter highlights the techniques of extracting features with relevant literature. The various AI models and techniques used for automatic sleep-stage scoring and identification of sleep are covered. The neural network models are generally built using convolution layers and pooling layers to identify the frequency bands in signal samples. The LSTM and RNN models are more useful for remembering the sequence of frequency bands so that they can identify the wrong placing and invalid time duration of a sleep stage in the continuous waveform. The chapter ends with a table narrating the models and comparison with other models on various parameters.

TABLE 2.1

Significant Parameters of Models

Model	Dataset	Pre-processing	Feature Set	Techniques Adopted	Model Complexity	Results	Drawbacks
Bi-directional LSTM–CNN (Sleep staging by bidirectional long short-term memory convolution neural network)	EDF database in MIT-BIH 39 records from 20 subjects without any sleep disorder and not on medication to train and evaluate the model	Data are band-pass filtered to recognize and extract α wave (8~13 Hz), β wave (13~30 Hz), θ wave (4~8 Hz), δ wave (0.5~3 Hz), spindle wave (12~14 Hz), K complex wave (0.5~1 Hz), etc.	Manual scoring of 300 seconds EEG, EOG, and EMG, Frequency bands of each wave and statistical features, such as mean, variance, std. deviation, skewness.	The 5-class problem that is Wake, N1, N2, N3, and REM. LSTM model to remember the previous patterns. 10-fold cross-validation.	The amount of hidden nodes in each hidden layer of LSTM–RNN is set as 100.	Accuracy rates were 94.8%, 82.6%, 87.4%, 90.3%, and 86.6% for the classification of W, N1, N2, N3, and REM were accomplished.	The model is very complex and requires more training time.
A DL architecture for temporal sleep-stage classification using multivariate and multimodal time series	A MASS dataset consisting of 62 nights' records of different subjects. Low pass filtered at 30 Hz. The time series data is downsampled to a sampling rate of 128 Hz. A sequence of time series sleep signal segments of 30 seconds is given as input.	No separate pre-processing the linear spatial filtering for identifying virtual channels, convolution layer to capture spectral features, and the separate pipeline of these layers for EOG, EMG, and EEG channels.	Automatic scoring using a single DL network for EEG, EOG, and EMG signals to capture the frequency bands and temporal transitions of sleep signals.	Linear spatial filtering and convolution network for spectral features without temporal details i.e., $k=0$ and the same network with $k>0$ to capture time-domain features. The model training is done in two parts: first, it is trained to extract features without temporal information, and second, the model is trained for Softmax classifier.	11 layers, including three convolution layers followed by max-pool layers and a 50% dropout layer.	Wake state 85%. Performed well for other sleep stages with the inclusion of temporal features.	Performance is moderate for other sleep stages compared to the wake state with 85%.

(*Continued*)

TABLE 2.1 (*Continued*)
Significant Parameters of Models

Model	Dataset	Pre-processing	Feature Set	Techniques Adopted	Model Complexity	Results	Drawbacks
An attention-based DL approach for sleep-stage classification with single-channel EEG	Publicly available four different datasets are used for extensive experimentation Sleep-EDF-20, Sleep-EDF-78 SHS	Pre-processing using CNN called multi-resolution CNN with different kernel sizes to extract spatial features and temporal context layers to capture the interdependencies among features.	Frequency domain features – frequency bands of each sleep stage and transition states to indicate the interdependencies	2- CNN with max-pool layer with different kernel sizes to extract the features and another two convolution layers with average pooling to capture the interdependencies and a fully connected layer to classify with Softmax activation.	CNN with max pool and average pooling class-aware loss function.	The model gives an overall accuracy of 85.6 and an $F1$ score of 80.9 for the Sleep-EDF20 dataset.	The training time of the model is more.
Decision support system for sleep-stage classification	Single-channel EEG signals Sleep-EDF is an open source, benchmark, and extensively utilized database in sleep scoring literature. Eight Caucasian female and male subjects took part in the study. The subjects' ages ranged from 21 to 35 years.	TQWT technique is used for decomposing input signals into different sub-bands and generating a histogram for each sub-band that is unique for each sleep stage.	Sub-band histograms for each sleep stage considering each sub-band represents a sleep stage. Statistical moment features, such as mean (θ), variance ($\sigma 2$), skewness (ι), and kurtosis (ν).	Bootstrapping/bagging for classification leave-one-out cross-validation,	Number of trees from 1 to 300 for cases I–V. After about 20 decision trees, the out-of-box (OOB) error almost becomes constant.	Accuracy (%) R&K 76.39, 74.39, 81.87, 88.98, 99.02.	

(*Continued*)

TABLE 2.1 (*Continued*)
Significant Parameters of Models

Model	Dataset	Pre-processing	Feature Set	Techniques Adopted	Model Complexity	Results	Drawbacks
Multiple SVM for sleep-stage classification	EDF database from the PhysioNet website consisting of 61 male and female sleep datasets for 24 hours sampled at 100 Hz and decomposed into 60-second frames.	IIR Butterworth band-pass filters to filter the signals into different bands.	The frequencies and amplitudes of alpha, beta, theta, and y sub-bands during normal conditions are evaluated using cutoff frequency and pass band and stopband frequencies.	SVMs with one-vs-all classification technique.	k-kernels for k classes for classification with cross-validation.	Achieves 92.43%, 93.69%, 94.36, 96.55, and 99.75 accuracy for 2-state to 6- state classification of sleep stages on Sleep-EDF database.	Training time is more as it uses one-vs-all.
Bi-directional LSTM-CNN (sleep staging by bidirectional long short-term memory convolution neural network)	EDF database in MIT-BIH 39 records from 20 subjects without any sleep disorder and not on medication to train and evaluate the model.	Data are band-pass filtered to recognize and extract α wave ($8\sim13$ Hz), β wave ($13\sim30$ Hz), θ wave ($4\sim8$ Hz), δ wave ($0.5\sim3$ Hz), spindle wave ($12\sim14$ Hz), K complex wave ($0.5\sim1$ Hz), etc.	Manual scoring of 300 sec EEG, EOG, and EMG. Frequency bands of each wave and statistical features, such as mean, variance, std. deviation, skewness.	A 5-class problem is Wake, N1, N2, N3 and REM. LSTM model to remember the previous patterns 10-fold cross-validation.	The amount of hidden nodes in each hidden layer of LSTM–RNN is set as 100.	Accuracy rates of 94.8%, 82.6%, 87.4%, 90.3%, and 86.6% for the classification of W, N1, N2, N3, and REM were accomplished.	The model is very complex and requires more training time.

(Continued)

TABLE 2.1 (*Continued*)
Significant Parameters of Models

Model	Dataset	Pre-processing	Feature Set	Techniques Adopted	Model Complexity	Results	Drawbacks
A DL architecture for temporal sleep-stage classification using multivariate and multimodal time series	A MASS dataset consisting of 62-night records of different subjects. Low pass filtered at 30 Hz. The time series data is downsampled to a sampling rate of 128 Hz, each time. Sequence of time series sleep signal segments of 30 seconds is given as input.	No separate pre-processing. The linear spatial filtering for identifying virtual channels, convolution layer to capture spectral features, and the separate pipeline of these layers for EOG, EMG, and EEG channels.	Automatic scoring using a single DL network for EEG, EOG, and EMG signals to capture the frequency bands and temporal transitions of sleep signal.	Linear spatial filtering and convolution network for spectral features without temporal details i.e., $k=0$ and the same network with $k>0$ to capture time domain features. The model training is done in two parts: first, it is trained to extract features without temporal information, and second, the model is trained for Softmax classifier.	11 layers, including 3 convolution layers followed by max pool layers and a 50% dropout layer.	Wake state with 85%. Performed well for other sleep stages with the inclusion of temporal features.	Performance is moderate for other sleep stages compared to wake state with 85%.
Attention-based DL approach for sleep-stage classification with single-channel EEG	Publicly available four different datasets are used for extensive experimentation Sleep-EDF-20, Sleep-EDF-78, Sleep Heart Health Study (SHHS).	Pre-processing using CNN called MR-CNN with different kernel size to extract spatial features and temporal context layers to capture the inter dependencies among features.	Frequency domain features – frequency bands of each sleep stage and transition states to indicate the interdependencies.	2- CNN with max-pool layer with different kernel sizes to extract the features and another two convolution layers with average pooling to capture the interdependencies and a fully connected layer to classify with Softmax. activation.	CNN with max-pool and average pooling. Class-aware loss function.	Model gives an overall accuracy of 85.6% and $F1$ score of 80.9 for Sleep-EDF20 dataset.	Training time of the model is more.

(*Continued*)

TABLE 2.1 (*Continued*)
Significant Parameters of Models

Model	Dataset	Pre-processing	Feature Set	Techniques Adopted	Model Complexity	Results	Drawbacks
Decision support system for sleep-stage classification	Single-channel EEG signals sleep-EDF is an open source, benchmark, and extensively uti- lized database in sleep scoring literature [21–24]. Eight Caucasian female and male subjects took part in the study. The subjects' ages ranged from 21 to 35 years	TQWT technique is used for decomposing input signal into different sub-bands and generating histogram for each sub-band that is unique for each sleep stage.	Sub-band histograms for each sleep stage, considering each sub-band represents a sleep stage. Statistical moment features, such as mean (θ), variance $(\sigma 2)$, skewness (ι), and kurtosis (ν).	Boot strapping/bagging for classification leave-one-out cross-validation	Number of trees from 1 to 300 for cases I–V. Fig. 5 manifests that after about 20 decision trees, the OOB error almost becomes constant.	Accuracy (%) R&K 76.39, 74.39, 81.87, 88.98, 99.02	
Multiple SVM for sleep-stage classification	EDF database from PhysioNet website consisting of 61 male and female sleep dataset for 24 hours sampled at 100 Hz and decomposed into 60-second frames.	IIR Butterworth band-pass filters to filter the signals into different bands	The frequencies and amplitudes of alpha, beta, theta, and y sub-bands during normal condition are evaluated using cutoff frequency and pass band and stop band frequencies.	SVMs with one-vs-all classification technique.	k-kernels for k classes for classification with cross-validation.	Achieves 92.43%, 93.69%, 94.36%, 96.55%, and 99.75% accuracy for 2-state to 6- state classification of sleep stages on Sleep-EDF database.	Training time is more as it uses one-vs-all.

REFERENCES

Abad, V.C.; Guilleminault, C. (2003). Diagnosis and treatment of sleep disorders: a brief review for clinicians. *Dialogues in Clinical Neuroscience*, 5(4), 371–388. https://doi.org/10.31887/DCNS.2003.5.4/vabad

Aboalayon, K.A.I.; Faezipour, M. (2014). Multi-class SVM based on sleep stage identification using EEG signal. In *2014 IEEE Healthcare Innovation Conference (HIC)*, Seattle, WA, pp. 181–184. https://doi.org/10.1109/HIC.2014.7038904

Aboalayon, K.A.I.; Faezipour, M.; Almuhammadi, W.S.; Moslehpour, S. (2016). Sleep stage classification using EEG signal analysis: a comprehensive survey and new investigation. *Entropy*, 18, 272. https://doi.org/10.3390/e18090272

Acharya, U.R.; Sudarshan, V.K.; Adeli, H. et al. (2016). A novel depression diagnosis index using nonlinear features in EEG signals. *European Neurology*, 74(1–2), 79–83.

Acharya,U.R.; Bhat, S.; Faust, O.; Adeli, H.; Chua, E.C.P.; Lim, W.J.E.; Koh, J.E.W. (2015). Nonlinear dynamics measures for automated EEG-based sleep stage detection. *European Neurology*, 74, 268–287. https://doi.org/10.1159/000441975

Ahmed, B.; Redissi, A.; Tafreshi, R. (2009). An automatic sleep spindle detector based on wavelets and the teager energy operator. In *Proceedings of the Annual International Conference of the IEEE Engineering in Medicine and Biology Society*, IEEE, Minneapolis, MN, pp. 2596–2599.

Alam, M.R.; Sameni, R. (2020). Automatic wake-sleep stages classification using electroencephalogram instantaneous frequency and envelope tracking, bioRxiv.05.13.092841; https://doi.org/10.1101/2020.05.13.092841

Al-Meer, M.H.; Al Mamun, M.D.A. (2019). Deep learning in classifying sleep stages. *Thirteenth International Conference on Digital Information Management (ICDIM)*. IEEE. https://doi.org/10.1109/ICDIM.2018.8846973

Anuradha, K.; Sairam, N. (2011). Classification of images using Jaccard co-efficient and higher-order co-occurrences. *Journal of Theoretical and Applied Information Technology*, 34(1), 100–105. https://www.jatit.org/volumes/Vol34No1/15Vol34No1.pdf

Aserinsky, E.; Kleitman, N. (1953). Regularly occuring periods of eye motility, and concomitant phenomena, during sleep. *Science*, 118, 273–274.

Boostani, R.; Karimzadeh, F.; Torabi-Nami, M. (2016). A comparative review on sleep stage classification methods in patients and healthy individuals. *Computer Methods and Programs in Biomedicine*, 140, 77–91.

Bollu, P.C.; Manjamalai, S., Thakkar, M.; Sahota, P. (2018 Jan-Feb). Hypersomnia. *Missouri Medicine*;115(1), 85–91. PMID: 30228690; PMCID: PMC6139790.

Cao, W.; Luo, J.; Xiao Y. (2020). A review of current tools used for evaluating the severity of obstructive sleep apnea. *Nature and Science of Sleep*, 12, 1023–1031. https://doi.org/10.2147/NSS.S275252

Chambon, S.; Galtier, M.N.; Arnal, P.J.; Wainrib, G.; Gramfort, A. (2018). a deep learning architecture for temporal sleep stage classification using multivariate and multimodal time series. *IEEE Transactions on Neural Systems and Rehabilitation Engineering*, 26(4), 758–769. https://doi.org/10.1109/TNSRE.2018.2813138

Cunningham, P.; Delany, S.J. (2021). K-nearest neighbour classifiers - A tutorial. *ACM Computing Surveys*, 54(6), 25. https://doi.org/10.1145/3459665

Delimayanti, M.K.; Purnama, B.; Nguyen, N.G.; Faisal, M.R.; Mahmudah, K.R.; Indriani, F.; Kubo, M.; Satou, K. (2020). Classification of brainwaves for sleep stages by high-dimensional FFT features from EEG signals. *Applied Sciences*, 10(5), 1797. https://doi.org/10.3390/app10051797

Derk-Jan, D.; Edgar, D.M. (1999). Circadian and homeostatic control of wakefulness and sleep. In Zee, P.C.; Turek, F.W. (eds.), *Regulation of Sleep and Circadian Rhythms*. Springer, Berlin, Heidelberg, pp. 111–147

da Silveira, T.L.T.; Kozakevicius, A.J.; Rodrigues, C.R. (2016). Automated drowsiness detection through wavelet packet analysis of a single EEG channel. *Expert Systems with Applications*, 55, 559–565. ISSN 0957-4174. https://doi.org/10.1016/j.eswa.2016.02.041

Diykh, M.; Li, Y. (2016). Complex networks approach for EEG signal sleep stages classification. *Expert Systems with Applications*, 63, 241–248. https://doi.org/10.1016/j.eswa.2016.07.004

Eldele, E.; Chen, Z.; Liu, C.; Wu, M.; Kwoh, C.K.; Li, X.; Guan, C. (2021). An attention-based deep learning approach for sleep stage classification with single-channel EEG. *IEEE Transactions on Neural Systems and Rehabilitation Engineering*, 29, 809–818. https://doi.org/10.1109/TNSRE.2021.3076234. Epub 2021 May 5. PMID: 33909566.

Evgeniou, T.; Pontil, M. (2001). Support vector machines: theory and applications. In Paliouras, G., Karkaletsis, V., Spyropoulos, C.D. (eds.), *Machine Learning and Its Applications. ACAI 1999. Lecture Notes in Computer Science*, vol. 2049. Springer, Berlin, Heidelberg. https://doi.org/10.1007/3-540-44673-7_12

Fuller, P.M.; Gooley, J.J.; Saper, C.B. (2006). Neurobiology of the sleep-wake cycle: sleep architecture, circadian regulation, and regulatory feedback. *Journal of Biological Rhythms*, 21(6), 482–493. https://doi.org/10.1177/0748730406294627. PMID 17107938. S2CID 36572447.

Hafezi, M.; Montazeri, N.; Saha, S.; Zhu, K.; Gavrilovic, B.; Yadollahi, A.; Taati, B. (2020). Sleep apnea severity estimation from tracheal movements using a deep learning model. *IEEE Access*, 8, 22641–22649. https://doi.org/10.1109/access.2020.2969227

Hassan, A.R.; Bashar, S.K.; Bhuiyan, M.I.H. (2015). On the classification of sleep states by means of statistical and spectral features from single channel Electroencephalogram. In *2015 International Conference on Advances in Computing, Communications and Informatics (ICACCI)*, Kochi, India, pp. 2238–2243, https://doi.org/10.1109/ICACCI.2015.7275950

Hassan, A.R.; Subasi, A. (2017). A decision support system for automated identification of sleep stages from single-channel EEG signals. *Knowledge-Based Systems*, 128, 115–124, ISSN 0950-7051, https://doi.org/10.1016/j.knosys.2017.05.005. (https://www.sciencedirect.com/science/article/pii/S095070511730206X)

Hjorth, B. (1970). EEG analysis based on time domain properties. *Electroencephalography and Clinical Neurophysiology*, 29(3), 306–310.

Hochreiter, S.; Schmidhuber, J. (1997). Long short-term memory. *Neural Computation*, 15, 9(8), 1735–1780. https://doi.org/10.1162/neco.1997.9.8.1735. PMID: 9377276.

Iber, C.; Ancoli-Israel, S.; Chesson, A.; Quan, S.F., eds. (2007). *The Aasm Manual for the Scoring of Sleep and Associated Events: Rules, Terminology, And Technical Specification*, 1st ed. American Academy of Sleep Medicine, Westchester, IL.

Inoue, K.; Tsujihata, T.; Kumamaru, K.; Matsuoka, S. (2005). Feature extraction of human sleep EEG based on a peak frequency analysis. *IFAC Proceedings*, 38, 1059–1064.

Jebelli, H.; Hwang, S.; Lee, S. (2018). EEG signal-processing framework to obtain high-quality brain waves from an off-the-shelf, wearable EEG device. *Journal of Computing in Civil Engineering*, 32(1), 04017070.

Krueger, J.M.; Frank, M.G.; Wisor, J.P.; Roy, S. (2015). Sleep function: toward elucidating an enigma. *Sleep Medicine Reviews*, 28, 46–54. https://doi.org/10.1016/j.smrv.2015.08.005. ISSN 1087–0792. PMC 4769986. PMID 26447948.

Lopes, T.; da Silveira, T.; Kozakevicius, A.; Rodrigues, C. (2017). Single-channel EEG sleep stage classification based on a streamlined set of statistical features in wavelet domain. *Medical & Biological Engineering & Computing*, 55(2), 343–352. https://doi.org/10.1007/s11517-016-1519-4

Mohammed, D.; Yan, L. (2016). Complex networks approach for EEG signal sleep stages classification. *Expert Systems with Applications*, 63, 241–248. ISSN 0957-4174. https://doi.org/10.1016/j.eswa.2016.07.004

Mostafa, S.S.; Mendonça, F.; Ravelo-García, A.G.; Morgado-Dias, F. (2019). A systematic review of detecting sleep apnea using deep learning. *Sensors (Basel, Switzerland)*, 19(22), 4934. https://doi.org/10.3390/s19224934

PhysioNet. (2018). The Sleep-Edf Database. (Accessed on 19 November 2018); Available online: https://www.physionet.org/physiobank/database/sleep-edf/

Rechtschaffen, A.; Kales, A. eds. (1968). *A Manual of Standardized Terminology, Techniques and Scoring System of Sleep Stages in Human Subjects*. Brain Information Service/Brain Research Institute, University of California, Los Angeles.

Ronzhina, M.; Janousek, O.; Kolarova, J. et al. (2012). Sleep scoring using artificial neural networks. *Sleep Medicine Reviews*, 16, 251–263.

Supratak, A.; Dong, H.; Wu, C.; Guo, Y. (2017). DeepSleepNet: A model for automatic sleep stage scoring based on raw single-channel EEG. *IEEE Transactions on Neural Systems and Rehabilitation Engineering*, 25(11), 1998–2008.

Thorpy, M. (1999). Classification of sleep disorders. In Chokroverty, S. (ed.). *Sleep Disorders Medicine*. Butterworth Heinemann, Woburn, MA, pp. 287–300.

Thorpy, M. (2000). Classification of sleep disorders. In Kryger, M.H., Roth, T., Dement, W.C. (eds.). *Principles and Practice of Sleep Medicine*, 3rd ed. WB Saunders, Philadelphia, PA, pp. 547–557.

Xu, Z.; Yang, X.; Sun, J.; Liu, P.; Qin, W. (2020). Sleep stage classification using time-frequency spectra from consecutive multi-time points. *Frontiers in Neuroscience*, 14, 14. https://doi.org/10.3389/fnins.2020.00014

Yildirim, O.; Baloglu, U.B.; Acharya, U.R. (2019). A deep learning model for automated sleep stages classification using PSG signals. *International Journal of Environmental Research and Public Health*, 16(4), 599. https://doi.org/10.3390/ijerph16040599

Zee, P.C.; Turek, F.W. (1999). Introduction to sleep and circadian rhythms. In Zee, P.C., Turek, F.W. (eds.), *Regulation of Sleep and Circadian Rhythms*. CRC Press, Boca Raton, FL, pp. 1–17.

Zhang, Y.; Wang, B.; Jing, J.; Zhang, J.; Zou, J.; Nakamura, M. (2017). A comparison study on multidomain EEG features for sleep stage classification. *Computational Intelligence and Neuroscience*, 2017(4574079), 8. https://doi.org/10.1155/2017/4574079

3 Recent Trends in EEG-Based MI and SSVEP Brain-Computer Interface Applications

A Review

Sheikh Farhana Binte Ahmed, Saiful Islam Leon, Jarina Akter, Maisha Anjum, Nazmus Sakib, and Md. Kafiul Islam

3.1 INTRODUCTION

Electrophysiological changes that happen in the brain due to different tasks and cognitive actions can be monitored by capturing the electrical signals generated inside the brain. Millions of neurons fire in the brain while a human being does any sort of activity, either physical or mental. Electroencephalography [1], i.e., EEG, is a popular non-invasive technique by which these brain signals can be recorded by placing electrodes on the surface of the scalp. The EEG signals have fine temporal resolution, which allows them to be used in different applications, namely, brain-computer interface (BCI) or brain-machine interface (BMI). A variety of real-world brain-computer applications [2] are in vogue, and day-by-day, it is being used for a variety of purposes. Brain signals nowadays are not only being used for the rehabilitation [3] of the physically disabled but also for improved lifestyle aspects also [4,5].

The focus of this chapter is to explore the EEG-based steady state visually evoked potential-BCI (SSVEP-BCI) and motor imagery-BCI (MI-BCI). The brain signals used to run the commands in a computer can be generated by both using stimulation and without stimulation. When a person spontaneously generates a brain signal to control a device, it is known as MI-BCI. On the other hand, when a potential in the brain is evoked due to the application of steady visual stimuli to run commands to a machine, it is called SSVEP-BCI.

Section 3.2 outlines the motivation along with a detailed description of EEG and BCI. Section 3.3 consists of the procedure of this review, i.e., which keywords were used in which database, along with the inclusion-exclusion criteria. Section 3.4 explains the brain signals SSVEP and MI, along with the several stages starting from preliminary signal acquisition to final classification for the target applications. Finally, Section 3.5 discusses the summary and draws the conclusion.

DOI: 10.1201/9781003252092-4

3.2 EEG AND BCI

3.2.1 EEG

EEG is used to capture the electrical signals produced inside the brain due to different activities done by the subject. It is highly popular due to its less cost compared to other modalities, its non-invasiveness, and its comparatively higher temporal resolution. Traditionally, EEG was captured in a restrained environment where the subject was not permitted to move. The devices were mostly wired and built-in mega-scale. But in the modern nano-scale world, nowadays portable wireless EEG headsets alongside built-in sensors are available as consumer-grade devices at affordable prices, whereas some of them do not even require a license to operate [6,7]. A graphical representation of the EEG wired data acquisition setup is presented in Figure 3.1.

EEG signals are divided into sub-bands. These sub-bands are significant when considering using them for different applications according to their characteristics [8]. These are shown in Figure 3.2.

3.2.2 BCI

BCI [9] is capable of translating human thoughts into actions by artificial means [10]. It refers to a non-neural or non-muscular medium of conveying commands between the human brain and an external computer device. Here, a computer or another

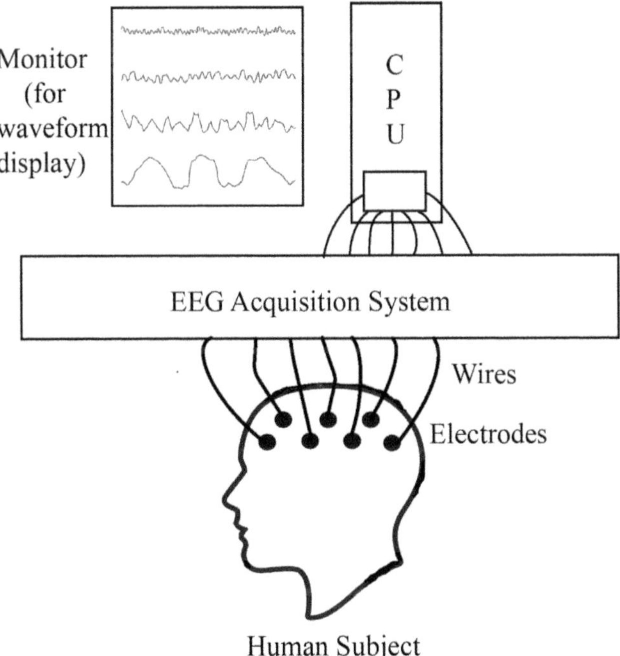

FIGURE 3.1 EEG wired data acquisition setup.

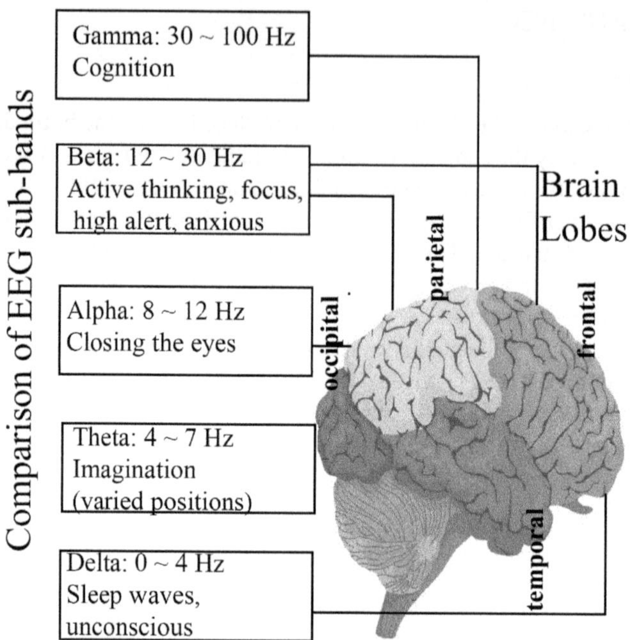

FIGURE 3.2 EEG frequency subbands, their origin, and the corresponding mental situation.

source can generate a stimulus, i.e., a signal or image, as an instruction and the brain, in turn, responds with a signal being generated inside the brain. If this brain signal is captured and sent to an external device for control or to a computer for further analysis, then it is known as an open-loop BCI. On the other hand, if this captured signal is sent to the computer and then the computer generates the next stimuli by re-adjusting parameters, then it is known as a closed-loop BCI [11]. Figure 3.3 represents the general process of a BCI application by a block diagram. Here, the raw EEG data is generated from the subject via placing surface electrodes by either providing stimuli or spontaneously (i.e., without stimuli). Then this data is preprocessed and denoised by different filtering algorithms. Then features required for executing the application are extracted and selected, and then passed to classifiers for final stage classification.

Figure 3.3 shows a generic classification of different types of BCI based on different approaches. EEG-based BCI can be broadly classified into different categories depending on (i) EEG recording technique, (ii) EEG signal type, and (iii) mode of operation. This chapter focuses on the second category, i.e., BCI depending on the type of EEG signal (Figure 3.4).

3.2.3 Advantages of EEG-Based BCI

BCI applications require brain signals to be captured, and EEG is one of the most portable [12] and low cost systems to do it. EEG signals have a higher temporal resolution, which allows them to be used in different applications [13]. This gives EEG an edge over other brain signal recording techniques such as MRI, fMRI, fNIRS, etc.

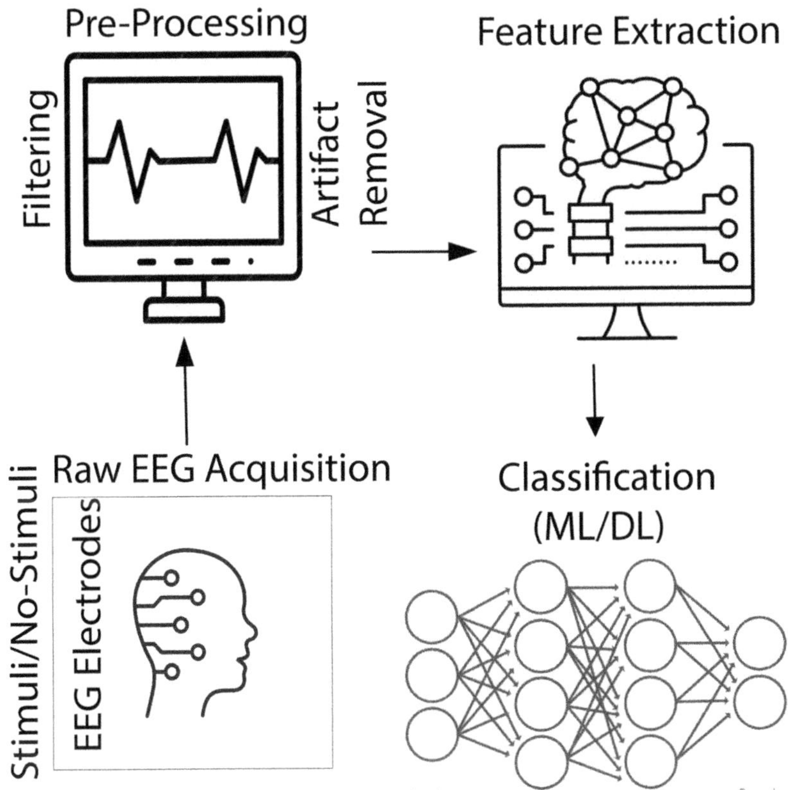

FIGURE 3.3   Generic block diagram of an EEG-based brain computer interface system.

MRI and fMRI require huge size equipment compared to EEG. On the other hand, fMRI provides high spatial resolution, but it has inadequate temporal sampling. On the other hand, EEG offers a significant temporal resolution (in ms). Contrarily, it also suffers from substandard localization of signal sources [14]. Electrocorticography (ECoG [15]) has higher temporal and spatial resolution than scalp EEG. It also does not suffer from the attenuation of signals by the skull and scalp. But electrocortico-gram is an invasive procedure, and most patients are not interested to go through it due to the higher surgical risks associated with it. All these facts motivate us to explore the potential of BCI applications using MI and SSVEP utilizing scalp EEG, which is a non-invasive brain signal recording technique.

3.3   REVIEW METHODOLOGY

A systematic review has been performed on the publications in the last five years (2017 AD–2021 AD) on the research progress of BCI applications using MI and SSVEP, where brain signals are acquired by EEG technique.

We have at first identified five databases IEEE, Frontiers, MDPI, ScienceDirect, and Springer, and used the search strings (EEG) AND (BCI) AND (Review) in the

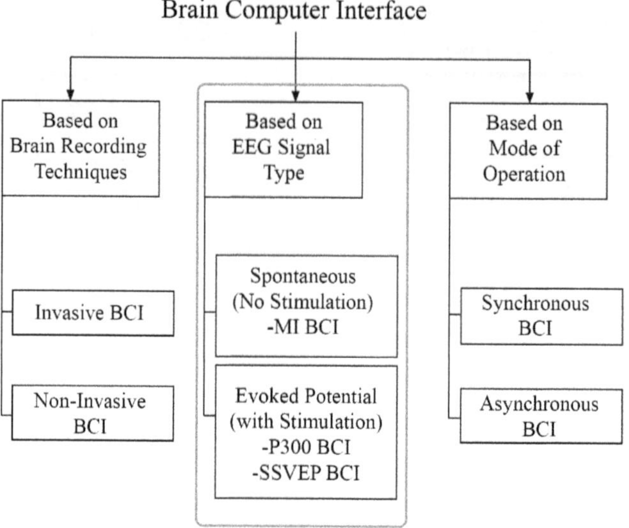

FIGURE 3.4   BCI classification based on different approaches.

metadata (i.e., title, abstract, and keywords) as mentioned in Figure 3.5 to find relevant review papers in the aforementioned year range. This table shows the databases and keywords that were used to search the papers for major brain SSVEP and MI. The number of relevant papers is also mentioned for each type of brain signal.

The inclusion/exclusion criteria are given in Table 3.1.

A comparison between this review and existing reviews in the literature on EEG-based BCI is shown in Table 3.2.

3.4   RESULTS AND ANALYSIS

The focus of this chapter is to analyze the recent works on the two types of BCI based on EEG signal type: evoked potential BCI, namely, SSVEP, and spontaneous BCI, namely, MI. These are detailed in the subsequent sections.

3.4.1   SSVEP-EEG-BASED BCIs

SSVEP, a paradigm in which external stimulation, either visual, auditory, or somatosensory, is applied to the subject. When a visual stimulus is applied on the retina at certain frequencies, electrical signals are generated in the brain at the same or multiple frequencies as the visual stimulus. This technique is used in EEG for research on vision and attention. The general block diagram showing the SSVEP-based BCI is manifested in Figures 3.6.

A 10–20 international protocol is the standard for EEG electrode placement. In all articles, this system is adopted for recording the EEG data. Figure 3.7 shows the channel selection strategy of SSVEP-based EEG-BCIs where mostly the use of occipital and parietal lobes is observed. The name of each electrode is a combination of a number and a letter. The letters O, P, T, F, and C stand for the different lobes of

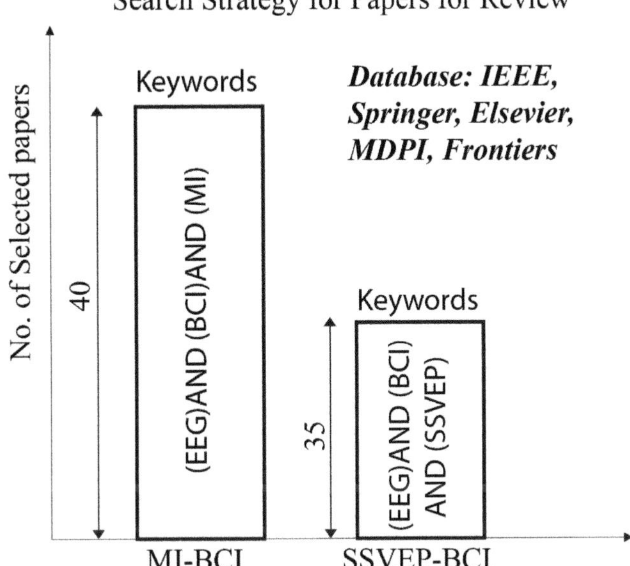

FIGURE 3.5   Search strategy for papers for review.

TABLE 3.1

Criterions Regarding Inclusion and Exclusion for Selecting Articles of This Review

Topic	Include	Exclude
Year	2017–2021	Any paper outside this time range
Language	English	Any language other than English
Content Type	Journal, Review Article, Chapter	Conference Paper, Book, Reference Work Entry
Discipline	Computer Science, Engineering (Biomedical Engineering and Bioengineering, Biotechnology, Signal Processing)	Biomaterials, Biomedicine, Business and Management, Environment, Medicine and Public Health, Neurology, Neurosciences, Pharmacy, Philosophy, Rehabilitation Medicine

---

the brain, i.e., occipital, parietal, temporal, frontal, and central, respectively. These letters refer to the part of the brain where electrodes are placed. The even numbers indicate the right hemisphere, while the odd numbers point to the left hemisphere [36]. These are shown via the anatomy of a human brain in Figure 3.8.

While the EEG signal is captured, it is likely to select the channels on the basis of the origin of the dominant signal. Table 3.3 shows the summary of the SSVEP-based EEG datasets where some research works used commercially available headsets

TABLE 3.2

Comparative Analysis between Existing Reviews and This Work

Reference/Year	Covered Area
[16]/2021	Direct Sense BCI
[17]/2020	SSVEP
[18]/2021	Signal acquisition and processing (not application oriented)
[19]/2021	Emotion Recognition
[20]/2018	MI
This work	SSVEP, MI

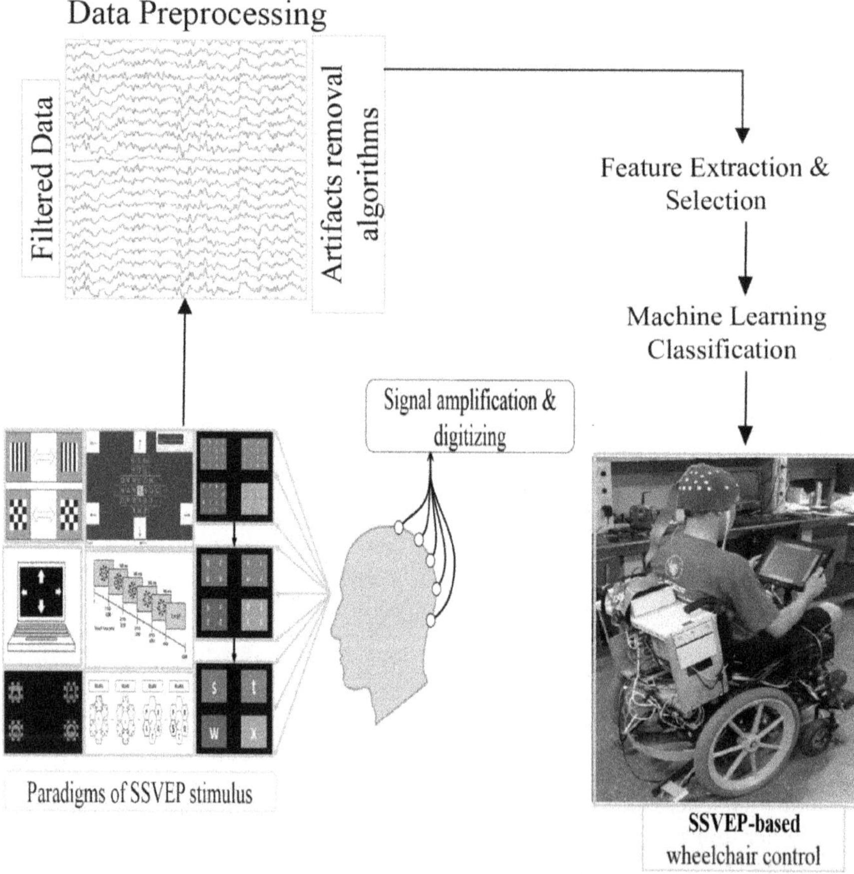

FIGURE 3.6   Graphical representation of a SSVEP-EEG signal-based BCI application.

TABLE 3.3

Channel Selection Strategy

References	No. of Subject	EEG Device/No. of Channels	Flickering Freq.
[21]	10	NuAmp/30	250 Hz
[22]	21	Biosemi/33	2,048 Hz
[23]	7	SAHARAsys/16	256 Hz
[24]	11	SynAmps2/64	1,000 Hz
[25]	13	BrainAmp DC amplifier/BCI2000 software	250 Hz
[26]	12	BioSemi/32	2,048 Hz
[27]	4	Custom-designed headset/8	500 Hz
[28]	22	Synamp2/ –	1,000 Hz
[29]	8	Custom-designed headset/Not mentioned	128 Hz
[30]	35	Open source data/Not mentioned	1,000 Hz
[31]	20	Synamps2/13	1,000 Hz
[32]	35	Synamps2/64	1,000 Hz
[33]	10	Enobio20/Not Mentioned	500 Hz
[34]	8	Bioradio/10	250 Hz
[35]	16	NuAmps/40 SynAmps2/64 (for SSMVEP)	1,000 Hz

while others used customized headsets too. Both high-density and low-density headsets are used having many channels and fewer channels respectively. The flickering frequencies also vary on the basis of applications. From Table 3.4, it is noticeable that almost all the authors collected the signals from those electrodes, which refer to the parietal and occipital lobes. SSVEP signals show the maximal amplitude and SNR in the parietal and occipital areas of the brain [38] and help to get the highest accuracies as well. As noted in Ref. [39], the occipital lobe part of the brain plays a vital role in the SSVEP-based BCI. Again, two different VEP signals, namely, SSVEP and SSMVEP, can be used to analyze BCI classification [40]. They acquired the signals with two different devices and considered different channels for each signal. The channel selection is shown in Table 3.5.

In Ref. [21], the common feature analysis (CFA) method was proposed to find out the inherent common features from a group of EEG data trials as natural reference signals for SSVEP recognition and improving the BCI performance. They compared the CFA-based method with canonical correlation analysis (CCA) and multiway canonical correlation analysis (MCCA). According to Ref. [21], CCA and MCCA have less optimal accuracy during SSVEP recognition for lack of features and do not completely rely on training data. In Ref. [23], the authors did their comparative analysis on three approaches ((Filter bank, Welch's method, and short time Fourier transform (STFT)) of feature extraction to extract power spectral density (PSD) features to implement the BCI command. To estimate PSD, the filter bank helps by setting bandpass filters to separate the input signal into different segments where each one carries a single frequency sub-band of the original signal. STFT helps to reduce the artifacts that are at the boundary. For both STFT and Welch's methods, the Hamming window was used for data windowing.

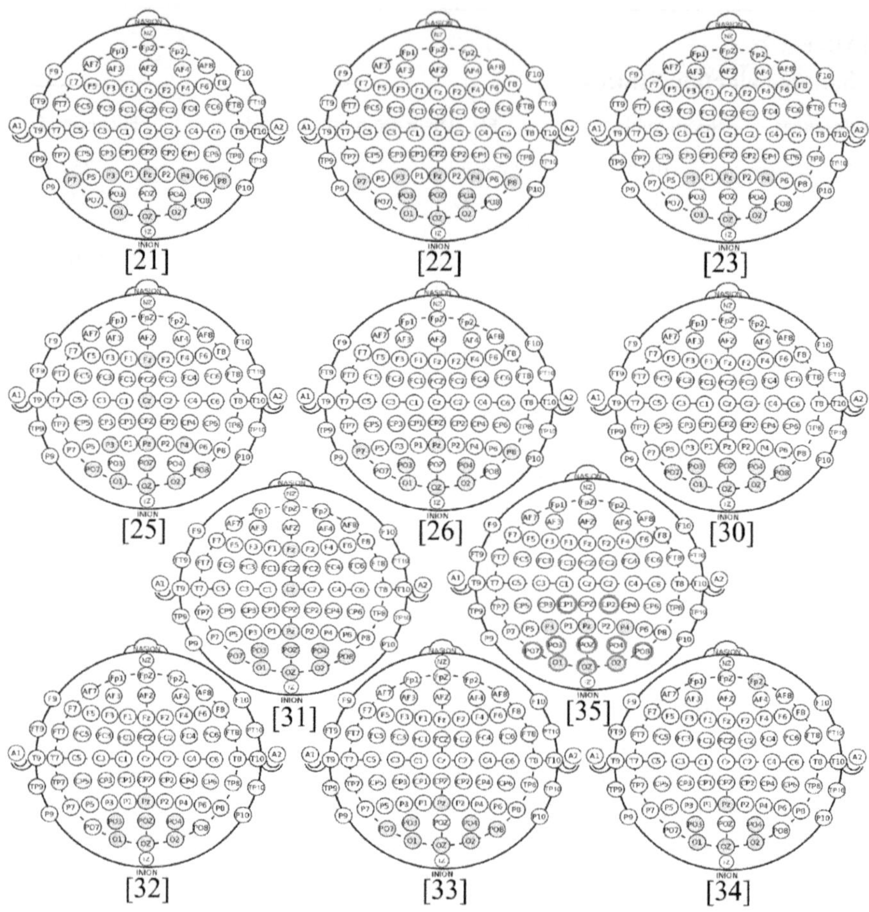

FIGURE 3.7 Channel selection of a SSVEP-EEG signal-based BCI application.

In Ref. [43], CCA and multivariate synchronization index (MSI) methods were proposed for feature extraction. The CCA method helps detect SSVEP signals of multichannel. MSI helps to identify the level of synchronization between the mixed versus reference signals for recognizing the stimulus frequency. In Figure 3.9, the classification accuracy of different algorithms on SSVEP-based EEG-BCI has been shown. Here it is seen that Support Vector Machine (SVM) outperforms other classifiers in terms of performance evaluation.

In Ref. [23], 95% is the average accuracy, which was obtained from the Welch method and incremental wrapper configuration. In Ref. [43], 82.7% accuracy for the face and 76% for the vase. In Ref. [48], 92.91, 98.95, and 94.50% accuracies have been obtained by using the SVM classifier along with the FBCSP algorithm, which had frequencies of 12, 15, and 20 Hz. They compared the SVM and LDA classifiers that showed SVM performed better than LDA. In Ref. [35], there is 80% accuracy for the Bayesian classifier and 90.4% for the SVM. In Ref. [28], the author achieved 89.83% accuracy for

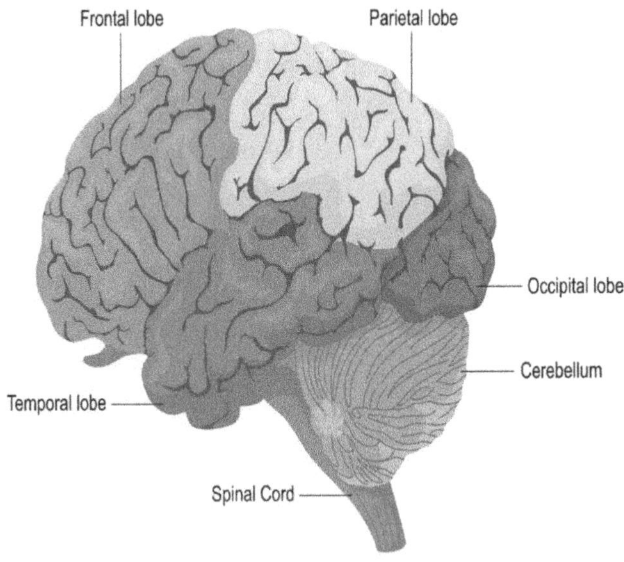

FIGURE 3.8 Human brain anatomy [37].

TABLE 3.4
Signal Preprocessing for BCI using SSVEP-based EEG

Preprocessing Methods		Research Papers	Filter's Frequency Range
Notch filter		[22,23,41]	58–62 Hz, 60 Hz, 50 Hz
Bandpass	Forward-Backward Butterworth	[21]	4–45 Hz
	Butterworth	[23]	5–60 Hz
	FIR filter	[42]	1–40 Hz
	–	[25]	0.1–45 Hz
	–	[43]	3–60 Hz
	–	[24]	6–28 Hz
	–	[26]	1–60 Hz
	IIR	[28]	7–90 Hz
	Zero phase IIR	[22]	2–54 Hz
	–	[29]	6–13 Hz
	–	[31]	0.1–200 Hz
	–	[32]	7–90 Hz
	FIR	[44]	1–50 Hz
	Butterworth	[33]	3–50 Hz
	Butterworth	[45]	–
	–	[46]	0.1–100 Hz
	Common Average Reference	[23]	
ICA	–	[24]	–
	Fast ICA and ICA	[47]	–
Chebyshev Type I	–	[41]	6–90 Hz

TABLE 3.5

Feature Extraction for BCI Using SSVEP-Based EEG

References	Selected Method
[21]	CFA
[23]	Filter bank, Welch's method, STFT
[25–27,33,43]	CCA
[43]	MSI
[34,48]	CSP
[29,40]	FFT

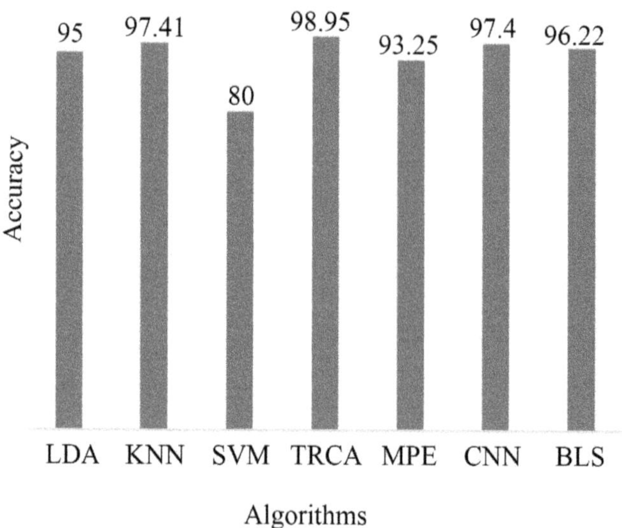

FIGURE 3.9 Performance evaluation metric (accuracy) for classification of SSVEP-EEG-based BCI.

a speller while considering the ensemble TRCA classification algorithm. In Ref. [25], 93.25% accuracy was reached by using MPE fusion. They have compared their results with those of other classifiers such as NBC, GSVM, LDA, and LSVM. They used different feature extraction methods, such as SWLDA for P300 and CCA for SSVEP. In Ref. [26], the researcher achieved around 90% accuracy by multi-class linear discriminant analysis (MLDA) along with the CCA feature extraction method. The ITR was 40.8, 51.4, and 65.2 bpm for the data lengths of 4, 3, and 1s, respectively. In Ref. [31], the author considered the SWLDA, ECCA, and TRCA classification algorithms and achieved the highest accuracy with TRCA. The best accuracy was 81.67% with an ITR 172.46 bpm for cue-guided spelling. In Ref. [29], the author used 1-D CNN for the classification along with the FFT feature extraction method with various numbers of points and achieved

97.4% accuracy with an ITR 49 bpm (bits/min). In Ref. [30], the researcher reached 86 and 77% accuracy while using DCNN and PodNet, respectively. In Ref. [24], the author applied the double-partial least-squares (D-PLS) algorithm and achieved around 90% for the 3.5s window and 93.9% for the 5s window. In Ref. [40], the author applied various classification algorithms on SSVEP and SSMVEP to compare these two signals. They achieved the highest accuracy with SSVEP while considering LPVG-based BLS, and the accuracy was 96.22%. In Ref. [32], the researcher considered different data lengths for classification. They combined a few feature extraction methods to get the desired accuracy through a linear SVM classifier. ECCA, FBCCA, and TRCA algorithms were used as feature extraction methods. Different data lengths gave different accuracies, but the best result was 98.4% for the 3s window with combined FBCCA and TRCA, and the rate at which information got transferred was 88.3 bits/min. In Ref. [49], a classification process was implemented on both offline and online data with the extended MSI (EMSI) algorithm. For the online process, the accuracy was 92.8% with an ITR 37.4 bits/min. During offline analysis, they considered various data lengths. The accuracy gets better with increasing data length, i.e., 82.5% with 2s and 90.8% with 4s window.

3.4.2 MI-EEG-Based BCI

A BCI is an environment where neural signals are collected from the brain and utilized as command signals for operating an electrical device. Any kind of limb movement, literal, or imagery, initiates varying patterns of ERS, which indicates an increase in the power of the rhythm. It also initiates ERD, i.e., power levels of the rhythms in the EEG signals generated from the region of the sensory-motor cortex of the brain get decreased. MI-BCI uses neural signals generated during imagination of limb movement and utilizes the signals as commands to operate the various electrical devices in numerous application fields [20,50]. Figure 3.10 shows a general block diagram of MI-EEG signal- based BCI applications.

The alpha and beta rhythms (8–30 Hz) have the most prominent activity during MI [51]. Hence, it is ideal to filter the alpha and beta rhythms for further processing. This is done in the preprocessing stage, where various filters and artifact removal methods are applied to the raw EEG signal to enhance the classification accuracy. The raw EEG data collected contains both valuable information along with unnecessary frequency bands and contaminations. Data acquisition for research and study faces many challenges and limitations. Datasets are publicly available, while many researchers create their own datasets. Preprocessing needs to be done before valuable information and features are identified, collected, and further utilized. For online applications, high-density EEG is not preferable. The bulkiness of the EEG headset as well as the computational time for signal processing get reduced [52]. Such methods and techniques are summarized in Figure 3.11 using a pie-chart where the mostly used signal processing methods and their corresponding references are grouped together. Band Pass Filter (BPF) is a commonly used filtering technique in all types of EEG based applications. Figure 3.12 shows the cut-off frequencies of MI-EEG based BCI applications in recent literature.

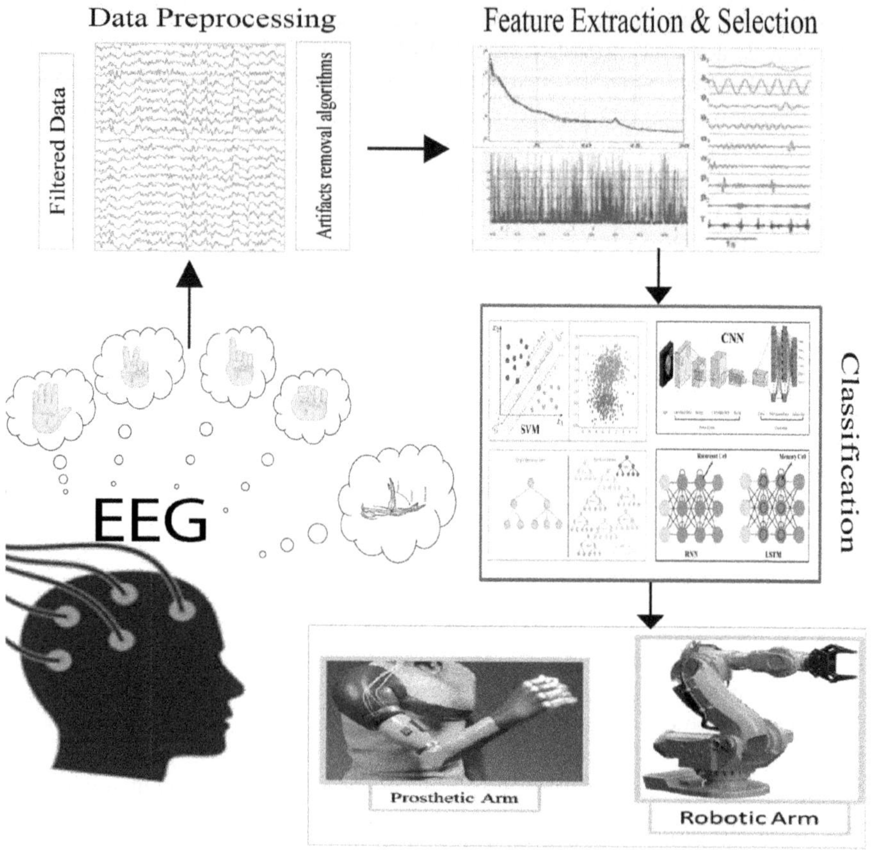

FIGURE 3.10   General block diagram of a MI-EEG signal-based BCI application.

There has been extensive ongoing research in the field of MI-BCI. Different forms of techniques to extract features and classification have been studied. The research is aimed to reducing the complexity of these techniques due to the instability of EEG signals [53]. Different artifacts introduced into the EEG signal reduce classification accuracy. This may also result in false positive commands during online applications. It is crucial to evaluate performance after classification to understand the reliability and suitability of the processed signal. MI-BCI is used for the purpose of rehabilitation of movement-locked patients, controlling wheelchairs and robots, for applications in military fields, special industrial areas, and much more [54–57].

Datasets are collected online and offline based on the purpose of the system. The offline dataset is the dataset acquired first in a controlled environment and stored for use. It is required for experimenting with the proposed BCI system as well as for training the system initially before it operates online. Online data collection is simultaneously processed and classified into commands in real-life applications. Some of the research works used public datasets i.e. which are freely accessible for all as shown in Table 3.6. On the other hand, many researchers generate their own dataset which are not made available in the internet as listed in Table 3.7.

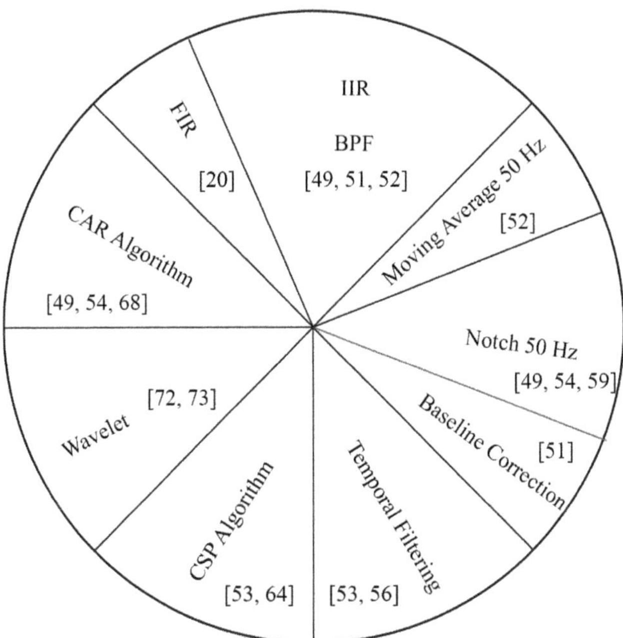

FIGURE 3.11   Signal preprocessing method for EEG-based MI-BCI.

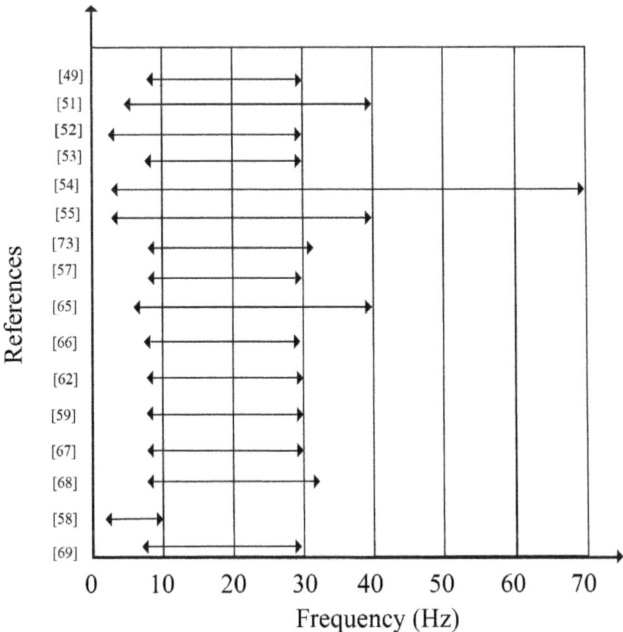

FIGURE 3.12   BPF range in signal preprocessing method for EEG-based MI-BCI.

TABLE 3.6

Dataset (Public) for BCI Using MI-based EEG

References	Sub	Fs	Data Length and Trials	Device	MI Task
Wadsworth dataset [52]	3	160 Hz	10 sessions per subject, 30 minutes each, and six runs per session, per run consists 32 trials (Session 1–6 used to train classifier) (Session 7–10 is unlabelled) update rate (to control target): 10 times/sec	64 channels, electrode on the right ear is used as reference (amplification 20,000; bandpass 0.1–60 Hz)	Control vertical cursor while it moves from left to right on video screen. The target (cursor) appears at four different positions in the beginning.
BCI2000 dataset [58,59]	109	160 Hz	14 trials 1 minutes: eyes open 2 minutes: 4 different tasks, repeated three times 1 minutes: eyes closed	64-channel, 10-10 system, using the BCI2000 system (excluding Nz, TP9, TP10, P9, F10, FT9, F9, FT10, A1, A2, and P10)	Task 1: opening and closing of the left or right fist. Task 2: imagine Task 1. Task 3: opening and closing of both the fists or feet. Task 4: imagine Task 3 Baseline, eyes open Baseline, eyes closed
BCI Competition IV 2A [20,54,58, 60–62]	9	250 Hz	MI activity = 3s Total 6s data with short break in the end.2 sessions per subject, 288 trials per session	22 Ag/AgCl electrodes, 3.5 cm inter-electrode distance, amplifier sensitivity is 100 µV,reference- left mastoid ground-right mastoid as 22 EEG channels, 3 EOG channels,	Imagining to move left hand, right hand, feet, and tongue

(Continued)

TABLE 3.6 (*Continued*)

Dataset (Public) for BCI Using MI-based EEG

References	Sub	Fs	Data Length and Trials	Device	MI Task
BCI Competition IV 2B [54,58,63,64]	9 (right handed)	250 Hz	5 sessions per subject (2 sessions without feedback, 3 sessions with feed back) (without feedback) MI activity-3s (with feedback) Total trial length-7.5s with short break afterwards.	3 EEG channels (bipolar), ground-Fz dynamic range for the screening is ±100 μV and for the feedback sessions is ±50 μV 3 EOG channels, monopolar, (left mastoid is reference), dynamic range of ±1 mV	Thinking to move left hand and right hand, 2 class
BCI Competition III A [50]	3	250 Hz	60 EEG channels (1–50 Hz), 60 trials per class	64-channel EEG amplifier from Neuroscan, reference-left mastoid and ground-right mastoid	Imagine to move left hand, right hand, foot, and tongue
BCI Competition III dataset V [51]	3	512 Hz	32 EEG channels (DC-256 Hz), each task performed randomly for 15s	Biosemi system, 32 integrated electrodes in cap, International 10–20 system	MI of left hand andright hand, generation of words with random letters
BCI Competition III dataset IVa [63]	5	1,000 Hz	280 trials per subject	BrainAmp amplifier,128 channel, International 10/20-system	MI of right hand, foot

TABLE 3.7

Dataset (Private) for BCI Using MI-Based EEG

References	Subjects	Fs	Data Length and Trials	Device	MI Task
[51]	5 female and 5 male subjects (24.9 ± 2.3 years) Previously worked with MI BCI high-pass filter at 0.5 Hz, a low-pass filter at 100 Hz, and a notch filter at 50 Hz.	512 Hz	Trial length-8s MI activity (3.25s – 7s = 3.75s) C3, Cz, or C4 channels studied.	Data were recorded with two g.USBamps (Guger Technologies OEG, Graz, Austria). 32 Ag/ AgCl-electrodes. Reference electrode: left mastoid; ground: the right mastoid.	Subjects could move the car on screen to the left by performing feet MI and to the right by performing right-hand MI.
[52]	5 subjects (3 males, average age of 25.5 9.7 years) with previous BCI experience per session has 4 runs of 20 trials for each pair of tasks.	1,000 Hz	Total-11s (includes 1 sec intertrial interval) MI activity = 4s 17 electrodes utilized (FC3, FC1, FCz, FC2, FC4, C5, C3, C1, Cz, C2, C4, C6, CP3, CP1, CPz, CP2, CP4)	64 channels, 10–20 electrode system using a SynAmpsRT amplifier (Neuroscan Compumedics, Singen, Germany)	Flexion and extension (FE) and supination and pronation (SP) *MI tasks were paired together and randomized within each run*
[55]	10 healthy male subjects, Age range is 22–26 years, 40 MI trials per direction Online exp-4 session and 160 trials per subject	512 Hz	Trial length-21–24 s. (MI task from 4s–12s) MI activity = 8s	Novel design of EEG device-dry electrodes, consists of a pre-amplifier unit, a, Bluetooth transmission unit and a microcontroller unit. Wireless integrated-circuit-based acquisition module with dimensions $55.08 \times 38.8 \times 5\,mm^3$ approximately. Commercial 700 mAh Li-ion battery for power supply.	Left hand and right-hand movements.

(Continued)

TABLE 3.7 (*Continued*)

Dataset (Private) for BCI Using MI-Based EEG

References	Subjects	Fs	Data Length and Trials	Device	MI Task
[56]	Total 32 healthy subjects Hybrid-Group : 16 subjects (15 male/1 female, age of 24.4 ± 2.3 years) Control-group: 15 subjects (15 male/1 female, age of 25.6 ± 2.3 years)	250 Hz	MI activity $= 4.5s - 8s = 3.5s$ Control group: total 120 trials Hybrid group: total 240 trials	64-channel, 10/20 system, SynAmps2 system (Neuroscan, U.S.A.). Reference electrode positioned on the vertex, the ground electrode positioned on the forehead.	The hybrid group performed four mental tasks randomly instructed (i.e., L MI, R-MI, L-SAO, and R-SAO), L-SAO is left hand somatosensory attentional orientation. R-SAO is right hand somatosensory attentional orientation.
[52]	11 subjects, 11 subject - hand opening/closing. 10 subjects- wrist flexion/ extension. 5 subjects - forearm pronation/supination.	250 Hz	Trial length-7 seconds 8 sessions, per session 8 run, 20 trials per run MI activity-4 seconds C3, C4, C3, F3, Fz, F4, P3, Pz, P4, T7 and T8 channels used.	G.Nautilus headset, 16 Ag/AgCl electrodes, 10/20 system	Hand opening/closing, wrist flexion/extension and forearm pronation/ supination movements
[50]	12 healthy subjects	128 Hz	10s data per subject. 4s MI. 180 trials in 3 sessions.	EEG headset (Emotiv Flex), 32 channels, signal resolution of 14 bits, and the connectivity of 2.4 GHz	Left, right and stop MI.
[50]	9 subjects (healthy)	250 Hz	MI activity-3 seconds One session per subject, 12 runs, 10 trials per run, 120 trials per session.	32 channels, 120 trials per session, using g. Nautilus portable EEG acquisition system from g.tec, Ag/AgCl wet electrode reference-right mastoid, and the ground - Fz.	MI-adduction, reach forward, outreach, and back stretch of the upper limb with the right-arm shoulder joint as the axis.

The number of subjects for the dataset varies from study to study. However, the more the number of subjects, the more reliable the experiment results are. In many cases, the subjects are new to BCI. They are trained before the experiment is initiated to get familiar with the process. Training the subjects has shown improvement in classification accuracy. For acquiring the datasets, the researchers must gain permission from the respectable authorities, ensure that the participants clearly understand the procedure, any side effects, and the outcome of the experiment, and have their consent henceforth. The dataset acquisition must follow the codes of conduct and ethics.

Among the publicly available datasets, the BCI competition datasets are widely used for research. Some studies used the BCI competition dataset to train the BCI system offline and locally collected data for online applications. The BCI competition is one of the most widely used publicly available datasets, as seen from the literature review in Tables 3.8 and 3.9.

The volunteers who provide data are ensured to be physically and mentally healthy. Healthy subjects are required to provide data to study the application of MI-BCI systems in aircraft, construction robots, and military applications. However, if the proposed design is for rehabilitation purposes or for application in the medical field, then datasets might be collected from patients or people with disabilities.

To collect data, it is to be ensured that the electrodes are placed properly on the scalp. Uneven positions of electrodes can introduce artifacts into the signal. The volunteers are instructed to perform MI, which can usually be hand and feet movements. Furthermore, there can be tongue imagery, imagery of the hand's rotational movement. The MI information may later be used to direct a cursor, control a simple game on the video screen, a robotic arm, hovering aircraft, and many more.

TABLE 3.8

Feature Extraction for MI using EEG-based BCI

References	Feature Extraction Method
[57,63,66,69–73],	CSP
[56,74,75]	FB-CSP
[59]	CBN
[76]	SCSSP
[67]	MFBCSP
[77]	SBCSP
[86]	Correlation matrix and coherence matrix
[82]	Time domain power and Clough-Tocher interpolation-based imaging (TPCT imaging method) (10-fold CV) + mVGG (modified Visual Geometry Group Network)
[78]	SwTDA
[80]	FAWT multidimensional scaling (MDS)
[84]	Time-varying signed distance (TSD)
[79]	Tensor Decomposition Algorithm
[68]	Temporal convolutional network (TCN)

TABLE 3.9

Classifier Models for MI Using EEG-Based BCI

References	Classifier Model/Class Size
[63,69,71,80,74,78]	LDA/4
[66]	Fisher's LDA/4
[72]	Stacked Regularized LDA/4
[59,75]	SVM/4
[73]	SVM/3
[81]	SVM/2
[82]	DCNN/4
[60]	HF-CNN/3
[62]	CNN-SSAE/2
[83]	CNN/2
[76]	NBPW/4
[55]	ANN/4
[57]	Feed Forward NN/4
[84]	QDA/4
[61]	clsSRC2/2
[77]	Fuzzy Fusion/2
[56]	Bagging Ensemble Classifier/4
[67]	SVM/–

EEG headsets are readily available in markets like g.USBamps (Guger Technologies OEG, Graz, Austria) with 32 Ag/AgCl-electrodes, SynAmpsRT amplifier (Neuroscan Compumedics, Singen, Germany) with 64 electrodes, BrainAmp, BrainProduct GmbH, Germany (amplifier), and many more are available. The electrodes are to be placed according to the international 10–20 system. Not all the channels recorded by the electrodes are utilized, but rather only the ones that lie over the motor cortex region of the brain are used for further processing. For the EEG data acquisition, some of the electrodes are considered the ground for other channels. The reference and ground electrodes can be placed on the mastoids, on the vertex, or on the forehead according to preference.

The sampling frequency of the recorded data ranges from 160 to 1,000 Hz. The higher the sampling frequency, the more valuable information recorded. However, the computational time is also increased with a higher sampling frequency. In many cases, the recorded EEG data is downsampled to lower frequencies, such as 125, 160, 200 Hz, etc., for processing.

The trial length of the data per subject usually varies from 8 to 12 seconds. The MI activity is commonly recorded for 3–4s. However, the time period does not have a fixed range and can vary as per the study requirements. The longer the time length, the more information will be recorded.

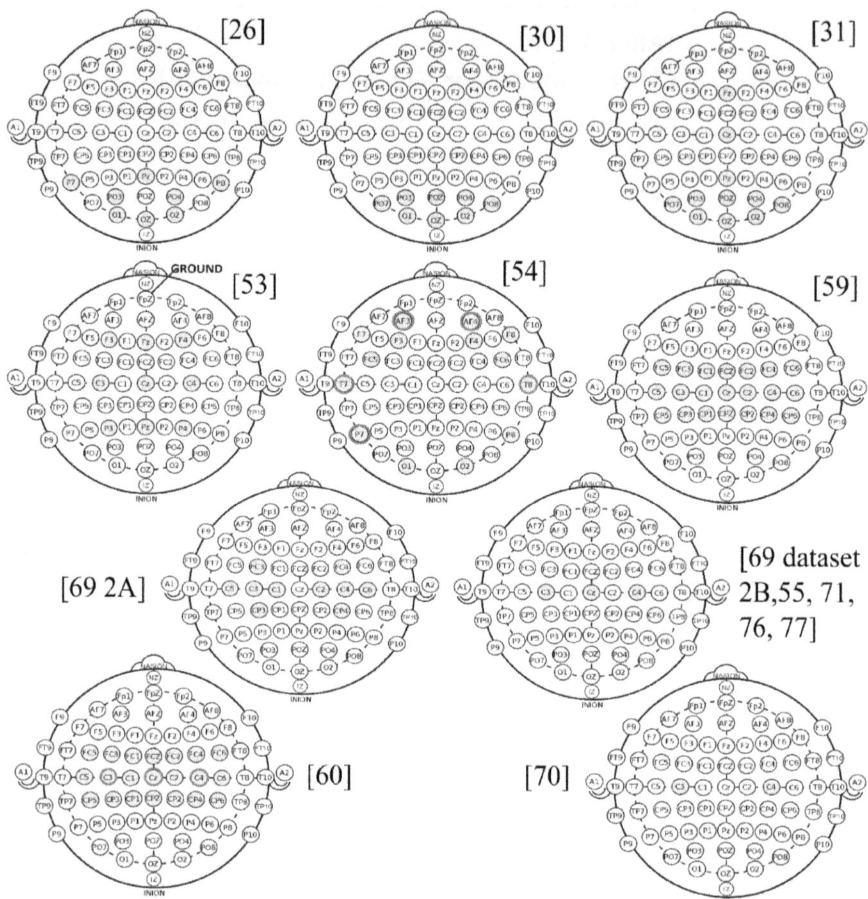

FIGURE 3.13 Channel selection strategy for EEG-based MI-BCI.

The raw EEG signals get contaminated with biological and non-biological arti-facts. The common biological artifacts are eye blinking artifacts, unintentional motion artifacts, and muscle movement during chewing or swallowing, etc. Whereas common non-biological artifacts are spikes due to powerline interference, incorrect electrode placement, and many more [58,65].

Usually, the EEG data is amplified and recorded at a high frequency and later down-sampled to reducing computational cost, as done in Ref. [50]. The 50 and 60 Hz powerline interference is mainly removed by applying the notch filter [57,66]. Almost all the authors have applied the bandpass filter to separate the rhythm related to MI. The Butterworth bandpass filter is widely used to separate the rhythm related to MI for further processing. The analog bandpass filter is also quite common among the bandpass filters (Figure 3.13).

The EEG headset can have many electrodes to acquire EEG data. But for MI-BCI, only the electrodes placed on the scalp near the motor cortex region can provide valuable MI-related information. Therefore, in many cases, the authors use selective channels for data acquisition while ignoring the remaining channels. From the literature review, it is seen that almost all the authors used the channels detected from the central region of the brain, denoted by 'C'. The most important channels are seen to be Cz, C3, and C4, which have been used in all research except in Ref. [56]. Figure 3.13 shows the channel selection strategy for EEG based MI-BCI. In Ref. [67], the authors used iterative multi-objective optimization for channel selection (IMOCS). The IMOCS method can reduce the computational complexity of the BCI system due to the high-dimensional features involved in MI. The performance of ICMOS proved an average classification accuracy of about 80% from the evaluated data of 35 participants. Other than the channels in the central, the frontal and parietal temporal regions have also been utilized. In some cases, all the channels have been utilized [63,64,68,69].

The most commonly used feature extraction method is the common spatial patterns (CSP) method [57,63,66,69–71,72,73]. Another common method is the FB-CSP [56,74,75]. Researchers have also used modified forms of the CSP method, such as separable SCSSP, MFBCSP, and SBCSP [67,76,77].

In MI-BCI applications, the classifier is also the most crucial and final stage where different tasks of MI are identified. Table 3.10 demonstrates the list of classifiers that were proposed in different literature. The commonly used classifier models are LDA, SVM, CNN, ANN, and NN.

For 4 class and 2 class, MI-BCI authors of Refs. [63,69,71,74,78,80] proposed a LDA classifier. The authors of Refs. [66] and [72] used Fisher's LDA and Stacked Regularized LDA, respectively, for MI-BCI task classification. SVM was proposed in Refs. [59,69,73,75] for 4 class, 3 class, and 2 class MI-BCI applications. Even SVM was used for classifying the MI-based cursor movement [67]. DCNN for 4 class MI-BCI [82], HF-CNN for 3 class MI-BCI [60], CNN-SSAE [85] and CNN [83] for 2 class MI-BCI were proposed.

Besides, other classifiers such as Naïve Bayes Parzen window (NBPW) [76], ANN [55], feed forward NN [57], quadrative discriminant analysis (QDA) [84], clsSRC2 [61], Bagging ensemble classifier [56], and fuzzy fusion [77] models were proposed to classify different sizes of MI tasks. Figure 3.14 shows a comparative illustration for classification accuracy of different hybrid algorithms at running brain-computer interface applications using motor-imagery signals acquired by Electroencephalogram technique.

The minimum classification accuracy percentage is obtained in Ref. [71], which is 71.6% for one subject among three others. The percentage classification accuracy for the other two subjects is 83.3 and 78.3%, respectively. However, the accuracy percentage is calculated for offline data. From a literature review, the minimum percentage accuracy acquired for online data is 73.08% in Ref. [60]. However, the percentage accuracy for the online data is 82.55%. In Ref. [80], all eight subjects performed the tasks accurately within three minutes. The data was collected and processed in real time as well. The highest level of accuracy reached for offline data is in Ref. [58]. In Ref. [58], the performance was also evaluated by obtaining a confusion matrix of 4 different methods for further comparison and kappa values obtained for proper and

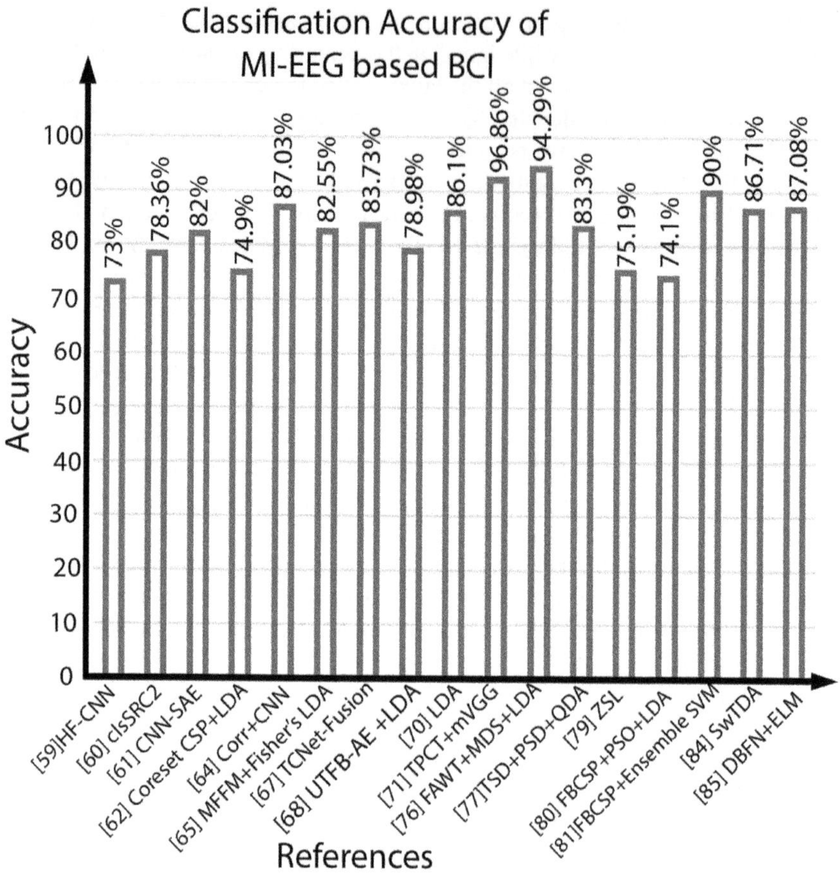

FIGURE 3.14   Performance evaluation metric (accuracy) for classification of MI-EEG-based BCI.

improper electrode positions. Kappa values are also obtained in Ref. [50], for the first dataset, it is 0.9, and for the other, it is 0.66. Moreover, some of the research works evaluate the performance of the proposed system by comparing approaches using different other techniques.

Application: Rigorous studies have been done on the applications of MI BCI. In most cases, it has been proven to be an effective tool to control the BCI. In Ref. [55], two off-the-shelf quadcopters, AR Drone 2.0 and Parrot Bebop 2 were controlled with MI commands consisting of MI of the left hand, right hand, left and right elbows, and finger movements. The authors in Ref. [56] experimentally controlled the NAO robot movements with MI-BCI. The experiment aimed to study the effect of MI-BCI to control robots, keeping in mind that it can aid patients with "gradual freezing syndrome". The authors in Ref. [74] practiced the application of MI-BCI in neurorehabilitation by proposing a novel processing stage consisting of temporal filter banks, for feature extraction, a common spatial pattern algorithm is used, and particle swarm optimization is used for the feature selection method

TABLE 3.10

Classification Result for MI Using EEG-Based BCI

References	Selected Method Result
[72]	Binary: 79% Multiclass: 74% (kappa)
[57]	100% task completion within short time
[59]	BCI III III2A: 0.9 BCI IV 2A: 0.66 (Kappa coefficients) Multiclass
[71]	Hybrid Modality: 86.1 ± 7.6
[55]	classification accuracy of 98.8% for 14-channel and 84.5% 5-channel system
[74]	average offline and online performances were of $76.2\% \pm 7.6\%$ and 70 ± 6.7, respectively
[86]	400 samples: 73.64 ± 4.01 150 samples: 75.03 ± 3.37 with ensemble learning by integrating 91 Corr+CNN classifier a high accuracy of 87.03% was achieved
[82]	Dataset 1 = 88.62%, Dataset 2 = 92.28%, Dataset 3 = 96.86%
[60]	Dataset 1: ME: 0.73 ($\pm$0.04) MI: 0.65 ($\pm$0.09), Dataset 2: ME: 0.52 ($\pm$0.03) MI:0.51($\pm$0.04)
[78]	Dataset A: 86.71%, Dataset B: 84.4%
[69]	Dataset 1: 92.20 ± 9.36, Dataset 2: 81.52 ± 13.72
[61]	Dataset 1: CSP: 78.20% RCSP: 78.36%, Dataset 2: CSP: 58.66% RCSP: 59.08%
[73]	$91.81\% \pm 7.01\%$
[62]	Mean 86.41%. SD 1.6%
[63]	Average classification 0.706. Using traditional classification method, Avg. classification is 0.704. This shows proposed algorithm has similar classification accuracy but higher computational efficiency and suitable for online computation.
[80]	The maximum accuracy (ACC) of 94.29% using BCI Dataset III,
[84]	The accuracy of the classifier was found to be 83.3%, 71.6%, and 78.3%, res
[56]	EEG classification accuracy up to 78.29%, and the accuracy of NAO robot action is up to 86.33%,
[75]	$79.1\% \pm 1.85\%$ Accuracy % ($\pm$ SD %)
[66]	"Offline data-82.55% average accuracy Online data-73.08%"
[79]	Average classification accuracy: 87.08%, variance: 5.96
[68]	Classification accuracy of 83.73% on BCI Competition IV-2a dataset, and an accuracy of 94.41% on the High Gamma Dataset.
[69]	Average classification accuracy is 78.98% using SJTU dataset. BCI competition dataset-Kappa value of 0.60 (highest by comparison to other methods). Highest accuracy compared to TBS, CSP + SVM, NMWF, and PSD technique) TBS-tensor-based scheme NMWF-non-negative multi-way factorization PSD-power spectrum analysis

of the EEG signals. The participants of this experiment were both healthy subjects and subjects with paralyzed hands after suffering strokes. The experiment used the 10 × 10 validation, followed by average offline and online performances of $76.2\% \pm 7.6\%$ and $70\% \pm 6.7\%$. In Ref. [57], the authors combined the eye gaze information using an eye tracker device along with MI-BCI to form a system for grasping and dropping objects in desired positions accurately by controlling a robotic arm at most within three minutes. The eye tracking device confirms the intent of the user and, furthermore, the MI of the user to completely avoid any false positives. In Ref. [79], the authors proposed a design with a tensor decomposition method to analyze DBFN to achieve high accuracy for MI-BCI classification. The method allows analyzing signals and activity patterns of brain regions, such as epilepsy pathology, emotion recognition, and strong inclination, to be used to control a robotic arm in the BCI paradigm. In Ref. [75], a system design for teleoperation of construction robots using EEG-based MI-BCI with a hands-free control system has been proposed. The design uses machine learning and an ensemble algorithm to control an unmanned ground vehicle robot. The potential application of the design is that unmanned robots can be controlled to carry construction materials in accident-prone construction sites.

3.5 DISCUSSION AND CONCLUSION

EEG signal is popularly used in driving BMIs due to their non-invasiveness, low cost, high temporal resolution, portable equipment, and the availability of wearable and wireless headsets and caps. Although the use of EEG-based BMI is rising, EEG signals are prone to challenges and issues as to reliability. This paper critically reviews the EEG-based BCI for two control signals: SSVEP and MI.

After the relevant journals for each of these control signals with specific keywords were extracted from the five selected research databases, they were listed according to datasets, signal processing methods, channel selection strategy, feature extraction method, classifier models, and classification results. For SSVEP signals, dominant signals arise from the parietal and occipital lobes, whereas for MI signals, the central region of the brain plays a significant role. Hence, in the case of designing low-density EEG headsets, these regions must be covered for the respective signal-specific applications. The notch filters are used to removing the power line interference from the raw EEG. Different types of bandpass filters are implemented for extracting the specific bands of the EEG. Among the different public datasets for MI-BCI, the most widely used is BCI competition dataset IV 2A and 2B. A number of privately generated datasets also exist in the literature. For the feature extraction method, CCA is mostly used for SSVEP signals and CSP for MI signals. For classification, the TRCA method tops in accuracy for both SSVEP-BCI and MI-BCI, with a classification accuracy of 98.95%.

In conclusion, EEG signals can be used for different types of BCI applications. Day-by-day, the multitude of this usage is diversifying. Some of the crucial challenges in this paradigm is to select relevant preprocessing and denoising methods, as well as to extract and select features. Then one needs to choose a suitable classification method to get accurate results. This chapter explores these topics.

ACKNOWLEDGMENT

The Biomedical Instrumentation and Signal Processing Lab (BISPL-IUB) at Independent University, Bangladesh, for its support and motivation.

APPENDIX

Acronym/Abbreviation	Full Meaning
ANN	artifical neural network
APF	adaptive predictor filter
BCI	brain computer interface
BMI	brain machine interface
CBN	common Bayesian network
CCA	canonical correlation analysis
CFA	common feature analysis
CNN	convolutional neural network
CSP	common spatial pattern
DWT	discrete wavelet transform
ECG/EKG	electrocardiography
ECoG	electrocorticography
EEG	electroencephalography
EMD	empirical mode decomposition
EMG	electromyography
EOG	electrooculography
ERP	event-related potential
FAWT	flexible analytic wavelet transforms
FB	filter bank
FFT	fast Fourier transform
ICA	independent component analysis
KNN	K-nearest neighbor
MDS	multi-dimensional scaling
MFBCSP	modified filter bank common spatial pattern
MI	motor imagery
MSI	multivariate synchronization index
mVGG	modified Visual Geometry Group network
PCA	principal component analysis
PSD	power spectral density
SBCSP	sub-band common spatial pattern
SCSSP	separable common spatial-spectral patterns
SSVEP	steady state visual evoked potential
STFT	short time Fourier transform
SVM	support vector machine
SWT	stationary wavelet transform
SwTDA	spectrum-weighted tensor discriminant analysis
TCN	temporal convolutional network
TPCT	time domain power and Clough-Tocher interpolation-based imaging
TSD	time-varying signed distance
WT	wavelet transform

REFERENCES

1. C. D. Binnie and P. F. Prior, "Electroencephalography," *J. Neurol. Neurosurg. Psychiatry.*, vol. 57, no. 11, pp. 1308–1319, 1994.
2. M. M. Moore, "Real-world applications for brain-computer interface technology," *IEEE Trans. Neural Syst. Rehabil. Eng.*, vol. 11, no. 2, pp. 162–165, 2003, 10.1109/TNSRE.2003.814433
3. R. Mane, T. Chouhan, and C. Guan, "BCI for stroke rehabilitation: Motor and beyond," *J. Neural Eng.*, vol. 17, no. 4, p. 041001, 2020, doi: 10.1088/1741–2552/aba162
4. F. S. Rawnaque et al., "Technological advancements and opportunities in neuromarketing: A systematic review," *Brain Inform.*, vol. 7, no. 1, p. 10, 2020, doi: 10.1186/s40708-020-00109-x
5. J. L. Soler-Dominguez and C. Gonzalez, "Using EEG and gamified neurofeedback environments to improve E-sports performance: Project neuroprotrainer," *VISIGRAPP 2021- Proc. 16th Int. Jt. Conf. Comput. Vision, Imaging Comput. Graph. Theory Appl.*, vol. 1, no. Visigrapp, pp. 278–283, 2021, doi: 10.5220/001031450278028.
6. J. W. Y. Kam et al., "Systematic comparison between a wireless EEG system with dry electrodes and a wired EEG system with wet electrodes," *Neuroimage*, vol. 184, pp. 119–129, 2019, https://doi.org/10.1016/j.neuroimage.2018.09.012
7. P. Sawangjai, S. Hompoonsup, P. Leelaarporn, S. Kongwudhikunakorn, and T. Wilaiprasitporn, "Consumer grade EEG measuring sensors as research tools: A review," *IEEE Sens. J.*, vol. 20, no. 8, pp. 3996–4024, 2020, doi: 10.1109/JSEN.2019.2962874
8. J. S. Kumar and P. Bhuvaneswari, "Analysis of electroencephalography (EEG) signals and its categorization: A study," *Procedia Eng.*, vol. 38, pp. 2525–2536, 2012, doi: 10.1016/j.proeng.2012.06.298
9. M. Van Gerven et al., "The brain-computer interface cycle," *J. Neural Eng.*, vol. 6, no. 4, p. 041001, 2009, doi: 10.1088/1741–2560/6/4/041001
10. A. Ortiz-Rosario and H. Adeli, "Brain-computer interface technologies: From signal to action," *Rev. Neurosci.*, vol. 24, no. 5, pp. 537–552, 2013, doi: 10.1515/revneuro-2013–0032
11. S. Aggarwal and N. Chugh, "Ethical implications of closed loop brain device: 10-year review," *Minds Mach.*, vol. 30, no. 1, pp. 145–170, 2020, doi: 10.1007/s11023-020-09518-7
12. U. Seneviratne and W. J. D'Souza, "Ambulatory EEG," *Handb. Clin. Neurol.*, vol. 160, pp. 161–170, 2019, doi: 10.1016/B978-0-444-64032-1.00010-2
13. B. Burle, L. Spieser, C. Roger, L. Casini, T. Hasbroucq, and F. Vidal, "Spatial and temporal resolutions of EEG: Is it really black and white? A scalp current density view," *Int. J. Psychophysiol.*, vol. 97, no. 3, pp. 210–220, 2015, doi: 10.1016/j.ijpsycho.2015.05.004
14. G. Mele, C. Cavaliere, V. Alfano, M. Orsini, M. Salvatore, and M. Aiello, "Simultaneous EEG-fMRI for functional neurological assessment," *Front. Neurol.*, vol. 10, pp. 00848, 2019, doi: 10.3389/fneur.2019.00848
15. C. Guger, C. Kapeller, H. Ogawa, R. Prückl, J. Grünwald, and K. Kamada, *Electrocorticogram Based Brain-Computer Interfaces*, 2nd ed., no. 1. Elsevier B.V., Amsterdam, Netherlands, 2018.
16. C. T. Lin and T. T. N. Do, "Direct-sense brain-computer interfaces and wearable computers," *IEEE Trans. Syst. Man, Cybern. Syst.*, vol. 51, no. 1, pp. 298–312, 2021, doi: 10.1109/TSMC.2020.3041382
17. Y. Zhang, S. Q. Xie, H. Wang, and Z. Zhang, "Data analytics in steady-state visual evoked potential-based brain-computer interface: A review," *IEEE Sens. J.*, vol. 21, no. 2, pp. 1124–1138, 2021, doi: 10.1109/JSEN.2020.3017491
18. U. Salahuddin and P. X. Gao, "Signal generation, acquisition, and processing in brain machine interfaces: A unified review," *Front. Neurosci.*, vol. 15, pp. 1–21, 2021, doi: 10.3389/fnins.2021.728178

19. P. R. Bhise, S. B. Kulkarni, and T. A. Aldhaheri, "Brain computer interface based EEG for emotion recognition system: A systematic review," *2nd International Conference on Innovative Mechanisms for Industry Applications (ICIMIA 2020): Conference Proceeding*, Piscataway, NJ, March 2020, pp. 327–334, 2020, doi: 10.1109/ICIMIA48430.2020.9074921

20. P. Wierzgała, D. Zapała, G. M. Wojcik, and J. Masiak, "Most popular signal processing methods in motor-imagery BCI: A review and meta-analysis," *Front. Neuroinform.*, vol. 12, p. 78, 2018, https://doi.org/10.3389/fninf.2018.00078

21. A. Widmann, E. Schröger, and B. Maess, "Digital filter design for electrophysiological data - a practical approach," *J. Neurosci. Methods*, vol. 250 pp. 34–46, 2015, doi: 10.1016/j.jneumeth.2014.08.002

22. S. Park, H. S. Cha, and C. H. Im, "Development of an online home appliance control system using augmented reality and an SSVEP-based brain-computer interface," *IEEE Access*, vol. 7, pp. 163604–163614, 2019, doi: 10.1109/ACCESS.2019.2952613

23. S. N. Carvalho et al., "Comparative analysis of strategies for feature extraction and classification in SSVEP BCIs," *Biomed. Signal Process. Control*, vol. 21, pp. 34–42, 2015, doi: 10.1016/j.bspc.2015.05.008

24. S. Ge, R. Wang, Y. Leng, H. Wang, P. Lin, and K. Iramina, "A double-partial least-squares model for the detection of steady-state visual evoked potentials," *IEEE J. Biomed. Heal. Informatics*, vol. 21, no. 4, pp. 897–903, 2017, doi: 10.1109/JBHI.2016.2546311

25. E. Yin, T. Zeyl, R. Saab, T. Chau, D. Hu, and Z. Zhou, "A hybrid brain - computer interface based on the fusion of P300 and SSVEP scores," *IEEE Trans. Neural Syst. Rehabil. Eng.*, vol. 23, no. 4, pp. 693–701, 2015, doi: 10.1109/TNSRE.2015.2403270

26. A. Maye, D. Zhang, and A. K. Engel, "Utilizing retinotopic mapping for a multi-target SSVEP BCI with a single flicker frequency," *IEEE Trans. Neural Syst. Rehabil. Eng.*, vol. 25, no. 7, pp. 1026–1036, 2017, doi: 10.1109/TNSRE.2017.2666479

27. E. Erkan and M. Akbaba, "A study on performance increasing in SSVEP based BCI application," *Eng. Sci. Technol. Int. J.*, vol. 21, no. 3, pp. 421–427, 2018, doi: 10.1016/j.jestch.2018.04.002

28. M. Nakanishi, Y. Wang, X. Chen, Y. Te Wang, X. Gao, and T. P. Jung, "Enhancing detection of SSVEPs for a high-speed brain speller using task-related component analysis," *IEEE Trans. Biomed. Eng.*, vol. 65, no. 1, pp. 104–112, 2018, doi: 10.1109/TBME.2017.2694818

29. T. H. Nguyen and W. Y. Chung, "A single-channel SSVEP-based BCI speller using deep learning," *IEEE Access*, vol. 7, pp. 1752–1763, 2019, doi: 10.1109/ACCESS.2018.2886759

30. J. J. Podmore, T. P. Breckon, N. K. N. Aznan, and J. D. Connolly, "On the relative contribution of deep convolutional neural networks for SSVEP-based bio-signal decoding in BCI speller applications," *IEEE Trans. Neural Syst. Rehabil. Eng.*, vol. 27, no. 4, pp. 611–618, 2019, doi: 10.1109/TNSRE.2019.2904791

31. M. Xu, J. Han, Y. Wang, T. P. Jung, and D. Ming, "Implementing over 100 command codes for a high-speed hybrid brain-computer interface using concurrent P300 and SSVEP features," *IEEE Trans. Biomed. Eng.*, vol. 67, no. 11, pp. 3073–3082, 2020, doi: 10.1109/TBME.2020.2975614

32. J. Zhao et al., "Decision-making selector (DMS) for integrating CCA-based methods to improve performance of SSVEP-based BCIs," *IEEE Trans. Neural Syst. Rehabil. Eng.*, vol. 28, no. 5, pp. 1128–1137, 2020, doi: 10.1109/TNSRE.2020.2983275

33. Z. Duan, C. Liu, Z. Lu, J. Chen, Y. Li, and H. Wang, "Research on steady-state visual evoked brain–computer interface based on moving stimuli," *Biomed. Signal Process. Control*, vol. 70, p. 102982, 2021, doi: 10.1016/j.bspc.2021.102982

34. M. Rashid et al., "A hybrid environment control system combining EMG and SSVEP signal based on brain-computer interface technology," *SN Appl. Sci.*, vol. 3, no. 9, p. 782, 2021, doi: 10.1007/s42452-021-04762-7

35. H. Soltani, Z. Einalou, M. Dadgostar, and K. Maghooli, "Classification of SSVEP-based BCIs using genetic algorithm," *J. Big Data*, vol. 8, no. 1, pp. 1–11, 2021, https://doi.org/10.1186/s40537-021-00478-y

36. Y. Peng, C. M. Wong, Z. Wang, A. C. Rosa, H. T. Wang, and F. Wan, "Fatigue detection in SSVEP-BCIs based on wavelet entropy of EEG," *IEEE Access*, vol. 9, pp. 114905–114913, 2021, doi: 10.1109/ACCESS.2021.3100478

37. "BrainView Cortical Functions – BrainView," *Brainview*, 2022. [Online]. Available: https://www.brainview.com/s_science_cortical_functions.html. [Accessed: 13-Sep-2022].

38. X. Chen, Y. Wang, S. Gao, T.-P., Jung, X. Gao, "Filter bank canonical correlation analysis for implementing a high-speed SSVEP-based brain–computer interface," *J. Neural Eng.* vol. 12, no. 4, p. 046008, 2015.

39. I. Kramberger, Z. Kacic, and G. Donaj, "Binocular phase-coded visual stimuli for SSVEP-based BCI," *IEEE Access*, vol. 7, pp. 48912–48922, 2019, doi: 10.1109/ACCESS.2019.2910737

40. Z. Gao, W. Dang, M. Liu, W. Guo, K. Ma, and G. R. Chen, "Classification of EEG signals on VEP-based BCI systems with broad learning," *IEEE Trans. Syst. Man, Cybern. Syst.*, vol. 51, no. 11, pp. 7143–7151, 2021, doi: 10.1109/TSMC.2020.2964684

41. Y. Li, J. Xiang, and T. Kesavadas, "Convolutional correlation analysis for enhancing the performance of SSVEP-based brain-computer interface," *IEEE Trans. Neural Syst. Rehabil. Eng.*, vol. 28, no. 12, pp. 2681–2690, 2020, doi: 10.1109/TNSRE.2020.3038718

42. K. Lin, X. Chen, X. Huang, Q. Ding, and X. Gao, "A Hybrid BCI speller based on the combination of EMG envelopes and SSVEP," *Appl. Inform.*, vol. 2, no. 1, pp. 1–12, 2015, doi: 10.1186/S40535-014-0004-0

43. R. M. G. Tello, S. M. T. Müller, M. A. Hasan, A. Ferreira, S. Krishnan, and T. F. Bastos, "An independent-BCI based on SSVEP using figure-ground perception (FGP)," *Biomed. Signal Process. Control*, vol. 26, pp. 69–79, 2016, doi: 10.1016/j.bspc.2015.12.010

44. H. Y. Zhang, C. E. Stevenson, T. P. Jung, and L. W. Ko, "Stress-induced effects in resting EEG spectra predict the performance of SSVEP-based BCI," *IEEE Trans. Neural Syst. Rehabil. Eng.*, vol. 28, no. 8, pp. 1771–1780, 2020, doi: 10.1109/TNSRE.2020.3005771

45. D. Zhao, T. Wang, Y. Tian, and X. Jiang, "Filter bank convolutional neural network for SSVEP classification," *IEEE Access*, vol. 9, pp. 147129–147141, 2021, doi: 10.1109/ACCESS.2021.3124238

46. K. Zhang et al., "Weak feature extraction and strong noise suppression for SSVEP-EEG based on chaotic detection technology," *IEEE Trans. Neural Syst. Rehabil. Eng.*, vol. 29, pp. 862–871, 2021, doi: 10.1109/TNSRE.2021.3073918

47. I. Rejer and Ł. Cieszyński, "Independent component analysis for a low-channel SSVEP-BCI," *Pattern Anal. Appl.*, vol. 22, no. 1, pp. 47–62, 2019, doi: 10.1007/s10044-018-0758-4

48. B. Asheri et al., "Enhancing detection of steady-state visual evoked potentials using frequency and harmonics of that frequency in OpenVibe," *Biomed. Eng. Adv.*, vol. 2, p. 100022, 2021, doi: 10.1016/J.BEA.2021.100022

49. S. Park, H.-S. Cha, and C.-H. Im, "Development of an online home appliance control system using augmented reality and an SSVEP-based brain–computer interface," *IEEE Access*, vol. 7, pp. 163604–163614, 2019, doi: 10.1109/ACCESS.2019.2952613

50. A. Singh, A. A. Hussain, S. Lal, and H. W. Guesgen, "A comprehensive review on critical issues and possible solutions of motor imagery based electroencephalography brain-computer interface," *Sensors 2021*, vol. 21, no. 6, p. 2173, 2021, doi: 10.3390/S21062173

51. K. W. Ha and J. W. Jeong, "Motor imagery EEG classification using capsule networks," *Sensors 2019*, vol. 19, no. 13, p. 2854, 2019, doi: 10.3390/S19132854

52. M. K. Islam, P. Ghorbanzadeh, and A. Rastegarnia, "Probability mapping based artifact detection and removal from single-channel EEG signals for brain–computer interface applications," *J. Neurosci. Methods*, vol. 360, p. 109249, 2021, doi: 10.1016/J.JNEUMETH.2021.109249

53. F. Li, F. He, F. Wang, D. Zhang, Y. Xia, and X. Li, "A novel simplified convolutional neural network classification algorithm of motor imagery EEG signals based on deep learning," *Appl. Sci.*, vol. 10, no. 5, p. 1605, 2020, doi: 10.3390/APP10051605

54. J. Cantillo-Negrete, R. I. Carino-Escobar, P. Carrillo-Mora, D. Elias-Vinas, and J. Gutierrez-Martinez, "Motor imagery-based brain-computer interface coupled to a robotic hand orthosis aimed for neurorehabilitation of stroke patients," *J. Healthc. Eng.*, vol. 2018, p. 1624637, 2018, doi: 10.1155/2018/1624637

55. A. Vijayendra, S. Kumaar, R. M. Vishwanath, and S. N. Omkar, "A performance study of 14-channel and 5-channel EEG systems for real-time control of unmanned aerial vehicles (UAVs)," *Proc. -2nd IEEE Int. Conf. Robot. Comput. IRC 2018*, vol. 2018, pp. 183–188, 2018, doi: 10.1109/IRC.2018.00040

56. Y. Guo, M. Wang, T. Zheng, Y. Li, P. Wang, and X. Qin, "NAO robot limb control method based on motor imagery EEG," *Proc. -2020 Int. Symp. Comput. Consum. Control. IS3C 2020*, vol. 141, pp. 521–524, 2020, doi: 10.1109/IS3C50286.2020.00141

57. H. Wang, X. Dong, Z. Chen, and B. E. Shi, "Hybrid gaze/EEG brain computer interface for robot arm control on a pick and place task," *Proc. Annu. Int. Conf. IEEE Eng. Med. Biol. Soc. EMBS*, vol. 2015, pp. 1476–1479, 2015, doi: 10.1109/EMBC.2015.7318649

58. A. Jafarifarmand and M. A. Badamchizadeh, "Artifacts removal in EEG signal using a new neural network enhanced adaptive filter," *Neurocomputing*, vol. 103, pp. 222–231, 2013, doi: 10.1016/J.NEUCOM.2012.09.024

59. L. He, D. Hu, M. Wan, Y. Wen, K. M. Von Deneen, and M. Zhou, "Common Bayesian network for classification of EEG-based multiclass motor imagery BCI," *IEEE Trans. Syst., Man, Cybern. Syst.*, vol. 46, no. 6, pp. 1–12, 2015.

60. J. H. Jeong, B. H. Lee, D. H. Lee, Y. D. Yun, and S. W. Lee, "EEG classification of forearm movement imagery using a hierarchical flow convolutional neural network," *IEEE Access*, vol. 8, pp. 66941–66950, 2020, doi: 10.1109/ACCESS.2020.2983182

61. V. P. Oikonomou, S. Nikolopoulos, and I. Kompatsiaris, "Robust motor imagery classification using sparse representations and grouping structures," *IEEE Access*, vol. 8, pp. 98572–98583, 2020, doi: 10.1109/ACCESS.2020.2997116

62. J. Yang, Z. Ma, J. Wang, and Y. Fu, "A novel deep learning scheme for motor imagery EEG decoding based on spatial representation fusion," *IEEE Access*, vol. 8, pp. 202100–202110, 2020, doi: 10.1109/ACCESS.2020.3035347

63. E. Netzer, A. Frid, and D. Feldman, "Real-time EEG classification via coresets for BCI applications," *Eng. Appl. Artif. Intell.*, vol. 89, p. 103455, 2020, doi: 10.1016/J.ENGAPPAI.2019.103455

64. Q. Zhang, B. Guo, W. Kong, X. Xi, Y. Zhou, and F. Gao, "Tensor-based dynamic brain functional network for motor imagery classification," *Biomed. Signal Process. Control*, vol. 69, p. 102940, 2021, doi: 10.1016/J.BSPC.2021.102940

65. R. Chatterjee, A. Datta, and D. K. Sanyal, "Ensemble learning approach to motor imagery EEG signal classification," *Mach. Learn. Bio-Signal Anal. Diagnostic Imaging*, vol. 2019, pp. 183–208, 2019, doi: 10.1016/b978-0-12–816086-2.00008-4

66. L. Hu, J. Xie, C. Pan, X. Wu, and D. Hu, "Multi-feature fusion method based on WOSF and MSE for four-class MI EEG identification," *Biomed. Signal Process. Control*, vol. 69, p. 102907, 2021, doi: 10.1016/J.BSPC.2021.102907

67. V. S. Handiru and V. A. Prasad, "Optimized Bi-objective EEG channel selection and cross-subject generalization with brain-computer interfaces," *IEEE Trans. Human-Machine Syst.*, vol. 46, no. 6, pp. 777–786, 2016, doi: 10.1109/THMS.2016.2573827

68. Y. K. Musallam et al., "Electroencephalography-based motor imagery classification using temporal convolutional network fusion," *Biomed. Signal Process. Control*, vol. 69, p. 102826, 2021, doi: 10.1016/J.BSPC.2021.102826

69. R. Tang, Z. Li, and X. Xie, "Motor imagery EEG signal classification using upper triangle filter bank auto-encode method," *Biomed. Signal Process. Control*, vol. 68, p. 102608, 2021, doi: 10.1016/J.BSPC.2021.102608

70. H. Raza, H. Cecotti, Y. Li, and G. Prasad, "Adaptive learning with covariate shift-detection for motor imagery-based brain–computer interface," *Soft Comput.*, vol. 20, no. 8, pp. 3085–3096, 2016, https://doi.org/10.1007/s00500-015-1937-5

71. L. Yao et al., "A stimulus-independent hybrid BCI based on motor imagery and somatosensory attentional orientation," *IEEE Trans. Neural Syst. Rehabil. Eng.*, vol. 25, no. 9, pp. 1674–1682, 2017, doi: 10.1109/TNSRE.2017.2684084

72. L. F. Nicolas-Alonso, R. Corralejo, J. Gomez-Pilar, D. Álvarez, and R. Hornero, "Adaptive stacked generalization for multiclass motor imagery-based brain computer interfaces," *IEEE Trans. Neural Syst. Rehabil. Eng.*, vol. 23, no. 4, pp. 702–712, 2015, doi: 10.1109/TNSRE.2015.2398573

73. L. Duan et al., "Zero-shot learning for EEG classification in motor imagery-based BCI system," *IEEE Trans. Neural Syst. Rehabil. Eng.*, vol. 28, no. 11, pp. 2411–2419, 2020, doi: 10.1109/TNSRE.2020.3027004

74. J. Cantillo-Negrete, R. I. Carino-Escobar, P. Carrillo-Mora, D. Elias-Vinas, and J. Gutierrez-Martinez, "Motor imagery-based brain-computer interface coupled to a robotic hand orthosis aimed for neurorehabilitation of stroke patients," *J. Healthc. Eng.*, vol. 2018, p. 1624637, 2018, doi: 10.1155/2018/1624637

75. Y. Liu, M. Habibnezhad, and H. Jebelli, "Brain-computer interface for hands-free teleoperation of construction robots," *Autom. Constr.*, vol. 123, p. 103523, 2021, doi: 10.1016/J.AUTCON.2020.103523

76. A. S. Aghaei, M. S. Mahanta, and K. N. Plataniotis, "Separable common spatio-spectral patterns for motor imagery BCI systems," *IEEE Trans. Biomed. Eng.*, vol. 63, no. 1, pp. 15–29, 2016, doi: 10.1109/TBME.2015.2487738

77. S. L. Wu et al., "Fuzzy Integral with Particle Swarm Optimization for a Motor-Imagery-Based Brain-Computer Interface," *IEEE Trans. Fuzzy Syst.*, vol. 25, no. 1, pp. 21–28, 2017, doi: 10.1109/TFUZZ.2016.2598362

78. S. Huang, Y. Chen, T. Wang, and T. Ma, "Spectrum-weighted tensor discriminant analysis for motor imagery-based BCI," *IEEE Access*, vol. 8, pp. 93749–93759, 2020, doi: 10.1109/ACCESS.2020.2995302

79. Q. Zhang, B. Guo, W. Kong, X. Xi, Y. Zhou, and F. Gao, "Tensor-based dynamic brain functional network for motor imagery classification," *Biomed. Signal Process. Control*, vol. 69, p. 102940, 2021, doi: 10.1016/j.bspc.2021.102940

80. Y. You, W. Chen, and T. Zhang, "Motor imagery EEG classification based on flexible analytic wavelet transform," *Biomed. Signal Process. Control*, vol. 62, p. 102069, 2020, doi: 10.1016/J.BSPC.2020.102069

81. M. K. I. Molla, A. Al Shiam, M. R. Islam, T. Tanaka, T. Tanaka, and T. Tanaka, "Discriminative feature selection-based motor imagery classification using EEG signal," *IEEE Access*, vol. 8, pp. 98255–98265, 2020, doi: 10.1109/ACCESS.2020.2996685

82. M. A. Li, J. F. Han, and L. J. Duan, "A novel MI-EEG imaging with the location information of electrodes," *IEEE Access*, vol. 8, pp. 3197–3211, 2020, doi: 10.1109/ACCESS.2019.2962740

83. O. Y. Kwon, M. H. Lee, C. Guan, and S. W. Lee, "Subject-independent brain-computer interfaces based on deep convolutional neural networks," *IEEE Trans. Neural Networks Learn. Syst.*, vol. 31, no. 10, pp. 3839–3852, 2020, doi: 10.1109/TNNLS.2019.2946869

84. G. S. Gupta, G. B. Dave, P. R. Tripathi, D. K. Mohanta, S. Ghosh, and R. K. Sinha, "Brain computer interface controlled automatic electric drive for neuro-aid system," *Biomed. Signal Process. Control*, vol. 63, p. 102175, 2021, doi: 10.1016/j.bspc.2020.102175

85. J. Yang, Z. Ma, J. Wang, and Y. Fu, "A novel deep learning scheme for motor imagery EEG decoding based on spatial representation fusion," *IEEE Access*, vol. 8, pp. 202100–202110, 2020, doi: 10.1109/ACCESS.2020.3035347

86. X. Ma, S. Qiu, W. Wei, S. Wang, and H. He, "Deep channel-correlation network for motor imagery decoding from the same limb," *IEEE Trans. Neural Syst. Rehabil. Eng.*, vol. 28, no. 1, pp. 297–306, 2020, doi: 10.1109/TNSRE.2019.2953121

4 Recent Trends in EEG-Based P300, Neuromarketing, and E-Sports Brain-Computer Interface Applications
A Review

Sheikh Farhana Binte Ahmed,
Mehedi Hasan, Md. Tawhid Islam Opu,
Faisal Bin Shahin, Md. Ahsan-Ul Kabir Shawon,
Tasnuva Faruk, and Md. Kafiul Islam

4.1 INTRODUCTION

Electroencephalography (EEG) captures electric signals of the brain, which allows us to measure the electrophysiological changes in the brain. The brain wave pattern is different for different tasks and cognitive actions, including states of rest and sleep. EEG [1] is a non-invasive recording of brain signals where the electrodes are mounted on the scalp's surface. The method is less costly and has a relatively high temporal resolution; it is also popular. The EEG signal has many diverse applications, one of the most popular being brain-computer interface (BCI) or brain-machine interface (BMI) applications [2]. Brain signals nowadays are not only being used for the rehabilitation [3] of the physically disabled but also for improved lifestyle aspects such as neuromarketing [4] and E-sports engineering [5]. This paper aims to address the recent studies conducted on these topics.

Section 4.2 consists of the procedure of this review, i.e., the keywords used as search strings in different databases, along with the inclusion-exclusion criteria. Section 4.3 explains the brain signal P300 and its applications in neuromarketing and E-sports engineering. Also, several stages have been explored, from preliminary signal acquisition to final classification for the target applications. Finally, Section 4.4 discusses the summary and conclusion.

DOI: 10.1201/9781003252092-5

4.2　REVIEW METHODOLOGY

A systematic review was performed on the publications in the last five years (2017 AD–2021 AD) on the research progress of BCI applications using brain signals acquired by EEG technique. The inclusion/exclusion criteria are given in Table 4.1.

Table 4.2 shows the database and keywords that were used to search the papers for P300 and applications such as neuromarketing and E-sports engineering. We have identified five databases IEEE, Frontiers, MDPI, ScienceDirect, and Springer and used the search strings in the metadata (i.e., title, abstract, and keywords) as mentioned in Table 4.2 to find relevant review papers in the year range as mentioned. The number of relevant papers is also mentioned for each type of brain signal.

TABLE 4.1

Inclusion and Exclusion Criteria for Selecting Articles of This Review

Topic	Include	Exclude
Year	2017–2021	Any paper outside this time range
Language	English	Any language other than English
Content Type	Journal, Review Article, Chapter	Conference Paper, Book, Reference Work Entry
Discipline	Computer Science, Engineering (Biomedical Engineering and Bioengineering, Biotechnology, Signal Processing)	Biomaterials, Biomedicine, Business and Management, Environment, Medicine and Public Health, Neurology, Neurosciences, Pharmacy, Philosophy, Rehabilitation Medicine

TABLE 4.2

Search Strategy for Papers for Review

Brain Signals/ Application- Based BCI	Search Strategy		
	Database	Keywords	No. of Paper Selected
P300-BCI	IEEE, Springer, Elsevier, Frontiers, MDPI	(EEG)AND(BCI) AND(P300)	23
Neuromarketing-BCI	IEEE, Springer, Elsevier, Frontiers, MDPI	(EEG)AND(BCI) AND(Neuromarketing)	25
eSports -BCI	IEEE, Springer, Elsevier, Frontiers, MDPI	(EEG)AND(BCI) AND(sports)	4

4.3 RESULTS AND ANALYSIS

Different brain signals are used to drive BCI applications. Among them, P300 is a brain signal with prominent applications. These interfaces have paved the way for modern neuromarketing and E-sports engineering concepts. These are presented in detail in the subsequent sections of the chapter.

4.3.1 P300-EEG-BASED BCI

BCI is a term that refers to a system that acts as a command from the human brain to the computer and also vice versa. Patients with neuromuscular illnesses may utilize the BCI system for everyday communication and rehabilitation. A general BCI system comprises the following components: a stimulus presentation paradigm, a signal acquisition system, a signal processing unit, and a controller for controlling the external device (Figure 4.1).

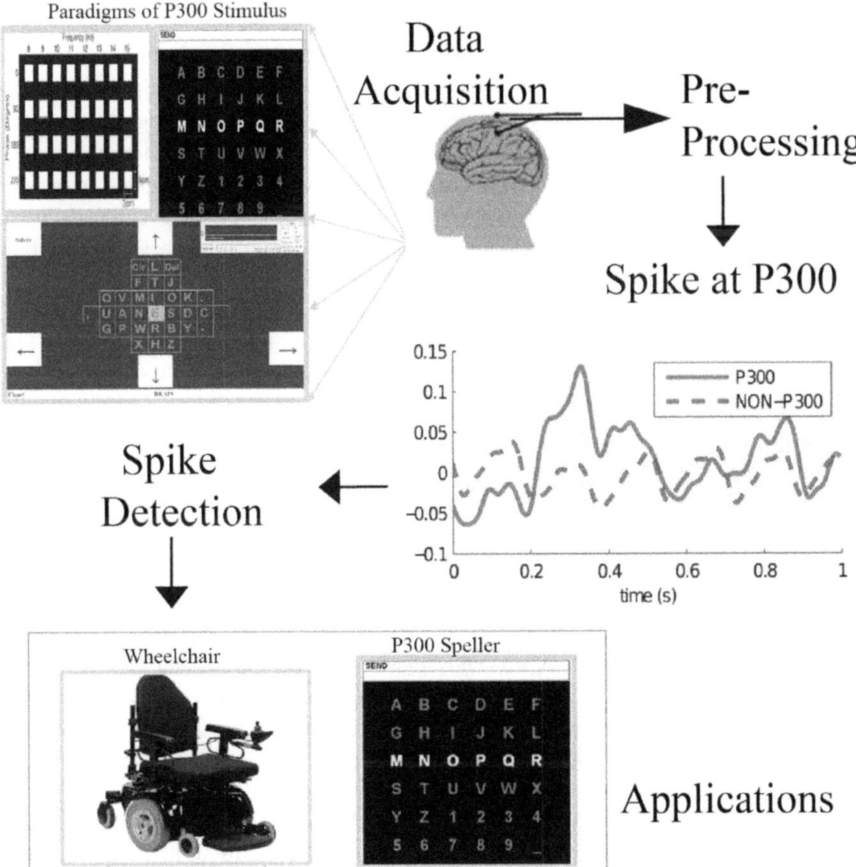

FIGURE 4.1 General block diagram of a P300-EEG signal-based BCI application.

The BCI system is controlled by various EEG signals, and P300 is one of them [6]. The P300 signal is a form of event-related potential (ERP) that causes a brief surge in electrical activity in the brain. The P300 is typically quantified by its amplitude and latency, which vary significantly across people. With a delay of roughly 300 ms, it is the most prominent positive deflection in the EEG following the stimulus onset. Furthermore, P300 BCI systems may elicit P100, N200, and N400 ERP components [7]. This produced delay and its magnitude are subjective and vary depending on the electrodes' spatiotemporal locations and the user's psycho-physiological status during the stimulus [8]. Farwell and Donchin's P300-speller was an early version of the P300-BCI. A 6×6 matrix of 26 letters and ten numerals was shown in the P300-speller, and rows and columns flashed a predetermined number of times in a random sequence, referred to as the row-column pattern (RCP). Subjects in their research were instructed to discretely pay attention to the target and count the number of times the target flashed. In comparison to other regularly used BCI paradigms, P300 has the benefits of being simple enough for most subjects to execute successfully with little to no previous training [9] and, in some instances, allowing for online model modification to be observed without additional subjects' training data [10]. It has been extensively studied using neuroimaging methods such as EEG and functional magnetic resonance imaging (fMRI). During the oddball task, in which two kinds of stimulus (target and standard) are randomly delivered to people, the P300 is often induced by the presence of the target stimulus. The P300 is associated with various cognitive functions, including attention and decision-making. It is also used as a biomarker to assess how the brain can process information in individual subjects. This biomarker has been widely applied in various fields, including clinical diagnosis, cognitive neuroscience, and BCI. Previously, it was shown that many brain regions, including the prefrontal, frontal, and parietal, contribute significantly to forming the P300. In contrast, lesions in a specific component of these areas, such as the frontal lobe, may result in its deficiency, such as lower amplitude. The indicated brain activity in various bands, including delta, theta, and alpha, highly correlates with cognitive processes and the P300. The brain and its activities operate daily inside a large-scale complex network; as a result, information is processed between the brain's specialized, geographically scattered, yet functionally connected parts [11]. By and large, the P300 signal is acquired non-invasively. Environmental noise and other biosignals affect the EEG signal. For each character, repeated stimuli are employed, and the data are averaged to increase the signal-to-noise ratio (SNR) [6] (Table 4.3).

Various P300 stimuli display paradigms have been proposed by different authors. In the P300 data-gathering system, several paradigms and auditory symbols, such as triangles, centers, letters, numbers, images, and colors, are employed. Typically, P300 data is produced by applications such as left- and right-hand fingers, wheelchair control, home appliances, quasi-periodic fluctuation, web browsers, and multimedia players. People who have lost their visual function may apply tactile vibrations as stimuli for P300 [25].

In Figure 4.2, it highlights the selected channels for the P300-based EEG-BCI applications in international 10–20 format.

In Figure 4.3a, from the pie chart, we can see that most of the research works use a bandpass filter as a signal preprocessing technique. In Figure 4.3b, the cut-off frequency range for the bandpass filters is shown, which were used for BCI applications for P300-based EEG signals. Different signal processing methods are applied on the EEG signals to extract features for driving the P300-based EEG-BCI. Table 4.4 demonstrates such feature extraction methods and the corresponding selected features.

TABLE 4.3

Feature Extraction for BCI Using P300-Based EEG

References	Paradigm	Symbol	Flashing Time			Subject		Data	Trials
			Flashing	Pause	Inter-Character Interval	Healthy	disable		
[12]	–	–	100 ms	–	–	4	–	Self-generated	–
[11]	–	Triangle and center	500 ms	1s	–	24	–	Self-generated	150
[9]	2×3 matrix based	Appliances Symbol	120 ms	80 ms	5s	14	09	Self-generated	30
[13]	4×10 button matrix	Characters	100 ms	30 ms	70 ms	200	–	Self-generated	120
[14]	6×6 speller matrix	Characters	62.5 ms	–	125 ms	22	–	Self-generated	–
[15]	6×6 matrix	26 letters 10 numbers and red blue gray picture	–	–	–	12	–	Self-generated	–
[16]	2×2 matrix	pictures of various objects	100 ms	75 ms	700 ms	10	–	Self -generated	–
[17]	6×6 matrix	Character and numbers	100 ms	75 ms	2.1 s	–	–	IIb of BCI Competition II	–
[18]	6×6 matrix	Character and numbers	100 ms	75 ms	2.1 s	–	–	IIb of BCI Competition II	–
[7]	6×6 matrix	Character and numbers	–	–	–	116	–	2018 World Robot Conference (WRC) BCI Contest	4
[19]	6×6 matrix	Characters	62.5 ms	125.5 ms	–	55	–	Self-generated	15
[20]	–	Auditory and visual stimuli	–	125 ms	275 ms	8	–	–	–
[21]	6×6 character matrix	–	100 ms	75 ms	Randomly	–	–	BCI Competition III	–
[22]	6×6 RCP matrix	Characters	75 ms	–	100 ms	10	–	Self-generated	15

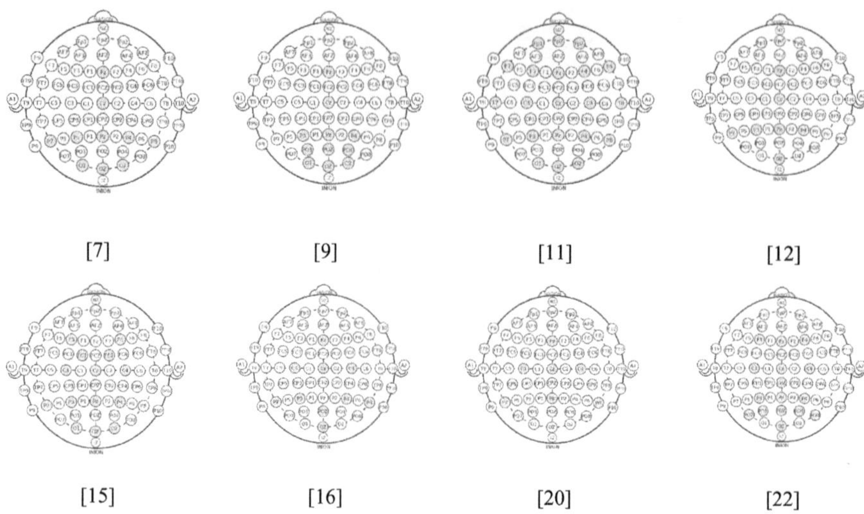

FIGURE 4.2   Channel selection strategy for BCI using P300-based EEG.

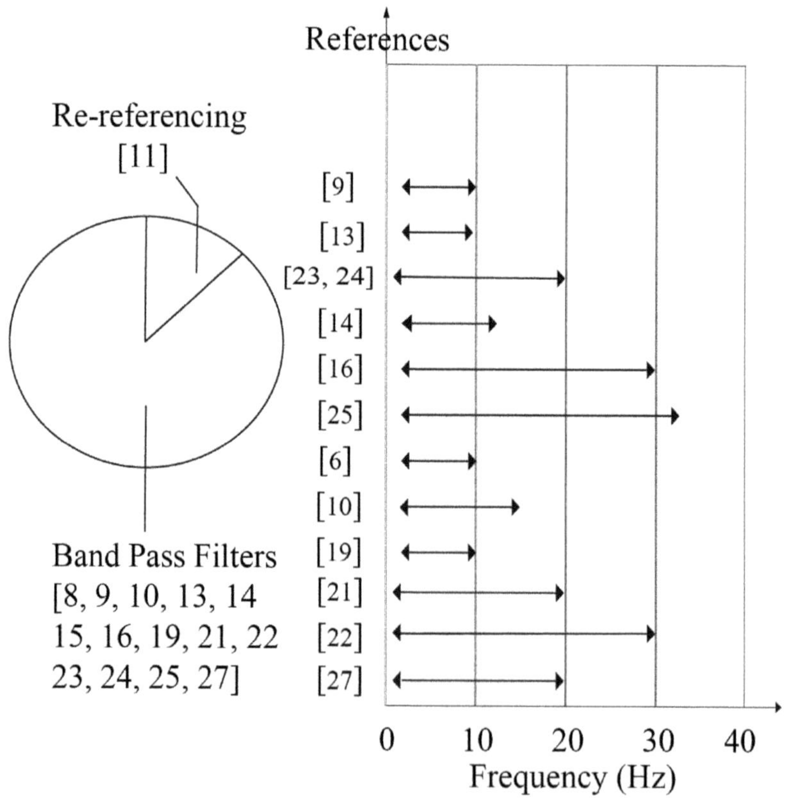

FIGURE 4.3   (a) Signal preprocessing techniques (b) bandpass filter cut-off frequency range.

TABLE 4.4

Signal Processing for P300-EEG-Based BCI

References	Extracted Features	Selected Features
[11,23]	k-medoid clustering algorithm	The Least absolute shrinkage and selection operator (Lasso)
[6,17]	ESVM	Fisher ratio (F-ratio)-based feature selection optimization phase, state-of-the-art classifiers
[10]	CSP, XDAWN	–
[19]	SWLDA	–
[28]	CCA	–

4.3.1.1 P300-EEG-Based BCI: Applications, Challenges, and Future Scopes

Patients with lower brain damage, such as a stroke or traumatic brain injury (TBI), may develop locked-in syndrome (LIS). Patients with LIS cannot move their limbs, which results in various complications, including highly restricted communication skills. However, it is possible to evaluate neurological impulses from LIS patients to improve communication capacities [12,24].

The P300 potential is generated while doing different cognitive functions, including attention and decision-making. It is also used as a biomarker to assess how much information can be processed by the brain in individual subjects. This biomarker has been widely utilized in various fields, including clinical diagnosis, cognitive neuroscience, and BCI [11].

Even while we are at rest, our brain is not inactive. At rest, spontaneous brain activity may represent the brain's capacity for effective information processing. It may be used to examine the pathophysiological processes behind many disorders, including epilepsy and Alzheimer's disease. Indeed, spontaneous activity (for example, spectral power and network measures) and task metrics contribute to our understanding of the P300. Apart from therapeutic uses, BCI technology has been tested and implemented in the realm of amusement games. Over the last decade, researchers have created several BCI-based video games in which BCI technology is utilized to give input, removing the need for intermediary devices entirely (mouse, keyboard, gamepad, and game controllers). The MindGomoku is a new BCI video game based on the P300. Created BrainArena, a multiplayer video game where two players may compete in a primary game [24]. Synchronous BCI implies that BCI users continually adapt to and make decisions in response to the BCI system. Several synchronous BCI spellers have been created recently. These systems are based on the SSVEP, the P300 potential, and a combination of the two. Synchronous BCI devices cannot determine the users' intentional control (IC) and non-control (NC) states. As a result, synchronous BCI is inappropriate for the majority of real-world applications. To overcome this constraint, the asynchronous system should be capable of distinguishing between the IC state (i.e., when the user pays attention to the stimuli) and the NC state (i.e., when the user ignores the stimuli). Numerous researchers have examined asynchronous BCIs, the P300 potential, and different hybrid signal combinations to develop an asynchronous data-collecting system for controlling household appliances in a realistic environment [9, 26]. Psychophysical studies suggested that color attention might activate visual circuits in the brain's occipital and temporal regions. N400 is associated with processing facial information in reaction to familiar faces. The factor "color" significantly altered the N400 peak values, presumably owing to the white backdrop. Additionally, a strong contrast of brightness tends to create a large amplitude. This may trigger unusually big P300 and N400, which may aid categorization [15].

A P300-based authentication paradigm in which images of various items are used as stimuli to elicit ERPs in the human brain is shown in [16]. Additionally, systems that detect P300 signals are not restricted to communication and control applications; other applications, such as a disguised information test for terrorist identification, have been created [10].

The stimulation process to generate the P300 signal can be very slow and exhausting for the subject. That is why it is suggested to make the number of stimulations on the subject as few times as possible, preferably a single trial. Also, it needs to be ensured that adequate detection of the P300 component is achieved. Classification within a subject refers to the detection of the P300 using information acquired in the calibration stage of the single subject. In contrast, cross-subject classification refers to the detection using information retrieved by many individuals [14].

Training machine learning algorithms to classify target vs. non-target P300 signals across participants has been difficult. This difficulty is primarily due to the inherent noise in electrode amplifiers, which results in a need for more distinguishing characteristics between raw target and non-target signals. Consequently, most BCIs are trained on domain-specific data that only generalizes to other users. Finally, establishing a common feature space for P300 signals across subjects while maintaining a low computational cost is critical for developing BCI prototypes that do not need subject-specific calibration. This study contributes to resolving this issue by demonstrating the viability of extracting common P300 traits from a collection of participants through deep learning [12].

System performance optimization remains an issue. A critical task for P300 spellers is to improve their performance in terms of character identification accuracy speed of operation [27] in online systems. In general, the performance of character recognition is highly dependent on the quality of the EEG data and the signal processing techniques used [23]. Before further processing, highly damaged epochs (with an amplitude of more than 100 V compared to baseline) were excluded as a noise reduction method. While epoch rejection improves classification accuracy, it also reduces bit rates when utilized in online P300 BCI systems due to data loss [17]. Concerning trials, there is a proper trade-off between these two parameters; increasing the number of trials improves accuracy but also increases spelling time. Decreasing the number of trials degrades accuracy but decreases spelling time. While current techniques for P300 categorization may enhance the ITR, they sacrifice accuracy by lowering the number of trials. Thus, optimizing the trade-off between accuracy and ITR in a limited number of trials is critical for practically adopting the P300 spellers [8].

4.3.2 EEG-Based BCI Application: Neuromarketing

The most known marketing strategy is the advertisement campaign, which promotes products and increases product sales and consumer awareness. Successful marketing strategies increase profit, but the success rate depends upon the consumption rate, consumer reviews, ratings, and, most importantly, consumers' actual preferences. Advertisements in newspapers and commercials on television are the most traditional marketing methodologies, which may fail to sell products; thus, manufacturing units may undergo losses because conventional marketing methodologies do not always predict consumers' purchasing preferences. Not only has BCI drawn attention to disabled patients but also to advanced viable economic solution areas such as neuromarketing, HMI, and monitoring of mental state. Neuromarketing is one of the most recent and useful strategies that can be used to investigate consumers' shopping preferences, including premarketing surveys. Using consumer neurophysiological data such as EEG, SST, fMRI, PET, MEG, and TMS to investigate preferences and purchasing behavior is defined as "neuromarketing," a highly demanded research field for its high potential. In the neuromarketing field, EEG is mainly used for research because of its high temporal resolution [29–31]. The authors of [32] have predicted consumers' preferences for different advertisements of mobile phone brands by spectral power of EEG. The authors also investigated the differences in consumers' shopping preferences based on different background colors and promotions. In the study of [33], two types of cosmetics advertisements were used to record EEG to investigate the preferences of fifteen female consumers on those cosmetic products. Consumer preferences such as like and dislike decisions were classified for shoe photographs by analyzing EEG signals [34]. Shopper's browsing attention and behavior of online shopping websites under a time limit were investigated by EEG recorded by a biosensor cap so that marketers may adopt showing the exciting catalogs of products to ensure shopper's attention [35]. The study of [31] predicts the premature video trailer skipping decisions of individuals from EEG recordings. The appearance of products controls the attention of consumers' purchase decisions, where ERPs from EEG data can be used to measure the affective preference of consumers [36].

When perception from the unconscious and conscious for a situation or object triggers, the process of both psychology and physiology is called emotion. Emotion is an essential aspect of human communication associated with decision-making, motivation, mood, personality, preferences, and other human interactions, which can be used for BCI applications such as neuromarketing if the physiological signal can be appropriately analyzed [37].

Emotions recorded from audio and video stimuli such as popular music videos and movie clips in the form of EEG data play an essential role in neuromarketing, where emotion correlates with marketing tasks. The process is the measurement of valence, dominance, and arousal from the EEG data to detect the consumer's preference or emotional state [38–41]. The efficiency of musical therapy can be distinguished [42] (Figure 4.4).

Moreover, EEG potential exploration for music preference recognition can pave the way for the development of BCI and neuromarketing [43]. Music preference considerations should be accountable during the design of BCI systems such as

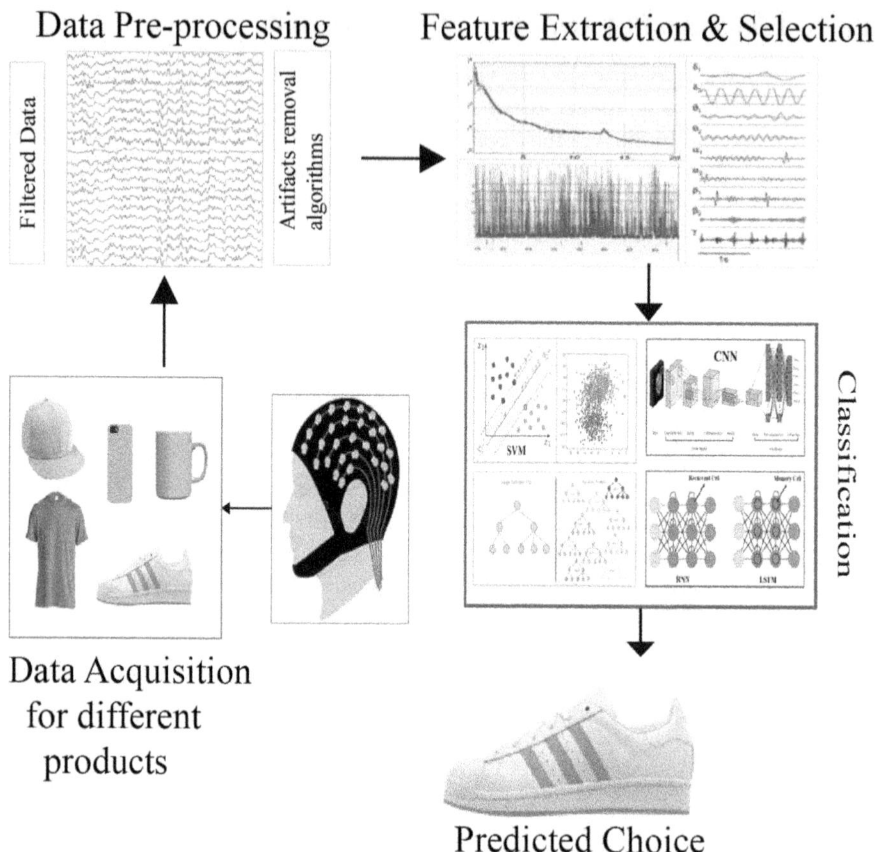

FIGURE 4.4 General block diagram of an EEG signal-based BCI application for neuromarketing.

neuromarketing, and the system can be useful for cognitive patients or patients with motor impairments [44]. The attitude of consumers toward branding smartphone products is classified with the help of EEG data and advanced machine learning algorithms, which is another doorway of neuromarketing [45].

For neuromarketing-based BCI applications, the acquisition of physiological data or selecting the proper dataset is one of the most challenging tasks. EEG datasets are the most popular dataset type for analyzing the preferences of consumers because of their inherent potential, such as high temporal resolution [30]. Table 4.5 shows the list of datasets provided, which have been used in several neuromarketing journals.

The widely used dataset is "DEAP- A Database for Emotion Analysis Using Physiological Signal," which was published in 2012 and is still very popular for different application-based neuromarketing analyses. The authors of [30,39,41,46–49] have utilized this data for their proposed research work. The DEAP dataset was recorded through a dedicated 3.2 GHz clock speed, Pentium 4 processor-based PC, and Biosemi-32 channel device with a recording sampling frequency of 512 Hz. AgCl electrodes were used and placed following the international 10–20 system. There

TABLE 4.5

Dataset for EEG-Based BCI on Neuromarketing

References	Dataset Title	Dataset Details
[30,37,39,41,46–49]	DEAP dataset	Biosemi-32 channel, Recording Fs=512 Hz AgCl Electrodes (10–20 system) 32 Subjects (16 F and 16 M) 40 Audio-Video Stimuli, 40 trials
[43,44	Own Dataset	EPOC-14 channel Recording Fs=2048 Hz, Down Sampling (to 128 Hz) Band-pass (0.16–85 Hz) and Notch (50 Hz and 60 Hz) 9 Subjects (2 F & 7 M), 75 Musical Stimuli, 540 trials
[42]	Own Dataset	Biosignal Amplifier-62 channel, Recording Fs=1200 Hz 20 Subjects (10 F and 10 M) 110 Thai-Musical Stimuli
[45]	Own Dataset	EPOC-14 channel Recording Fs=128 Hz 11 Subjects (7 F and 4 M) 20 smartphone image Stimuli
[29]	Own Dataset	EPOC+ 14 channel, Recording Fs=2048 Hz, Down Sampling (to 128 Hz) 40 Subjects (15 F and 25 M) 14 product, 3 types image Stimuli

were a total of 32 subjects (16 female and 16 male), and each participant had seen 40 audio-video stimuli in 40 trials during the recording of a dataset. Valence, arousal, dominance, like/dislike, and familiarity were rated on the dataset.

The authors of [29,42–45] have used their own recorded dataset, where the EPOC-14 channel device was mostly used, except for the authors of Biosemi [42].

Preprocessing is a noise removal task introduced to the main signal while recording. There are many types of noise, such as power line interference and different types of artifacts. Figure 4.5 shows that most of the authors used bandpass filters of different bandwidths as well as Notch filters of 50 Hz power line interference. The authors of [30,39,46,49] removed EOG artifacts by ICA from EEG signals. Most of the authors also used the down-sampling technique if the datasets were recorded at a high sampling frequency.

EEG channel selection is another useful technique of data processing that is done to find the most dominant channel or EEG band to get more accurate features for the classifier model. This technique also reduces the dimensionality of data. Figure 4.6 shows that most of the authors have selected different sets of channels from their chosen dataset.

The extraction of features from the dataset holds a crucial role in EEG-based neuromarketing, thus the BCI application [30]. It reduces the complexity and dimensionality of the original EEG dataset by extracting the statistical or attributive values.

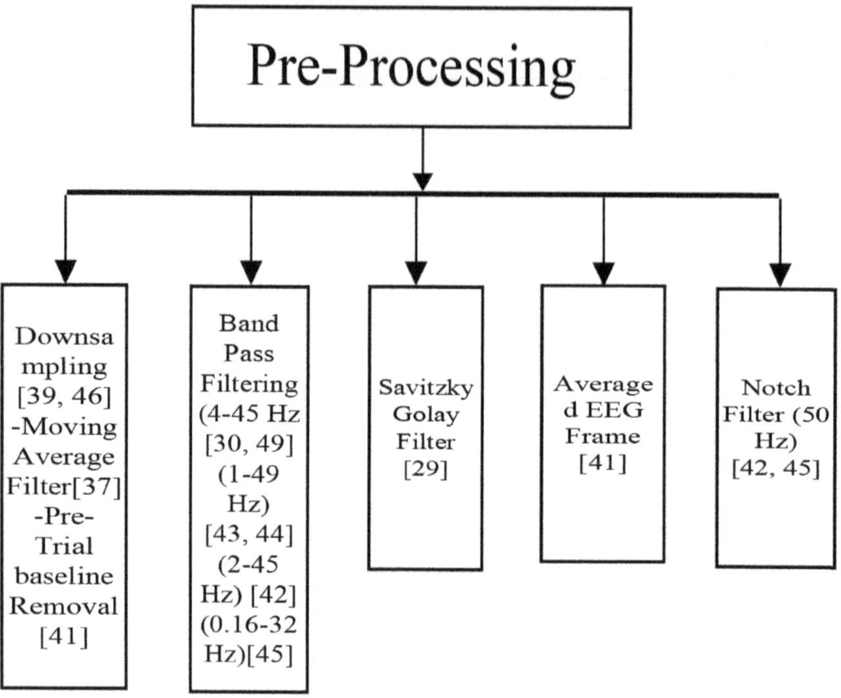

FIGURE 4.5   Signal preprocessing for EEG-based BCI on neuromarketing.

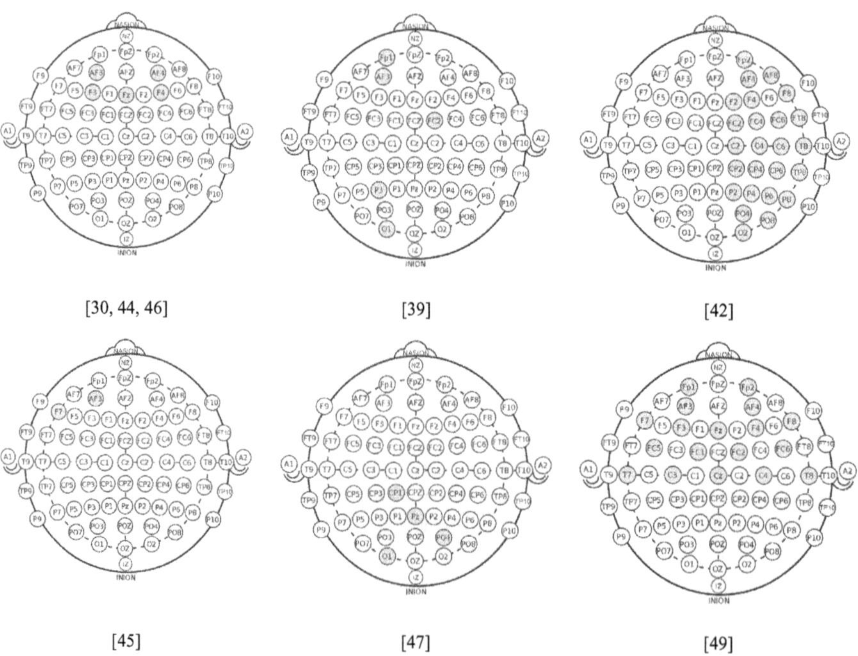

FIGURE 4.6   Channel selection for BCI – neuromarketing.

For classification purposes, raw data cannot be used because of its very large dimension and complexity [47]. Hence, the model will take a very high computational time and will provide very low performance. Most of the authors of Table 4.6 extracted PSD features from their datasets, whereas the authors of [45] and [29] extracted statistical features.

Not all the extracted features dominate the result. It is observed that some features may not be useful for the classifier, which emerges to select the features to minimize the computational time as well as to maximize the performance of the classifier. The authors of [37,39,42,43,48] selected all the features that were extracted from the datasets for their model, whereas other authors of Table 4.7 selected a few features from the extracted feature vectors for their classifier model to maximize their model's performance.

Classifier models are the final and crucial stage of the neuromarketing application, which take selected features and separate them into distinguished classes. There are several widely used classifiers, such as SVM, ANN, k-NN, CNN, and DNN. Different authors propose their model for their particular application and particular

---

TABLE 4.6

Feature Extraction and Feature Selection for BCI-Neuromarketing

References	Extracted Features	Selected Features
[35,46]	PSD Valence	Valence
[44]	F[Afb, wn, Rfb]	FV[Fbeta, Fgamma]
[37]	PSD; Spectral power asymmetry;	PSD; Spectral power asymmetry;
[43]	F[Afb, wn(i,j), Rfb(i)], FV[Fdelta, Falpha, Ftheta, Fbeta, Fgamma] dFV[Rp, NoR, Nl],rFV[Rp, NoR, Nl]	FV[freq. bands] dFV[Rp, NoR, Nl] rFV[Rp, NoR, Nl]
[42]	Fam; ResR; correlation(Fam,ResR); PSD(Left-Right hemisphere); PSD(Left-Right Frontal);	Fam; ResR; correlation(Fam,ResR); PSD(Left-Right hemisphere); PSD(Left-Right Frontal);
[45]	AR (Autoregressive); PCA; PCM;	PCA;
[29]	DWT M (Mean) SD (Standard deviation) EN (Energy) RMS	DWT
[47]	Time domain feature [Power (P), line length (L), RMS, First difference (D1), Second Difference (D2)] Frequency Domain feature [Peak Power, Dominant Frequency, Alpha power, Delta power, Total wavelet energy (TE)] Entropy based feature [Spectral Entropy, Shannon Entropy, Sample entropy]	Entropy-based feature [Spectral Entropy, Shannon Entropy, Sample entropy]
[48]	CWT	CWT
[39]	DWT	DWT
[49]	MSST & SST	MSST & SST
[41]	PSD; Logarithmic Energy; Linear Frequency Cepstral Coefficints; DWT;	DWT -db4;

TABLE 4.7
Classification for
BCI-Neuromarketing

References	Classifier Models
[46]	DTL (Fine Tuning)
[44]	TFD (ZAM)
[37]	Gaussian Naïve Bayes
[43]	TF (HHS)
[42]	SVM; RF;
[45,47]	ANN
[29]	HMM
[48]	AlexNet
[39]	MLPNN; k-NN;
[49]	Linear SVM
[30]	DNN
[41]	k-NN

dataset. The authors also compared different models to justify their proposal. The performance of the classifier is measured by several metrics, such as accuracy, sensitivity, specificity, precision, and recall. The reliability of the models has been mostly quantified by standard deviation, data validation, and ground truth table.

Table 4.8 demonstrates the proposed methods and models that have been used for particular applications with respect to class size by the authors. It also provides the classifier with accuracy, performance, and reliability for different class sizes. From the table, it is seen that most of the authors have shown accuracy results with different validation models, but reliability results have been shown in very few pieces of literature.

4.3.2.1 Neuromarketing BCI: Applications, Challenges, and Future Scopes

Neuromarketing can be used for several marketing strategies, predicting the success rate of marketing [29]. In the other applications of neuromarketing research, such as controlling social media videos and screening adult-contained videos to minimize the effect of those videos on teenagers, even the bad media entrance in the market can be controlled; harmful emotions can be detected [47]. Emotional activities such as musical appraisal, the efficiency of musical therapy, and the effect of proper advertisement background music and graphics have been predicted through neuromarketing research for the last decade [32,42,44].

More classifier models with more selective and robust features of EEG with other physiological data such as EOG, EKG, EMG, BP, body temperature, and GSR could be used to improve the marketing prediction analysis; thus, neuromarketing applications [29,39,47]. More comprehensive datasets for more emotion states, EEG sub-band analysis for emotional activities, and latency-related brain responses can be future research topics [39,43,49].

TABLE 4.8

Performance Metric for Classification for BCI-Neuromarketing

References.	Class Size	Results		
		Accuracy (%)	Performance	Reliability (SD %)
[46]	Like, Dislike	Hinge Cross [Acc-93%]	Rec-93% Prec-93%	–
		Binary Cross [Acc-93%]	Rec-93% Prec-94%	
[44]	Familiarity (LD); Familiar (LDF); Unfamiliar (LDUF);	LD [Acc-85.28% (12–15 s)]	–	±0.77%
		LDF [Acc-91.02% (7.5–10.5 s]		±1.45%
		LDF [Acc-87.10% (10–15 s)]		±1.84%
[37]	Low/High arousal; low/high valence; low/high liking;	Arousal [Acc-62%];	F1–58.3%	–
		Valence [Acc-57.6%];	F1–56.3%	–
		Liking [Acc-55.4%];	F1–50.2%	–
[43]	Like, Dislike	Acc-86.52%	–	±0.76
[42]	Favored, Non-Favored	Melody [Acc-75.2];	F1–71.09	Acc±2.45 F1±2.90
		Song [Acc-84.64];	F1–74.92	Acc±1.59 F1±2.80
[45]	Branded, Unbranded	Acc-72%	–	±3.79
[29]	Like Dislike	Acc- 70.33% (M) 63.56% (F)	–	–
[47]	Happy; Angry; Sad; Relaxing	Average [Acc-97.74%;]	Prec-94.83% Rec-95.61%	–
[48]	High valence (Happy emotion); Low valence (Sad emotion);	Valence Acc-87.5% (at epoch 10 & batch size 10)	–	–
[39]	Positive Emotion; Negative emotion;	MLPNN [Acc-77.14%]; k-NN [Acc-77.14%]	–	–
[49]	PVHAHD; PVHALD; PVLALD; PVLAHD; NVLALD; NVHALD; NVHAHD; NVLAHD;	(MSST) H.Acc-93%	–	–
[30]	Pleasant Unpleasant	Hinge Cross [Acc-94%]	Rec-94% Prec-94%	–
[41]	Dislike	Average Acc-98.6%	–	–

4.3.3   EEG-Based BCI Application: E-sports Engineering

A BCI built on EEG has the potential to improve virtual reality applications, primarily for gaming. Even understanding how gaming actions affect brainwave activity rhythms and variations in the consequences on various persons is critical for diagnosing gaming disorders. EEG can also compare the brain activity between an athlete and a non-athlete and a judgment being observed in their sporting actions.

Given the enormous need to develop intelligent systems along with local processing, this section reviews the highly advanced sensors targeted in the entertainment sector. These technologies are used in various tasks, such as monitoring the biological processes of humans, enhancing an individual's performance and rehabilitation, and adjusting motions and ergonomics. Also, it is a potential technique for improving the virtual reality world. Simultaneously, EEG data can be used to investigate gaming addiction using microstate characteristics.

An EEG sensor is an electronic device that measures the electrical activity of the brain. EEG sensors typically record the potential of the electrical signals in the time domain, which are generated by the firing of millions of neurons within the brain's scalp. These sensors detect the electrical current variations between the skin and the sensor electrode. Then the signals are amplified and bandpass filtered according to the mechanisms built inside the EEG headset devices. These devices can either operate on the principle of dry electrodes or wet electrodes. There are different types of wet EEG devices, as shown in [50].

The role of the brain while a person is engaged in different types of sports activities has been in discussion over the years. Some researchers have investigated how to optimize the performance of sports players by analyzing brain waves [51]. The sample size of the dataset is very important in different BCI applications especially considering real time applications. Table 4.9 shows the dataset sizes of the different BCI applications on E-sports.

In [52], resting-state EEG data were collected from 38 subjects. There were subjects of different categories, some having gaming disorders, while others were recreational players and also with healthy controls. The data were collected before the onset of the game. Then again, data was collected after playing a video game for 30 minutes. The microstate parameters were compared before and after playing the game. In [53] included 21 participants, including seven females who had an average age of 26 years. Eighteen participants were between the ages of 19 and 28. The three participants were 33, 38, and 44 years old, outside of this age range. Each subject was briefed about health precautions due to any radiation from the devices. A total of 20 participants, ten males

TABLE 4.9

Dataset for BCI-E-Sports

References	Sample Size
[52]	38
[53]	21
[54]	20
[55]	40

and ten females, with a combined age of 253 years, were recruited for this study. The recruitment targets must meet the following conditions mentioned in [54]. In [55], there were forty participants, 26 males and 14 females, aged from 18 to 45 years old. Different preprocessing methods were applied to the datasets to make the data suitable for use and to remove the artifacts. In [52], EEG recordings were made at a sampling rate of 1,000 Hz. The bandpass filter was set at 0.1–100 Hz, and all electrodes had a 10k impedance. First, the recordings were down-sampled to 500 Hz. The data was then filtered with a 1–30 Hz bandpass frequency and re-referenced to a shared average reference. Finally, independent component analysis (ICA) detected cardiac and muscular artifacts and then removed them. The global field power (GFP) of the preprocessed EEG data was determined for each participant. In [53], the bandpass area 1–20 Hz implemented a fourth-order linear phase response infinite impulse response (IIR) Butterworth filter as preprocessing. After that, they utilized a linear phase response IIR notch filter with a Q value of 35 at 50 Hz. The butter, iirnotch, and the filtfilt function, which perform zero-phase digital filtering, were used to create these filters in MATLAB. After that, the data were downsampled to 128 samples per second. In [54], Kernel principal component analysis (KPCA) was a crucial step in the data pretreatment and classification of the algorithm. In [55], using Ag/AgCl electrodes linked to a DC amplifier that digitalized the data at 1,000 Hz, EEG signals were obtained from the F3 and F4 sites on the scalp. Then it was bandpass filtered from 1 and 30 Hz. Eye blink artifacts were manually adjusted from continuous EEG data. Each 2-minute block was separated into 2-second epochs (75% overlap), with periods with artifacts higher than 75 µV excluded.

Table 4.10 indicates the lobes of the brain which are covered by the selected channels in the BCI E-Sports applications.

Table 4.11 mentions the selected features for executing the BCI E-sports applications.

TABLE 4.10

Channel Selection for BCI-E-Sports

References	Sample Size
[52]	A 64-channel Quick-cap device captured EEG data.
[53]	Reference: right earlobe; ground: scalp location
[54]	19 channels: covering the frontal, parietal, central, and occipital lobe; reference electrode: bilateral mastoid line
[55]	Reference: mastoids; ground: FPz

TABLE 4.11

Feature Extraction Selection for BCI-E-Sports

References	Extraction	Selection
[52]	EEG	Microstate
[53]	EEG	Event-Related Potential (ERP)
[54]	EEG signals during exercise fatigue is performed (Hilbert EEG).	μ rhythm and β rhythm
[55]	EEG	EEG Neurofeedback

TABLE 4.12

Classification for BCI-E-Sports

References	Extraction
[52]	Automatic Agglomerative Hierarchical Clustering (AAHC)
[53]	Cluster-Based Permutation Test
	Riemannian Minimum-Distance-To-Mean Classifier (RMDM)
[54]	SVM Classifier (Gaussian Kernel Function)
[55]	Mixed-Model ANOVA (Hanning Windowing Function)

TABLE 4.13

Results of Classification for BCI-E-Sports

References	Remarks
[52]	Significant changes occurred in microstates B and D but still need more research to concrete their results.
[53]	The classification accuracy is adequate on average.
[54]	This paper uses it to detect the condition of sports tiredness, with promising results.
[55]	long-term effects of neurofeedback training needed

Table 4.12 shows the classifiers used for classification of the BCI E-sports applications.

Table 4.13 shows the classification results of the classifiers used for classification of the BCI E-sports applications.

4.3.3.1 E-sports Engineering: Applications, Challenges, and Future Scopes

In [52], the authors analyzed the resting EEG in two states: before and after the game. This helped to analyze if the person is gaming addicted or not. Our findings show that gaming behavior inhibits or activates a specific brain region and reorganizes the total brain activity as measured by EEG microstates. In [53], authors compared the performance of an ordinary VR device (a smartphone) to a computer (PC)-based BCI. It was seen that when HMD is employed, correct ERPs are triggered, and the average classification accuracy is satisfactory. In [54] provides a method for interpreting EEG signals based on the MEMD method. The SVM classifier is utilized to classify the motor image EEG signals. The simulation results show that by using MEMD for feature extraction, the correct recognition rate, i.e., the accuracy rate, could reach 90%, which is much more significant than using a typical feature extraction algorithm. In [55] contains the first study to show that neurofeedback can increase endurance performance without requiring invasive brain stimulation. The findings from two different datasets show that, in order to positively affect endurance exercise performance, EEG-neurofeedback can be used to increase left frontal cortex activity.

4.4 DISCUSSION AND CONCLUSION

In conclusion, technological advancements allow different BCI applications to use P300 signals in EEG-based BCI. It is one of the most highly used EEG-based BCIs, including rehabilitation using assistive technology for locked-in syndrome patients. Although it needs less training than other EEG signal-based BCIs, the amount of fatigue induced due to the high concentration and mental effort during training phases remains a concern. Moreover, the suitability of the number of trials (i.e., single or multi) is also a topic of further research. These P300 signals play a role in the revolutionary concept of neuromarketing too. Neuromarketing helps to understand customer preferences, contributing to improved product design and efficient advertising. Also, it is imperative to consider ethical concerns and cross-cultural differences while incorporating this neuroscience with marketing strategy. Lastly, E-sports engineering is another very promising application of EEG-based BCI peripherals. More research needs to be done on this with benchmark datasets and validate the algorithms. Thus, this chapter reviews the current state of BCIs implemented using the electroencephalographic signals of the P300 alongside neuromarketing and E-sports engineering.

ACKNOWLEDGMENT

The Biomedical Instrumentation and Signal Processing Lab (BISPL-IUB) at Independent University, Bangladesh, for its support and motivation.

APPENDIX

Acronym/Abbreviation	Full Meaning
ANN	artificial neural network
APF	adaptive predictor filter
BCI	brain computer interface
BMI	brain machine interface
CBN	common Bayesian network
CCA	canonical correlation analysis
CFA	common feature analysis
CNN	convolutional neural network
CSP	common spatial pattern
DWT	discrete wavelet transform
EEG	electroencephalography
ECG/EKG	electrocardiography
ECoG	electrocorticography
EMD	empirical mode decomposition
EMG	electromyography
EOG	electrooculography
ERP	event-related potential
FAWT	flexible analytic wavelet transforms
FB	filter bank

FFT	fast Fourier transform
ICA	independent component analysis
KNN	k-nearest neighbor
MFBCSP	modified filter bank common spatial pattern
MDS	multi-dimensional scaling
MI	motor imagery
MSI	multivariate synchronization index
mVGG	modified visual geometry group network
PCA	principal component analysis
PSD	power spectral density
SBCSP	sub-band common spatial pattern
SCSSP	separable common spatial-spectral patterns
SSVEP	steady state visual evoked potential
STFT	short time Fourier transform
SVM	support vector machine
SWT	stationary wavelet transform
SwTDA	spectrum-weighted tensor discriminant analysis
TCN	temporal convolutional network
TPCT	time domain power and Clough-Tocher interpolation-based imaging
TSD	time-varying signed distance
WT	wavelet transform

REFERENCES

1. C. D. Binnie and P. F. Prior, "Electroencephalography," *Journal of Neurology, Neurosurgery & Psychiatry*, vol. 57, no. 11, pp. 1308–1319, 1994, doi: 10.1136/jnnp.57.11.1308.
2. M. M. Moore, "Real-world applications for brain-computer interface technology," *IEEE Trans. Neural Syst. Rehabil. Eng.*, vol. 11, no. 2, pp. 162–165, 2003, doi: 10.1109/TNSRE.2003.814433.
3. R. Mane, T. Chouhan, and C. Guan, "BCI for stroke rehabilitation: Motor and beyond," *J. Neural Eng.*, vol. 17, no. 4, p. 041001, 2020, doi: 10.1088/1741-2552/aba162.
4. F. S. Rawnaque et al., "Technological advancements and opportunities in Neuromarketing: a systematic review," *Brain Inform.*, vol. 7, no. 1, p. 10, 2020, doi: 10.1186/s40708-020-00109-x.
5. J. L. Soler-Dominguez and C. Gonzalez, "Using EEG and gamified neurofeedback environments to improve E-Sports performance: Project neuroprotrainer," In *Proceedings of the 16th International Joint Conference on Computer Vision, Imaging and Computer Graphics Theory and Applications (VISIGRAPP 2021) - Volume 1: GRAPP*, vol. 1, no. Visigrapp, pp. 278–283, 2021, https://doi.org/10.5220/0010314502780283
6. S. Kundu and S. Ari, "P300 based character recognition using convolutional neural network and support vector machine," *Biomed. Signal Process. Control*, vol. 55, p. 101645, 2020, doi: 10.1016/j.bspc.2019.101645.
7. J. Jin et al., "The study of generic model set for reducing calibration time in P300-based brain-computer interface," *IEEE Trans. Neural Syst. Rehabil. Eng.*, vol. 28, no. 1, pp. 3–12, 2020, doi: 10.1109/TNSRE.2019.2956488.
8. G. B. Kshirsagar and N. D. Londhe, "Weighted ensemble of deep convolution neural networks for single-trial character detection in devanagari-script-based P300 speller," *IEEE Trans. Cogn. Dev. Syst.*, vol. 12, no. 3, pp. 551–560, 2020, doi: 10.1109/TCDS.2019.2942437.

9. P. K. Shukla, R. K. Chaurasiya, S. Verma, and G. R. Sinha, "A thresholding-free state detection approach for home appliance control using P300-based BCI," *IEEE Sens. J.*, vol. 21, no. 15, pp. 16927–16936, 2021, doi: 10.1109/JSEN.2021.3078512.

10. J. M. C. Delgado, D. Achanccaray, E. R. Villota, and S. Chevallier, "Riemann-based algorithms assessment for single- and multiple-trial P300 classification in non-optimal environments," *IEEE Trans. Neural Syst. Rehabil. Eng.*, vol. 28, no. 12, pp. 2754–2761, 2020, doi: 10.1109/TNSRE.2020.3043418.

11. F. Li et al., "Reconfiguration of Brain Network between Resting-State and Oddball Paradigm," 2018, doi: 10.48550/ARXIV.1809.06676.

12. R. Sahay and C. G. Brinton, "Robust subject-independent P300 waveform classification via signal pre-processing and deep learning," *IEEE Access*, vol. 9, pp. 87579–87591, 2021, doi: 10.1109/ACCESS.2021.3089998.

13. W. Gao et al., "Learning invariant patterns based on a convolutional neural network and big electroencephalography data for subject-independent P300 brain-computer interfaces," *IEEE Trans. Neural Syst. Rehabil. Eng.*, vol. 29, pp. 1047–1057, 2021, doi: 10.1109/TNSRE.2021.3083548.

14. M. Alvarado-González, G. Fuentes-Pineda, and J. Cervantes-Ojeda, "A few filters are enough: Convolutional neural network for P300 detection," *Neurocomputing*, vol. 425, pp. 37–52, 2021, doi: 10.1016/j.neucom.2020.10.104.

15. X. Zhang, J. Jin, S. Li, X. Wang, and A. Cichocki, "Evaluation of color modulation in visual P300-speller using new stimulus patterns," *Cogn. Neurodyn.*, vol. 15, no. 5, pp. 873–886, 2021, doi: 10.1007/s11571-021-09669-y.

16. N. Rathi, R. Singla, and S. Tiwari, "A novel approach for designing authentication system using a picture based P300 speller," *Cogn. Neurodyn.*, vol. 15, no. 5, pp. 805–824, 2021, doi: 10.1007/s11571-021-09664-3.

17. L. Vařeka, "Evaluation of convolutional neural networks using a large multi-subject P300 dataset," *Biomed. Signal Process. Control*, vol. 58, p. 101837, 2020, doi: 10.1016/j. bspc.2019.101837.

18. S. Kundu and S. Ari, "A deep learning architecture for P300 detection with brain-computer interface application," *IRBM*, vol. 41, no. 1, pp. 31–38, 2020, doi: 10.1016/j. irbm.2019.08.001.

19. J. Lee, K. Won, M. Kwon, S. C. Jun, and M. Ahn, "CNN with large data achieves true zero-training in online P300 brain-computer interface," *IEEE Access*, vol. 8, pp. 74385–74400, 2020, doi: 10.1109/ACCESS.2020.2988057.

20. Z. Oralhan, "3D input convolutional neural networks for P300 signal detection," *IEEE Access*, vol. 8, pp. 19521–19529, 2020, doi: 10.1109/ACCESS.2020.2968360.

21. F. Li, X. Li, F. Wang, D. Zhang, Y. Xia, and F. He, "A novel P300 classification algorithm based on a principal component analysis-convolutional neural network," *Appl. Sci.*, vol. 10, no. 4, pp. 1–15, 2020, doi: 10.3390/app10041546.

22. V. Martínez-Cagigal, E. Santamaría-Vázquez, and R. Hornero, "Asynchronous control of P300-based brain-computer interfaces using sample entropy," *Entropy*, vol. 21, no. 3, p. 230, 2019, doi: 10.3390/e21030230.

23. S. Li, J. Jin, I. Daly, X. Wang, H. K. Lam, and A. Cichocki, "Enhancing P300 based character recognition performance using a combination of ensemble classifiers and a fuzzy fusion method," *J. Neurosci. Methods*, vol. 362, p. 109300, 2021, doi: 10.1016/j. jneumeth.2021.109300.

24. M. Li et al., "The mindgomoku: An online p300 bci game based on bayesian deep learning," *Sensors*, vol. 21, no. 5, pp. 1–19, 2021, doi: 10.3390/s21051613.

25. X. Han, J. Niu, and S. Guo, "A Tactile-based Brain Computer Interface P300 Paradigm Using Vibration Frequency and Spatial Location," *J. Med. Biol. Eng.*, vol. 40, no. 6, pp. 773–782, 2020, doi: 10.1007/s40846-020-00535-6.

26. T. Lee, M. Kim, and S. Kim, "Improvement of P300-based brain – computer balancing techniques," *Sensors*, vol. 20, no. 19, p. 5576, 2020, doi: 10.3390/s20195576.

27. M. Arican and K. Polat, "Pairwise and variance based signal compression algorithm (PVBSC) in the P300 based speller systems using EEG signals," *Comput. Methods Programs Biomed.*, vol. 176, pp. 149–157, 2019, doi: 10.1016/j.cmpb.2019.05.011.

28. J. D. C. Peguero, O. Mendoza-Montoya, and J. M. Antelis, "Single-option P300-BCI performance is affected by visual stimulation conditions," *Sensors (Switzerland)*, vol. 20, no. 24, pp. 1–22, 2020, doi: 10.3390/s20247198.

29. M. Yadava, P. Kumar, R. Saini, P. P. Roy, and D. Prosad Dogra, "Analysis of EEG signals and its application to neuromarketing," *Multimed. Tools Appl.*, vol. 76, no. 18, pp. 19087–19111, 2017, doi: 10.1007/s11042-017-4580-6.

30. M. Aldayel, M. Ykhlef, and A. Al-Nafjan, "Deep learning for EEG-based preference classification in neuromarketing," *Appl. Sci.*, vol. 10, no. 4, pp. 1–23, 2020, doi: 10.3390/app10041525.

31. A. Libert and M. M. Van Hulle, "Predicting premature video skipping and viewer interest from EEG recordings," *Entropy*, vol. 21, no. 10, p. 1014, 2019, doi: 10.3390/e21101014.

32. P. Golnar-Nik, S. Farashi, and M. S. Safari, "The application of EEG power for the prediction and interpretation of consumer decision-making: A neuromarketing study," *Physiol. Behav.*, vol. 207, pp. 90–98, 2019, doi: 10.1016/j.physbeh.2019.04.025.

33. D. Gabriel et al., "Emotional effects induced by the application of a cosmetic product: A real-time electrophysiological evaluation," *Appl. Sci.*, vol. 11, no. 11, p. 4766, 2021, doi: 10.3390/app11114766.

34. B. Yilmaz, S. Korkmaz, D. B. Arslan, E. Güngör, and M. H. Asyali, "Like/dislike analysis using EEG: Determination of most discriminative channels and frequencies," *Comput. Methods Programs Biomed.*, vol. 113, no. 2, pp. 705–713, 2014, doi: 10.1016/j.cmpb.2013.11.010.

35. D.-H. Shih, K.-C. Lu, and P.-Y. Shih, "Exploring shopper's browsing behavior and attention level with an EEG biosensor cap," *Brain Sciences,* vol. 9, no. 11, p. 301, 2019, doi: 10.3390/brainsci9110301.

36. F. Guo, X. Shuang Wang, W. Liu, and Y. Ding, "Affective preference measurement of product appearance based on event-related potentials," *Cogn. Technol. Work*, vol. 20, no. 2, pp. 299–308, 2018, doi: 10.1007/s10111-018-0463-5.

37. S. Koelstra et al., "DEAP: A database for emotion analysis; using physiological signals," *IEEE Trans. Affect. Comput.*, vol. 3, no. 1, pp. 18–31, 2012, doi: 10.1109/T-AFFC.2011.15.

38. G. Vecchiato et al., "How to measure cerebral correlates of emotions in marketing relevant tasks," *Cognit. Comput.*, vol. 6, no. 4, pp. 856–871, 2014, doi: 10.1007/s12559-014-9304-x.

39. M. S. Özerdem and H. Polat, "Emotion recognition based on EEG features in movie clips with channel selection," *Brain Inform.*, vol. 4, no. 4, pp. 241–252, 2017, doi: 10.1007/s40708-017-0069-3.

40. D. S. Naser and G. Saha, "Influence of music liking on EEG based emotion recognition," *Biomed. Signal Process. Control*, vol. 64, no. September 2020, p. 102251, 2021, doi: 10.1016/j.bspc.2020.102251.

41. F. Feradov, I. Mporas, and T. Ganchev, "Evaluation of features in detection of dislike responses to audio–visual stimuli from EEG signals," *Computers*, vol. 9, no. 2, pp. 1–11, 2020, doi: 10.3390/computers9020033.

42. S. Sangnark et al., "Revealing preference in popular music through familiarity and brain response," *IEEE Sens. J.*, vol. 21, no. 13, pp. 14931–14940, 2021, doi: 10.1109/JSEN.2021.3073040.

43. S. K. Hadjidimitriou and L. J. Hadjileontiadis, "Toward an EEG-based recognition of music liking using time-frequency analysis," *IEEE Trans. Biomed. Eng.*, vol. 59, no. 12, pp. 3498–3510, 2012, doi: 10.1109/TBME.2012.2217495.

44. S. K. Hadjidimitriou and L. J. Hadjileontiadis, "EEG-based classification of music appraisal responses using time-frequency analysis and familiarity ratings," *IEEE Trans. Affect. Comput.*, vol. 4, no. 2, pp. 161–172, 2013, doi: 10.1109/T-AFFC.2013.6.

45. A. Özbeyaz, "EEG-Based classification of branded and unbranded stimuli associating with smartphone products: Comparison of several machine learning algorithms," *Neural Comput. Appl.*, vol. 33, no. 9, pp. 4579–4593, 2021, doi: 10.1007/s00521-021-05779-0.

46. M. S. Aldayel, M. Ykhlef, and A. N. Al-Nafjan, "Electroencephalogram-based preference prediction using deep transfer learning," *IEEE Access*, vol. 8, pp. 176818–176829, 2020, doi: 10.1109/ACCESS.2020.3027429.

47. M. K. Ahirwal and M. R. Kose, "Audio-visual stimulation based emotion classification by correlated EEG channels," *Health Technol. (Berl).*, vol. 10, no. 1, pp. 7–23, 2020, doi: 10.1007/s12553-019-00394-5.

48. A. Mishra, P. Ranjan, and A. Ujlayan, "Empirical analysis of deep learning networks for affective video tagging," *Multimed. Tools Appl.*, vol. 79, no. 25–26, pp. 18611–18626, 2020, doi: 10.1007/s11042-020-08714-y.

49. P. Ozel, A. Akan, and B. Yilmaz, "Synchrosqueezing transform based feature extraction from EEG signals for emotional state prediction," *Biomed. Signal Process. Control*, vol. 52, pp. 152–161, 2019, doi: 10.1016/j.bspc.2019.04.023.

50. M. Soufineyestani, D. Dowling, and A. Khan, "Electroencephalography (EEG) technology applications and available devices," *Appl. Sci.*, vol. 10, no. 21, pp. 1–23, 2020, doi: 10.3390/app10217453.

51. L. Angius, A. R. Mauger, J. Hopker, A. Pascual-Leone, E. Santarnecchi, and S. M. Marcora, "Bilateral extracephalic transcranial direct current stimulation improves endurance performance in healthy individuals," *Brain Stimul.*, vol. 11, no. 1, pp. 108–117, 2018, doi: 10.1016/j.brs.2017.09.017.

52. L. Wang, X. Ding, W. Zhang, and S. Yang, "Differences in EEG microstate induced by gaming: A comparison between the gaming disorder individual, recreational game users and healthy controls," *IEEE Access*, vol. 9, pp. 32549–32558, 2021, doi: 10.1109/ACCESS.2021.3060112.

53. C. Y. Chen, J. Y. Yen, P. W. Wang, G. C. Liu, C. F. Yen, and C. H. Ko, "Altered functional connectivity of the insula and nucleus accumbens in internet gaming disorder: A resting state fMRI study," *Eur. Addict. Res.*, vol. 22, no. 4, pp. 192–200, 2016, doi: 10.1002/hbm.1058

54. A. P. Nichols and T. E. Holmes, "Nonparametric permutation tests for functional neuroimaging: a primer with examples," *Hum. Brain Mapping*, vol. 15, no. 1, pp. 1–25, 2002.

55. Z. Yang and H. Ren, "Feature extraction and simulation of EEG signals during exercise-induced fatigue," *IEEE Access*, vol. 7, pp. 46389–46398, 2019, doi: 10.1109/ACCESS.2019.2909035.

Section II

EEG – Signal Processing

5 Significance of Fourier Transform for Epileptic EEG Signals Analysis

Pooja, Sourav Maity, and Karan Veer

5.1 INTRODUCTION

Electroencephalogram (EEG) signals provide well-characterized brain pathological and physiological information by recording the electrical activity of cerebral cortex nerve cells (Aydemir, Tuncer, and Dogan 2020). An EEG signal behaves like the gold standard to diagnose brain abnormalities, especially epilepsy (Zhang, Chen, and Li 2020; Nagarajan, Ghosh, and Palumbo 2011). Epilepsy occurs due to an excess of neuronal discharge (Elgohary, Eldawlatly, and Khalil 2016). Traditional methods of detecting epilepsy are time-consuming. So, an efficient algorithm may help in reducing the workload by automatic seizure detection. Researchers make the field more focused by extracting features from epileptic signals.

As an essential signal for determining brain function, it can be described in five stages in terms of analysis methods. The first section is the acquisition of EEG signals. The second phase, called pre-processing, makes the signal noise or interference-free and helps in simplifying signal analysis. The movement that is not recorded from a cerebral signal is named noise (Kappel et al. 2017; Wang et al. 2017) and occurs due to a heartbeat artifact, an eye blink, and muscle movement. These artifacts are removed using the Butterworth filter (Tiwari et al. 2017), differential windowing (Joshi, Pachori, and Vijesh 2014), and the simple classifier (Raghu and Sriraam 2017) by reducing background waveforms. The third phase is of feature extraction of subsequent EEG signals which discriminate between different signals and decrease the vector dimension to reduce calculation complexity. Some generally used feature extraction techniques are phase correlation, non-linear features of Discrete Wavelet Transform (DWT) (Joshi, Pachori, and Vijesh 2014), Empirical Mode Decomposition (EMD), Common Spatial Pattern (CSP), and morphological (Bagheri et al. 2016) and statistical features (Hamad et al. 2016; Sharmila and Geethanjali 2016). Phase correlation predicts translational displacement (Parvez and Paul 2017). Non-linear features are based on DWT as entropy and sample entropy (Wang et al. 2018). The time-frequency pattern of an EEG signal is analyzed by decomposing the signal into a finite number of intrinsic mode functions (IMFs). These IMFs are used in a potential-based hierarchical agglomerative (PHA) algorithm (Belhadj et al. 2017; Riaz et al. 2016; Pachori and Bajaj 2011).

DOI: 10.1201/9781003252092-7

The spatial pattern is also significant for feature extraction where spatial filters are used to discriminate the class of signal (Lotte and Guan 2011). The fourth phase is the classification of extracted features using various classification approaches. Here, the classifier plays a significant role in attaining effective results. The primary goal of classification is to set the limit between classes. A classifier can work either by keeping the threshold value for a feature or by using machine learning algorithms (Shoka et al. 2019). Normally used classification techniques are the support vector machine, a linear discriminant analysis, the Gaussian mixture model, a decision tree, a logistic regression, an artificial neural network, a visibility graph, the K nearest neighbor, and ensemble and deep learnings. The last stage is to send the results to judgment devices or control external devices. Recently, various studies have been done to detect different brain disorders, most of them are oriented to a Brain-Computer Interface (BCI), a system that reads and interprets signals directly from patients and extracts some useful results from these input signals (Abdulkader, Atia, and Mostafa 2015; Shoka et al. 2019).

In all these phases of EEG signal analysis, the Fourier Transform (FT) has a significant role in feature extraction. It also extracts the power spectrum, frequency response functions, and various domain functions from time domain signals. FT can be described as a Continuous Time Fourier Transform (CTFT) and a Discrete Time Fourier Transform (DTFT). The need of FT has been increased in the last few decades due to a decrement in computer costs and an increment in the sophistication of measurement systems. The CTFT theory is helpful for theoretical work, but not appropriate for instrumentation techniques. So, the transform generally used is DTFT, where sampled versions of both the time and frequency domain are used. This version of the signal maintains duration limitations in both domains. More advanced versions of FT such as Fast Fourier Transform (FFT) and Short-time Frequency Transform (STFT) etc. are also used for EEG signal analysis. A feature represents a specific property, a functional component, and is a considerable measurement of a particular pattern of a signal. Features are extracted to reduce the information of loss of signal. For signals, it is also important to reduce the algorithm complexity and information processing. Nowadays, a number of methods are used to extract the features of an EEG signal such as FT, the Eigenvector method (EM), and the time-frequency distribution and auto-regressive method (ARM).

Different studies show various forms of the FT are applicable for sliding windows and feature extraction. In some cases, the signal decomposes into short segments, and then, the FT is applied, but in other cases, it is applied directly to attain the required results. This chapter shows how FT is helpful in EEG signal analysis. It also depicts the implementation of FT on a real-time EEG database available on Physionet (a publically available database website). The present work shows a variation in the results of EEG signal analysis when FT is applied and not applied. With different forms of FT, it also shows which form is essential for each specified task performed in the study. The study concluded on the electrical representation of brain signals and the role of FT in particular circumstances/tasks/activities (Figure 5.1).

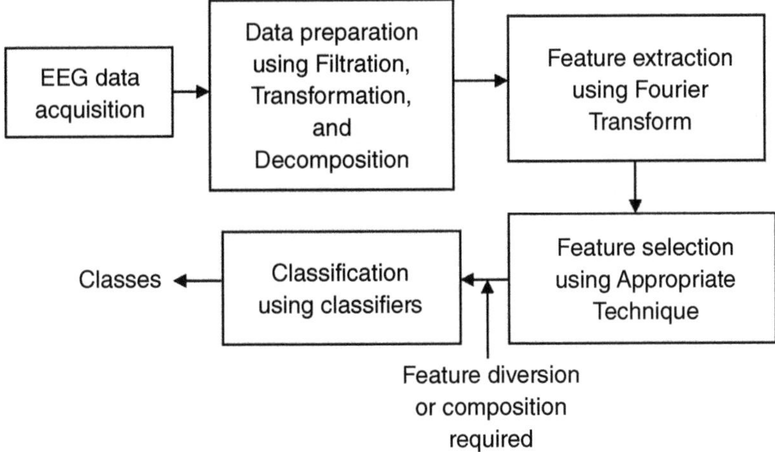

FIGURE 5.1 Diagram illustrating EEG data (Fourier Transform) processing steps.

5.2 FOURIER TRANSFORM

FT is an arithmetic operation that collects a time-oriented sample as an input and estimates the comprehensive offset cycle, rotational speed, and robustness for each feasible cycle in a specified pattern. The FT is implemented on waveforms that are primarily a function of time, area, etc. The FT disintegrates a waveform into sinusoids and furnishes different ways to display a waveform.

The FT of a function $f(x)$ is represented as:

$$f(x) = \int_{-\infty}^{\infty} F(k)e^{2\Pi ikx}dk \tag{5.1}$$

$$F(k) = \int_{-\infty}^{\infty} f(x)e^{-2\Pi ikx}dx \tag{5.2}$$

where $F(k)$ is acquired by applying inverse FT.

5.3 CONTINUOUS TIME FOURIER TRANSFORM (CTFT)

The Fourier analysis estimates the signals and systems in the frequency domain. The CTFT of $x(t)$ is represented as:

$$F(f) = \int_{-\infty}^{\infty} f(t)e^{-j2\Pi ft}dt \tag{5.3}$$

$$f(t) = \int_{-\infty}^{\infty} F(f)e^{j2\Pi ft} df \tag{5.4}$$

5.4 DISCRETE TIME FOURIER TRANSFORM (DTFT)

The DTFT is always periodic in nature. The DTFT of $x(n)$ is represented as:

$$A_k = \sum_{n=0}^{N-1} e^{-i\frac{2\Pi}{N}kn} a_n \tag{5.5}$$

Here, our signal is a_n for $n = 0 \ldots N-1$, and $a_n = a_n + jN$ for all n and j.

5.5 FAST FOURIER TRANSFORM (FFT)

Fast Fourier Transform (FFT) is a method that determines the DTFT of a series or its inverse (IDFT). The Fourier analysis transforms a bio-signal from its time domain to its frequency domain. It is represented as:

$$F(w) = \int_{-\infty}^{\infty} f(x)e^{-iwx} dx \tag{5.6}$$

$$f(w) = \frac{1}{2\Pi} \int_{-\infty}^{\infty} F(w)e^{iwx} dw \tag{5.7}$$

5.6 SHORT-TIME FOURIER TRANSFORM (STFT)

This is an FT that is applied to estimate the sinusoidal frequency and phase of a signal as it varies with respect to time. The process of estimating STFTs is to split up a larger signal into smaller sections of uniform length and then determine the FT individually on every smaller part. This discloses the Fourier spectrum on every smaller segment. It is represented as:

$$\text{STFT}\{x(t)\} = X(\Gamma, w) = \int_{-\infty}^{\infty} x(t)w(t-\Gamma)e^{-jwt} dt \tag{5.8}$$

5.7 POWER SPECTRUM

The power spectrum is often interpreted as the FT of the autocorrelation function. The power spectrum of a time series characterizes the dissemination of power into frequency constituents including the signal. Corresponding to a Fourier analysis, a signal can be disintegrated into a number of discrete frequencies on a continuous range. It is represented as:

$$PS(f) = \frac{1}{T} \int_0^T r_{xx}(t) e^{-j2\Pi mf_i t}\, dt \tag{5.9}$$

$$PS[m] = \sum_{n=1}^{N} r_{xx}[n] e^{-\frac{j2\Pi mn}{N}} \tag{5.10}$$

5.8 MEAN POWER

The estimation of mean power frequency is a method implemented in the assessment of the frequency shift. It is represented as:

$$MNP = \sum_{j=1}^{M} P_j / M \tag{5.11}$$

5.9 MEAN FREQUENCY

The mean frequency of a spectrum is evaluated as the sum of the product of the spectrogram intensity (in dB) and the frequency, divided by the total sum of spectrogram intensity. It is represented as:

$$MNF = \sum_{j=1}^{M} f_j P_j / \sum_{j=1}^{M} P_j \tag{5.12}$$

5.10 HOW FT IS HELPFUL FOR EEG SIGNALS

It is assumed that 70% of epileptic patients stay safe from seizures throughout their lives if they are treated at an early stage of the disorder. A few commonly used non-invasive methods to treat epilepsy are computed tomography, EEG signal, position emission tomography (PET), and magnetic resonance imaging (Anyanwu and Motamedi 2017) but a more frequently used technique to detect the brain disorder is electroencephalograph (Adeli, Zhou, and Dadmehr 2003; Liu et al. 1992; Boashash 2015). The recording of brain signals for epilepsy is done by trained persons as trainer fatigue can affect the result a lot and so various efforts toward automatic detection have been made. Liu et al. described a neonatal periodic discharge for epilepsy detection but this method is not accurate for all age groups (Liu et al. 1992). An EEG epileptic signal is classified by Kaya et al. (2014), Kumar, Kanhangad, and Pachori (2015), and Tiwari et al. (2017) by extracting local binary patterns (LBPs). Ictal and seizure-free signals are differentiated using fractional linear prediction in various EEG analysis methods (Joshi, Pachori, and Vijesh 2014). In Raghu and Sriraam (2017), Shannon entropy, spectral entropy, log-energy, and Renyi entropy are extracted; but frequency domain parameters are completely excluded.

An EEG signal is classified using FT to extract an EEG rhythm (Singh et al. 2016). On the other hand, EEG rhythms are also extracted using Discrete Cosine Transform (DCT) (Gupta, Singh, and Karlekar 2018). It can be said that due to the non-stationary behavior of EEG signals, frequency analysis becomes significant (Boashash 2015; Pachori and Sircar 2008; Tzallas, Tsipouras, and Fotiadis 2007). So FT and DCT are frequently used techniques to analyze the EEG signal in a frequency domain. Nowadays, few advanced methods of these conventional techniques have been designed by researchers. The Fourier-Bessel series is used by Gupta and Pachori (2019), Tzallas, Tsipouras, and Fotiadis (2009), and Hyvärinen et al. (2010) but doesn't give full information regarding time and frequency. The Pseudo-Wigner-Ville distribution method is applied by Tzallas et al. by exploring different smoothing windows (Tzallas, Tsipouras, and Fotiadis 2009) while STFT is used by Ocak (2008), Bhati, Pachori, and Gadre (2017). If the used window is short, the frequency resolution in the time domain will be poor making it difficult to obtain accurate information simultaneously both in time and frequency domains.

Few studies (Bhati et al. 2017; Peker, Sen, and Delen 2016; Subasi 2007) of seizure detection are oriented toward Wavelet Transform (WT) as WT provides variable window sizes. Wang et al. (2017), Peker, Sen, and Delen (2016) used a linear phase wavelet filter while features using wavelet coefficients like mean, median, minimum, and maximum are extracted by Subasi (2007), Peker, Sen, and Delen (2016). Subasi (2007) explored Discrete Wavelet Transforms (DWTs) to detect epileptic seizures. In Subasi, Kevric, and Abdullah Canbaz (2019), Khan, Rafiuddin, and Farooq (2012), EEG signals were classified using DWTs, which decompose the signal into different frequency bands. Normal and epileptic classes are differentiated using several feature extraction frameworks. Seizure and seizure-free events are classified using a wavelet-based approach and two features; median absolute deviation (MAD) and interquartile range (IQR). A Harmonic Wavelet Packet Transform (HWPT) breaks the EEG signal into subsequent levels in Rafiuddin, Khan, and Farooq (2011).

While implementing WT, choosing accurate mother wavelet and decomposition levels is a difficult task. Few empirical mode decomposition (EMD) based studies have been done to explore the non-stationary behavior of EEG signals (Alam and Bhuiyan 2013; Riaz et al. 2016; Sharma and Pachori 2015; Pachori and Patidar 2014). EMD decomposes non-stationary EEG signals into amplitude-modulated (AM) and frequency-modulated (FM) oscillating components (Huang et al. 1998) and these components are called intrinsic mode functions (IMFs). Seizure and seizure-free events were classified using the hidden Markov model (HMM). A modified approach of EMD depending upon peak selection criteria was used to decompose the epileptic signal (Kaleem, Guergachi, and Krishnan 2013). In Fu et al. (2014) and Oweis and Abdulhay (2011), the Hilbert-Huang transform with EMD was used to decompose the EEG signal and extract the instantaneous frequency (Fu et al. 2014, Oweis and Abdulhay 2011). This technique was found efficient in determining epileptic signals (Fu et al. 2014). In Flandrin, Torres, and Colominas (2011), the complete ensemble EMD (CEEMD), an advanced stage of an EMD, was used to break the signal into components, and statistical features were extracted from IMFs. In Alickovic, Kevric, and Subasi (2018), the authors found that EMD and WT were both used to decompose the signal for correct detection. Still, the EMD has many limitations like mode mixing, end effect artifacts, non-uniformity, and alignment of scale. The mode-mixing issue was solved by ensemble EMD (Hassan and Haque 2016), but this enhances the computation complexity.

The non-uniformity issue is solved by the multivariate EMD (Rehman and Mandic 2009). So, all these problems of EMD are solved by the Fourier decomposition method (FDM) which is based on the Fourier theory and is helpful for non-linear and uncertain time-series signals (Singh, Joshi, Pateny, and Saha 2016). FDM gives better time-frequency energy approximation than EMD. FDM is capable of distinguishing frequency bands effectively during the extraction of Fourier intrinsic band functions (FIBFs) (Singh 2018). FDM has been implemented in several studies to remove artifacts from biomedical signals (Singhal et al. 2020), time-series data modeling (Singhal et al. 2015), and gravitational wave analysis.

More frequently used feature extraction techniques are FT, WT, EMD, ensemble empirical mode decomposition (EEMD), CEEMD, FDM, and statistical analysis which gives a better understanding of the behavior of the signal.

5.11 SIGNIFICANCE OF FT ON A REAL-TIME EEG SIGNAL

A comparison of various existing studies with the BONN dataset to differentiate two-class problems is shown in Tables 5.1–5.3. This comparison shows that FT-based extracted features give more accurate results. In the CHB-MIT dataset in Table 5.4, healthy and seizure classes are differentiated and it also shows more accurate results. This means that FT plays a significant role in epilepsy analysis.

5.12 CONCLUSION

Due to the non-stationary behavior of EEG signals automatic detection of epilepsy is itself a challenge. Various automatic detection methods are available in literature but their accuracy discriminates them. This accuracy depends upon features

TABLE 5.1

Comparison of Healthy and Seizure EEG Signals from the BONN Dataset

Authors	Extracted Feature	Classification Techniques	Accuracy (%)
Rizon et al. (2020)	Relative band power features	KNN, SVM	96.1, 94.9
Subasi (2007)	Sub-band features	Mixture of experts	94.5
Subasi and Gursoy (2010)	Sub-band features	LDA, SVM	100
Kaya et al. (2014)	LBP	SVM	99.50
Fu et al. (2015)	Entropy and sub-band energy	SVM	99.85
Peker, Sen, and Delen (2016)	Statistical features	CVANN	100
Tiwari et al. (2017)	LBP	SVM	100
Mehla et al. (2021) (high-pass filtered EEG)	L^P norms	SVM	100
Mehla et al. (2021) (low-pass filtered EEG)	L^P norms	SVM	99.96

TABLE 5.2

Classification of Seizure-Free and Seizure EEG Signal from BONN Dataset

Authors	Extracted Feature	Classification Techniques	Accuracy (%)
Joshi, Pachori, and Vijesh (2014)	Error and signal energy	SVM	95.33
Kaya et al. (2014)	LBP	Bayes net	97.00
Pachori and Patidar (2014)	Ellipse area of IMFs	MLPNN	95.75
Kumar, Kanhangad, and Pachori (2015)	LBP	KNN	98.33
Tiwari et al. (2017)	LBP	SVM	99.45
Kaya et al. (2014)	Entropy	MLPNN	84.58
Raghu and Sriraam (2017)	LGS-based features	RF, LDA, ANN, KNN, SVM	100
Mehla et al. (2021)	L^P norms	SVM	99.89
Mehla et al. (2021)	L^P norms	SVM	99.96

TABLE 5.3

Classification of Non-seizure and Seizure EEG Signal from BONN Dataset

Authors	Extracted Feature	Classification Techniques	Accuracy (%)
Rafiuddin, Khan, and Farroq (2011)	Energy	ANN	97.73
Guo, Rivero, and Pazos (2010)	Approximate entropy (ApEn)	MLPNN	98.27
Kaleem, Guergachi, and Krishnan (2013)	Energy, amplitude spectrum	INN	98.20
Hassan and Haque (2016)	Statistical features	ANN	98.87
Vidyaratne and Iftekharuddin (2017)	Statistical features	ANN	99.33
Wang et al. (2017)	Spectral and fractal feature	RVM	99.8
Hassan, Subasi, and Zhang (2020)	Statistical features, Entropy	SVM	99.25
Vidyaratne and Iftekharuddin (2017)	LBP	SVM	99.31
Subasi, Kevric, and Abdullah Canbaz (2019)	Wavelet coefficient	SVM	99.38
Hassan, Subasi, and Zhang (2020)	Normal inverse Gaussian	Adaboost	99.2
V. Gupta and Pachori (2019)	Renyi entropy	Regression	98.6
Mehla et al. (2021)	L^P norms	SVM	99.96
Mehla et al. (2021)	L^P norms	SVM	99.97

and classification algorithms. This chapter explored efficient techniques for binary class EEG datasets. Conventional FT doesn't give much accuracy but advanced Fourier-based feature extraction approaches affect the accuracy. Extracted features also help in attaining the desired results. EMD, ensemble EMD, and complete ensemble EMD are better feature extraction techniques and FDM gives more accurate results than others.

TABLE 5.4

Comparison of Healthy and Seizure EEG Signals from the CHB-MIT Dataset

Authors	Extracted Feature	Classification Techniques	Accuracy (%)
Rafiuddin, Khan, and Farooq (2011)	IQR, MAD	LDA	99.50
Khan, Rafiuddin, and Farooq (2012)	Coefficient of variation, energy	LDA	91.80
Fergus et al. (2014)	Sub-band features	KNN	88
Alickovic, Kevric, and Subasi (2018)	Statistical features	KNN, SVM, RF	100
Dash, Kolekar, and Jha (2020)	PSD, variance, FD	HMM	99.60
Mehla et al. (2021)	L^p norms	SVM	99.94
Mehla et al. (2021)	L^p norms	SVM	99.71

REFERENCES

Abdulkader, S.N., A. Atia, and M. Mostafa. 2015. Brain Computer Interfacing: Applications and Challenges. *Egyptian Informatics Journal* 16, no. 2: 213–230. https://www.sciencedirect.com/science/article/pii/S1110866515000237.

Adeli, H., Z. Zhou, and N. Dadmehr. 2003. Analysis of EEG Records in an Epileptic Patient Using Wavelet Transform. *Journal of Neuroscience Methods* 123, no. 1: 69–87.

Alam, S.M.S., and M.I.H. Bhuiyan. 2013. Detection of Seizure and Epilepsy Using Higher Order Statistics in the EMD Domain. *IEEE Journal of Biomedical and Health Informatics* 17, no. 2: 312–318.

Alickovic, E., J. Kevric, and A. Subasi. 2018. Performance Evaluation of Empirical Mode Decomposition, Discrete Wavelet Transform, and Wavelet Packed Decomposition for Automated Epileptic Seizure Detection and Prediction. *Biomedical Signal Processing and Control* 39: 94–102. https://doi.org/10.1016/j.bspc.2017.07.022

Anyanwu, C., and Motamedi, G.K. 2017. Diagnosisand Surgical Treatmentof Drug-Resistant Epilepsy. *Brain Sciences* 8, no. 4: 49.

Aydemir, E., T. Tuncer, and S. Dogan. 2020. A Tunable-Q Wavelet Transform and Quadruple Symmetric Pattern Based EEG Signal Classification Method. *Medical Hypotheses* 134: 109519.

Bagheri, E., J. Jin, J. Dauwels, S. Cash, and M.B. Westover. 2016. Fast and Efficient Rejection of Background Waveforms in Interictal EEG. *ICASSP, IEEE International Conference on Acoustics, Speech and Signal Processing - Proceedings 2016-May*, New York: 744–748.

Belhadj, S., A. Attia, A.B. Adnane, Z. Ahmed-Foitih, and A.A. Taleb. 2017. Whole Brain Epileptic Seizure Detection Using Unsupervised Classification. *Proceedings of 2016 8th International Conference on Modelling, Identification and Control, ICMIC 2016*, Algiers, Algeria: 977–982.

Bhati, D., R.B. Pachori, and V.M. Gadre. 2017. A Novel Approach for Time–Frequency Localization of Scaling Functions and Design of Three-Band Biorthogonal Linear Phase Wavelet Filter Banks. *Digital Signal Processing: A Review Journal* 69: 309–322. https://doi.org/10.1016/j.dsp.2017.07.008

Bhati, D., M. Sharma, R.B. Pachori, and V.M. Gadre. 2017. Time–Frequency Localized Three-Band Biorthogonal Wavelet Filter Bank Using Semidefinite Relaxation and Nonlinear Least Squares with Epileptic Seizure EEG Signal Classification. *Digital Signal Processing: A Review Journal* 62, no. November: 259–273.

Boashash, B. 2015. *Time-Frequency Signal Analysis and Processing: A Comprehensive Reference.* Academic Press, Cambridge, MA.

Dash, D.P., M.H. Kolekar, and K. Jha. 2020. Multi-Channel EEG Based Automatic Epileptic Seizure Detection Using Iterative Filtering Decomposition and Hidden Markov Model. *Computers in Biology and Medicine* 116: 103571. https://doi.org/10.1016/j.compbiomed.2019.103571

Elgohary, S., S. Eldawlatly, and M.I. Khalil. 2016. Epileptic Seizure Prediction Using Zero-Crossings Analysis of EEG Wavelet Detail Coefficients. *CIBCB 2016 – Annual IEEE International Conference on Computational Intelligence in Bioinformatics and Computational Biology,* Chiang Mai, Thailand.

Fergus, P., D. Hignett, A.J. Hussain, and D. Al-Jumeily. 2014. An Advanced Machine Learning Approach to Generalised Epileptic Seizure Detection. *Lecture Notes in Computer Science (Including Subseries Lecture Notes in Artificial Intelligence and Lecture Notes in Bioinformatics) 8590 LNBI,* Springer, Cham: 112–118.

Flandrin, P., E. Torres, and M.A. Colominas. 2011. A Complete Ensemble Empirical Mode Decomposition Laboratorio de Se ˜ Nales y Din ́. *Amicas No Lineales, Universidad Nacional de Entre R ́ Laboratoire de Physique (UMR CNRS 5672), Ecole Normale Sup ` Erieure de* Lyon, France: 4144–4147.

Fu, K., J. Qu, Y. Chai, and Y. Dong. 2014. Classification of Seizure Based on the Time-Frequency Image of EEG Signals Using HHT and SVM. *Biomedical Signal Processing and Control* 13, no. 1: 15–22. https://doi.org/10.1016/j.bspc.2014.03.007

Fu, K., J. Qu, Y. Chai, and T. Zou. 2015. Hilbert Marginal Spectrum Analysis for Automatic Seizure Detection in EEG Signals. *Biomedical Signal Processing and Control* 18: 179–185. https://doi.org/10.1016/j.bspc.2015.01.002

Guo, L., D. Rivero, and A. Pazos. 2010. Epileptic Seizure Detection Using Multiwavelet Transform Based Approximate Entropy and Artificial Neural Networks. *Journal of Neuroscience Methods* 193, no. 1: 156–163. https://doi.org/10.1016/j.jneumeth.2010.08.030

Gupta, A., P. Singh, and M. Karlekar. 2018. A Novel Signal Modeling Approach for Classification of Seizure and Seizure-Free EEG Signals. *IEEE Transactions on Neural Systems and Rehabilitation Engineering* 26, no. 5: 925–935.

Gupta, V., and R.B. Pachori. 2019. Epileptic Seizure Identification Using Entropy of FBSE Based EEG Rhythms. *Biomedical Signal Processing and Control* 53: 101569. https://doi.org/10.1016/j.bspc.2019.101569

Hamad, A., E.H. Houssien, A.E. Hassanien, and A.A. Fahmy. 2016. Feature Extraction of Epilepsy EEG Using Discrete Wavelet Transform. *2016 12th International Computer Engineering Conference (ICENCO),* Cairo, Egypt: 190–195.

Hassan, A.R., and M.A. Haque. 2016. Epilepsy and Seizure Detection Using Statistical Features in the Complete Ensemble Empirical Mode Decomposition Domain. *IEEE Region 10 Annual International Conference, Proceedings/TENCON,* Macao, China: 1–6.

Hassan, A.R., A. Subasi, and Y. Zhang. 2020. Epilepsy Seizure Detection Using Complete Ensemble Empirical Mode Decomposition with Adaptive Noise. *Knowledge-Based Systems* 191: 105333. https://doi.org/10.1016/j.knosys.2019.105333

Huang, N.E., Z. Shen, S.R. Long, M.C. Wu, H.H. Snin, Q. Zheng, N.C. Yen, C.C. Tung, and H.H. Liu. 1998. The Empirical Mode Decomposition and the Hubert Spectrum for Nonlinear and Non-Stationary Time Series Analysis. *Proceedings of the Royal Society A: Mathematical, Physical and Engineering Sciences* 454, no. 1971: 903–995.

Hyvärinen, A., P. Ramkumar, L. Parkkonen, and R. Hari. 2010. Independent Component Analysis of Short-Time Fourier Transforms for Spontaneous EEG/MEG Analysis. *NeuroImage* 49, no. 1: 257–271. https://doi.org/10.1016/j.neuroimage.2009.08.028

Joshi, V., R.B. Pachori, and A. Vijesh. 2014. Classification of Ictal and Seizure-Free EEG Signals Using Fractional Linear Prediction. *Biomedical Signal Processing and Control* 9, no. 1: 1–5. https://doi.org/10.1016/j.bspc.2013.08.006

Kaleem, M., A. Guergachi, and S. Krishnan. 2013. EEG Seizure Detection and Epilepsy Diagnosis Using a Novel Variation of Empirical Mode Decomposition. *Proceedings of the Annual International Conference of the IEEE Engineering in Medicine and Biology Society, EMBS*, Osaka, Japan: 4314–4317.

Kappel, S.L., D. Looney, D.P. Mandic, and P. Kidmose. 2017. Physiological Artifacts in Scalp EEG and Ear-EEG. *Biomedical Engineering Online* 16, no. 1: 103.

Kaya, Y., M. Uyar, R. Tekin, and S. Yildirim. 2014. 1D-Local Binary Pattern Based Feature Extraction for Classification of Epileptic EEG Signals. *Applied Mathematics and Computation* 243: 209–219.

Khan, Y.U., N. Rafiuddin, and O. Farooq. 2012. Automated Seizure Detection in Scalp EEG Using Multiple Wavelet Scales. *2012 IEEE International Conference on Signal Processing, Computing and Control, ISPCC 2012*, Solan, India: 1–5.

Kumar, T.S., V. Kanhangad, and R.B. Pachori. 2015. Classification of Seizure and Seizure-Free EEG Signals Using Local Binary Patterns. *Biomedical Signal Processing and Control* 15: 33–40. https://doi.org/10.1016/j.bspc.2014.08.014

Liu, A., J.S. Hahn, G.P. Heldt, and R.W. Coen. 1992. Detection of Neonatal Seizures through Computerized EEG Analysis. *Electroencephalography and Clinical Neurophysiology* 82, no. 1: 30–37.

Lotte, F., and C. Guan. 2011. Regularizing Common Spatial Patterns to Improve BCI Designs: Unified Theory and New Algorithms. *IEEE Transactions on Biomedical Engineering* 58, no. 2: 355–362.

Mehla, V.K., A. Singhal, P. Singh, and R.B. Pachori. 2021. An Efficient Method for Identification of Epileptic Seizures from EEG Signals Using Fourier Analysis. *Physical and Engineering Sciences in Medicine* 44, no. 2: 443–456. https://doi.org/10.1007/s13246-021-00995-3

Nagarajan, L., S. Ghosh, and L. Palumbo. 2011. Ictal Electroencephalograms in Neonatal Seizures: Characteristics and Associations. *Pediatric Neurology* 45, no. 1: 11–16. https://doi.org/10.1016/j.pediatrneurol.2011.01.009

Ocak, H. 2008. Optimal Classification of Epileptic Seizures in EEG Using Wavelet Analysis and Genetic Algorithm. *Signal Processing* 88, no. 7: 1858–1867.

Oweis, R.J., and E.W. Abdulhay. 2011. Seizure Classification in EEG Signals Utilizing Hilbert-Huang Transform. *BioMedical Engineering Online* 10: 1–15.

Pachori, R.B., and V. Bajaj. 2011. Analysis of Normal and Epileptic Seizure EEG Signals Using Empirical Mode Decomposition. *Computer Methods and Programs in Biomedicine* 104, no. 3: 373–381. https://doi.org/10.1016/j.cmpb.2011.03.009

Pachori, R.B., and S. Patidar. 2014. Epileptic Seizure Classification in EEG Signals Using Second-Order Difference Plot of Intrinsic Mode Functions. *Computer Methods and Programs in Biomedicine* 113, no. 2: 494–502. https://doi.org/10.1016/j.cmpb.2013.11.014

Pachori, R.B., and P. Sircar. 2008. EEG Signal Analysis Using FB Expansion and Second-Order Linear TVAR Process. *Signal Processing* 88, no. 2: 415–420.

Parvez, M.Z., and M. Paul. 2017. Seizure Prediction Using Undulated Global and Local Features. *IEEE Transactions on Biomedical Engineering* 64, no. 1: 208–217.

Peker, M., B. Sen, and D. Delen. 2016. A Novel Method for Automated Diagnosis of Epilepsy Using Complex-Valued Classifiers. *IEEE Journal of Biomedical and Health Informatics* 20, no. 1: 108–118.

Rafiuddin, N., Y.U. Khan, and O. Farooq. 2011. Feature Extraction and Classification of EEG for Automatic Seizure Detection. *2011 International Conference on Multimedia, Signal Processing and Communication Technologies, IMPACT 2011*, Dhaka, Bangladesh: 184–187.

Raghu, S., and N. Sriraam. 2017. Optimal Configuration of Multilayer Perceptron Neural Network Classifier for Recognition of Intracranial Epileptic Seizures. *Expert Systems with Applications* 89: 205–221. https://doi.org/10.1016/j.eswa.2017.07.029

Rehman, N., and D.P. Mandic. 2009. Multivariate Empirical Mode Decomposition. *Proceedings of the Royal Society A* 466: 1291–1302.

Riaz, F., A. Hassan, S. Rehman, I.K. Niazi, and K. Dremstrup. 2016. EMD-Based Temporal and Spectral Features for the Classification of EEG Signals Using Supervised Learning. *IEEE Transactions on Neural Systems and Rehabilitation Engineering* 24, no. 1: 28–35.

Rizon, M., P. Krishnan, S. Yaacob, and A.P. Krishnan. 2020. EEG Based Drowsiness Detection Using Relative Band Power and Short Time Fourier Transform. *Proceedings of International Conference on Artificial Life and Robotics* 2020: 323–327.

Sharma, R., and R.B. Pachori. 2015. Classification of Epileptic Seizures in EEG Signals Based on Phase Space Representation of Intrinsic Mode Functions. *Expert Systems with Applications* 42, no. 3: 1106–1117. https://doi.org/10.1016/j.eswa.2014.08.030.

Sharmila, A., and P. Geethanjali. 2016. DWT Based Detection of Epileptic Seizure from EEG Signals Using Naive Bayes and K-NN Classifiers. *IEEE Access* 4: 7716–7727.

Shoka, A., M. Dessouky, A. El-Sherbeny, and A. El-Sayed. 2019. Literature Review on EEG Preprocessing, Feature Extraction, and Classifications Techniques. *Menoufia Journal of Electronic Engineering Research* 28, no. 1: 292–299.

Singh, P. et al. 2015. The Fourier Decomposition Method for Nonlinear and Nonstationary Time Series Analysis. *Proceedings of the Royal Society A* 473: 20160871.

Singh, P. 2018. Novel Fourier Quadrature Transforms and Analytic Signal Representation for Non-Linear and Non-Stationary Time Series Analysis. *Royal Society Open Science* 5: 181131.

Singh, P., S.D. Joshi, R.K. Patney, and K. Saha. 2016. Fourier-Based Feature Extraction for Classification of EEG Signals Using EEG Rhythms. *Circuits, Systems, and Signal Processing* 35, no. 10: 3700–3715.

Singhal, A., P. Singh, B. Fatimah, and R.B. Pachori. 2020. An Efficient Removal of Power-Line Interference and Baseline Wander from ECG Signals by Employing Fourier Decomposition Technique. *Biomedical Signal Processing and Control* 57: 101741. https://doi.org/10.1016/j.bspc.2019.101741

Singhal, A., P. Singh, B. Lall, and S.D. Joshi. 2020. Modeling and Prediction of COVID-19 Pandemic Using Gaussian Mixture Model. *Chaos Solitons Fractals* 138: 110023.

Subasi, A. 2007. EEG Signal Classification Using Wavelet Feature Extraction and a Mixture of Expert Model. *Expert Systems with Applications* 32, no. 4: 1084–1093.

Subasi, A., and M.I. Gursoy. 2010. EEG Signal Classification Using PCA, ICA, LDA and Support Vector Machines. *Expert Systems with Applications* 37, no. 12: 8659–8666. https://doi.org/10.1016/j.eswa.2010.06.065

Subasi, A., J. Kevric, and M. Abdullah Canbaz. 2019. Epileptic Seizure Detection Using Hybrid Machine Learning Methods. *Neural Computing and Applications* 31, no. 1: 317–325.

Tiwari, A.K., R.B. Pachori, V. Kanhangad, and B.K. Panigrahi. 2017. Automated Diagnosis of Epilepsy Using Key-Point-Based Local Binary Pattern of EEG Signals. *IEEE Journal of Biomedical and Health Informatics* 21, no. 4: 888–896.

Tzallas, A.T., M.G. Tsipouras, D.I. Fotiadis. 2007. Automatic Seizure Detection Based on Time-Frequency Analysis and Artificial Neural Networks. *Computational Intelligence a nd Neuroscience* 2007: 80510.

Tzallas, A.T., M.G. Tsipouras, and D.I. Fotiadis. 2009. Epileptic Seizure Detection in EEGs Using Time-Frequency Analysis. *IEEE Transactions on Information Technology in Biomedicine* 13, no. 5: 703–710.

Vidyaratne, L.S., and K.M. Iftekharuddin. 2017. Real-Time Epileptic Seizure Detection Using EEG. *IEEE Transactions on Neural Systems and Rehabilitation Engineering* 25, no. 11: 2146–2156.

Wang, D., D. Ren, K. Li, Y. Feng, D. Ma, X. Yan, and G. Wang. 2018. Epileptic Seizure Detection in Long-Term EEG Recordings by Using Wavelet-Based Directed Transfer Function. *IEEE Transactions on Biomedical Engineering* 65, no. 11: 2591–2599.

Wang, L., W. Xue, Y. Li, M. Luo, J. Huang, W. Cui, and C. Huang. 2017. Automatic Epileptic Seizure Detection in EEG Signals Using Multi-Domain Feature Extraction and Nonlinear Analysis. *Entropy* 19, no. 6: 1–17.

Zhang, T., W. Chen, and M. Li. 2020. Complex-Valued Distribution Entropy and Its Application for Seizure Detection. *Biocybernetics and Biomedical Engineering* 40, no. 1: 306–323. https://doi.org/10.1016/j.bbe.2019.10.006

6 Alternative Treatment with Non-Periodic Acoustic Stimulation for Pharmacoresistant Epileptic Patients
An Exploratory Study

Juliana Carneiro Gomes,
Marília Marinho de Lucena,
Jeniffer Emídio de Almeida Albuquerque,
Igor Tchaikovsky Mello de Oliveira,
Belmira Lara da Silveira Andrade da Costa,
Wellington Pinheiro dos Santos,
and Marcelo Cairrão

6.1 INTRODUCTION

Epilepsy is a condition characterized by excessive and uncontrolled neuronal activity. Normally, there is a balance between the excitation and inhibition of neurons in the central nervous system. However, epileptic brain neurons are dysfunctional and characterized by hyperexcessive or hypersynchronous activity. This scenario leads to at least one epileptic seizure (Berg, Berkovic, Brodie, Buchhalter, Cross, van Emde Boas, Engel, French, Glauser, Mathern, et al., 2010; Dubé, Molet, Singh-Taylor, Ivy, Maras, and Baram, 2015; Tóth, Hofer, Kandrács, Entz, Bagó, Eross, Jordán, Nagy, Sólyom, Fabó, et al., 2018).

There are many causes of epilepsy. Vascular diseases like strokes or bleeding, infections like meningitis, and traumas, for instance. Also, metabolic disorders, neoplasms, and autoimmune diseases can cause seizures. Furthermore, there are many idiopathic cases, which means that their etiology is unknown (Shorvon, Guerrini, Trinka, and Schachter, 2019; Shorvon, Andermann, and Guerrini, 2011; Sisodiya, Lin, Harding, Squier, and Thom, 2002).

An epileptic disorder is common and affects around 5% of the world population (Fisher, Cross, French, Higurashi, Hirsch, Jansen, Lagae, Moshé, Peltola,

DOI: 10.1201/9781003252092-8

Roulet Perez, et al., 2017). It is estimated that one-third of the patients are refractory to pharmacological treatment. In other words, it cannot stop seizures (Arrais, Modolo, Mogul, and Wendling 2021; Sisodiya et al. 2002). Moreover, half of them do not benefit from the surgical removal of the epileptic focus (Lee, Shon, and Cho, 2012). As a result, many patients live with neurobiological, cognitive, psychological, and social impairments (Fisher, Boas, Blume, Elger, Genton, Lee, and Engel Jr, 2005).

In studies with animal models such as rats (Cota, de Castro Medeiros, da Páscoa Vilela, Doretto, and Moraes, 2009; de Castro Medeiros, Cota, da Páscoa Vilela, Mourão, Massensini, and Moraes, 2012), it was verified that non-periodic electrical stimulation in deep brain structures, such as the amygdala and hippocampus, have an anticonvulsant effect. It led to a decrease in the number, duration, and severity of seizures. The aperiodic electrical stimulation is an unstructured temporal pattern. It is capable of destabilizing the rhythmic oscillation activity within reverberant neural circuits. Thereby, it acts on the ictogenesis, that is, the neurophysiological process of epileptic seizure generation, and also on the maintenance of epileptiform activity.

However, the application of this technique in humans is restricted as it requires surgical positioning of deep electrodes. Alternatively, this study seeks new forms of non-periodic stimuli with similar effects and possible insertion into clinical practice.

A type of stimulation that has been tested by many medical research groups is acoustic binaural beats (da Silva Junior, de Freitas, dos Santos, da Silva, Rodrigues, and Conde, 2019; Gálvez, Recuero, Canuet, and Del-Pozo, 2018; Perales, Riera, Ramis, and Guerrero, 2019; Perez, Dumas, and Lehmann, 2020). It can induce alterations of neuronal activity and brain functional states, modulating cortical activity. The literature has several applications of its use as an intervention technique for psychophysiological processes. Revealing results have been presented in combating anxiety (da Silva Junior et al., 2019), pain (Perales et al., 2019), and to stimulate relaxation (Perez et al., 2020). There are even studies to improve the memory of Parkinson's patients (Gálvez et al., 2018).

Thinking about this, we propose the development of an aperiodic binaural acoustic stimulation (ABAS) focusing on the treatment of epilepsy. This approach will be aligned with brain signals monitored by electroencephalography (EEG). In this way, it will be possible to monitor patients noninvasively and treat them painlessly and without further side effects.

In this context, this article will focus on the development of a non-periodic acoustic stimulus, in addition to recruiting patients with refractory epilepsy. After selecting patients, we will study the effect of the sound created on the electroencephalographic signals. For this, we will apply an EEG acquisition protocol, which aims to make the patient more susceptible to crises. We will call this the first acquisition of T0 signals. Then, the patient will hear the non-periodic stimulus for a period of 30 minutes. Finally, a new EEG acquisition will be made, in order to observe the acute effect of the sound on the physiological signals. We will call this second acquisition of T1. This same protocol will also be applied to the patients five days after this first assessment. In this case, we will make the third and fourth signals acquisition, here called T3 and T4. In this case, we will study the effect of the treatment sound after five days of continuous use. Finally, we will discuss these preliminary results and what they point to.

The structure of the subsequent sections is organized as follows: in Section 6.2, we comment on works related to binaural beats; in Section 6.3, we present the theoretical concepts necessary for a good understanding of this work; and in Section 6.4 we show the results and discussion. Finally, our conclusions and future works are described in Section 6.5.

6.2 RELATED WORKS

Several studies have shown the importance of binaural beats to induce alterations in neuronal activity. da Silva Jr. et al. (2019) showed the contribution of binaural beats stimulation in the reduction of anxiety and the modification of some psychological states, affecting the patient's cognition as a result. They applied 5 Hz binaural beats to six subjects and used an intelligent classifier and eLORETA in order to differentiate signals before and after 10 sessions of 20-minute acoustic stimulation. The study revealed modifications in high Beta and Theta brainwaves and also indicated neuromodulation in high Alpha brainwaves.

Gálvez et al. (2018), inspired by the effectiveness of musicotherapy in many diseases, investigated the influence of binaural beats applied to 14 patients with Parkinson's disease (PD). They designed a 10-minute beat masked by pink noise, in order to improve user experience, and presented these tones at 120 bpm (beats per minute). Their protocol consisted of two 10-minute sessions spaced by at least one week. An EEG was used to collect data before and after the administration of the stimuli. The authors concluded that binaural beats can support PD treatment, as a decrease in Theta activity and functional connectivity, and an improvement in working memory performance were observed.

In the work of Perales et al. (2019), researchers proposed a virtual reality system with multiple scenarios, combining visual, acoustic, and haptic stimulation. The main idea was to evaluate the user's pain perception through a self-assessment combined with the measurement of galvanic skin response (GSR). GSR is a typical marker of emotional states in humans, determined by sweat gland activity. In addition to bio-signals monitoring, the system provides acoustic stimuli, which is a binaural beat. The theory of the study is that binaural sounds can modulate the power of brain signals, which allows greater relaxation for the user. As a consequence, there is a reduction in electrodermal activity. The study consisted of two case studies. In the first one, ten students participated in two sessions in which they heard placebo monaural and binaural sounds. The second series of experiments consisted of assessing pain management in children. Eighteen children between 7 and 12 years old were selected and divided into two groups: a control or pain-free group, and a group of those who manifested pain. The authors concluded that binaural beats work better than non-binaural beats when we talk about meditation and relaxation. It was also possible to observe a decrease in the based pain line.

The study (Gkolias, Amaniti, Triantafyllou, Papakonstantinou, Kartsidis, Paraskevopoulos, Bamidis, Hadjileontiadis, and Kouvelas, 2020) also tested the application of binaural beats in order to reduce the perception of pain and the use of analgesics in patients with chronic pain. They realized a double-blind, randomized, crossover trial, and compared 5 Hz binaural beats with sham stimulation. The stimuli were applied while electroencephalographic signals were captured simultaneously. Parameters such as perceived pain, stress, and medication usage were analyzed. Finally, all three performance metrics had a significant reduction during and after the binaural beats stimulation. In addition, the mean EEG theta power at 5 Hz was significantly increased only during the binaural beats application.

6.3 MATERIALS AND METHODS

6.3.1 Brainwaves Monitoring with Electroencephalograph

For over 60 years, the EEG has been the routine exam for the diagnosis and follow-up of patients with epilepsy. It is a method that records the electrical activity of the brain from neuronal activity. The registration takes place through electrodes attached to the scalp with the aid of a conductive paste or gel. Generally, the signal occupies a range between 0 and 100 Hz, and an amplitude between 2 and 200 µV. However, relevant information is usually concentrated between 0.5 and 60 Hz with a mean amplitude of 50 µV (Niedermeyer, Froescher, and Fisher, 1985).

EEG signals have a relative frequency, morphology, and amplitude regularity, and they have a large amount of complex cerebral information. The EEG spectrum is normally subdivided into frequency bands that may be related to various physical and behavioral states. The main frequencies are the Alpha (8–13 Hz), Beta (14–30 Hz), Theta (4–7 Hz), and Delta (0.5–3.5 Hz) waves (Webster, 2009).

In order to standardize the acquisition of EEG signals, the international system 10–20 is used, which distributes 21 electrodes over the scalp. To determine the positioning, two reference points are used: Nasion, which is at the top of the nose, between both eyebrows and Inion, located at the base of the skull behind the head. From these points, the perimeters of the skull are measured in the transverse direction and median planes. Electrode positions are determined by dividing these perimeters at 10 or 20% intervals (Webster, 2009).

Brain signals can show epileptic markers called epileptiform discharges. They are divided into two states: Ictal (during seizures) and interictal (between seizures) (Engel, Pedley, and Aicardi, 2008; Niedermeyer et al., 1985). Nevertheless, the records analysis requires a long examination period in order to detect seizures. Studies have shown that the probability of catching a seizure during a routine 20-minute examination in a patient with one seizure per week is only 1% (Sundaram, Sadler, Young, and Pillay, 1999). Therefore, interictal signals are most commonly used. Interictal epileptiform discharges (IED) are elements that confirm the diagnosis of epilepsy within a clinical context and classify the disease depending on the projection of the epileptiform activity, in addition to providing a more precise location when compared to ictal discharges (Engel et al., 2008). The signals present in the interictal period are formed by spicules or spikes, acute or sharp waves, and complex spike waves. Thus, in order to facilitate the identification of these paroxysms, it becomes necessary to use protocols that make the patient more susceptible to abnormal activities (Hauser and Josephson, 2015; Malow, Kushwaha, Lin, Morton, and Aldrich, 1997).

6.3.2 BINAURAL BEATS

A type of stimulation that has found applications in areas of medicine is the acoustic binaural beats A binaural beat is a brain perception of a sound of a specific frequency. It is generated when two sine waves of slightly different frequencies are presented to each ear separately. As a result, the brain perceives a third illusory tone, corresponding to the absolute difference between both frequencies. For instance, it can be applied at a 114 Hz tone in the right ear, while a 124 Hz tone is applied in the left one. Then, inside the brain, the beat perception corresponds to a 10 Hz frequency (da Silva Jr. et al., 2019; Perales et al., 2019). The perception of the binaural beat is the result of the overlapping of the neuronal synapses that occur in subcortical stages of auditory processing. Especially in the upper olivary complex and inferior colliculus, there is information on the comparison of the right and left auditory inputs. This occurs before sound reaches the cortex and is as perceived as conscious (Perez et al., 2020).

These beats have been advertised to induce alterations of neuronal activity and brain functional states, being able to modulate cortical activity, depending on the selected frequencies. This hypothesis can be explained by the fact that the brain tries to adjust its brainwaves to the frequency of external stimuli. Thereby, the literature has several applications of its use as an intervention technique on psychophysiological processes. These works assume that sound modifies brain activities, involving, for this, the ascending reticular activating system.

6.3.3 PROPOSED METHOD

In this work, we propose the use of acoustic non-period stimulation as a complement in the treatment of pharmacoresistant epileptic patients. We believe that this type of stimulus is able to destabilize the rhythmic oscillation activity within reverberant neural circuits and promote the antiseizure effect.

In order to test the effectiveness of this method, we recruited refractory epileptic patients. In the first moment, they were evaluated with the Quality of Life 31 questionnaire. In the following, an EEG acquisition protocol was performed, with the objective of making the patient more sensitive and more susceptible to crises during the examination period. We call this first EEG assessment T0, which is the patient's basal state. Then, the patient listened to the non-periodic acoustic stimuli while he was sleeping. After a period of 20 minutes of listening to the stimulus, the patient was reevaluated with EEG. This second assessment we called T1. Finally, the patient was released to go home, where he could hear the sound for another three days. On the fifth day, the patient returned to be evaluated and the same process as on the first day was repeated, resulting in the T2 (before hearing the sound) and T3 (after hearing the sound) evaluations.

Thus, we collected four EEG assessments (T0, T1, T2, and T3) from 14 patients with refractory epilepsy. Based on these data, this work aims to evaluate the acute and short-term effects of non-periodic acoustic stimulus using machine learning. For this, we will compare the signals T0 and T1 (approach A) and then we will compare the signals T0, T1, T2, and T3 (approach B). Our methodology consists of feature

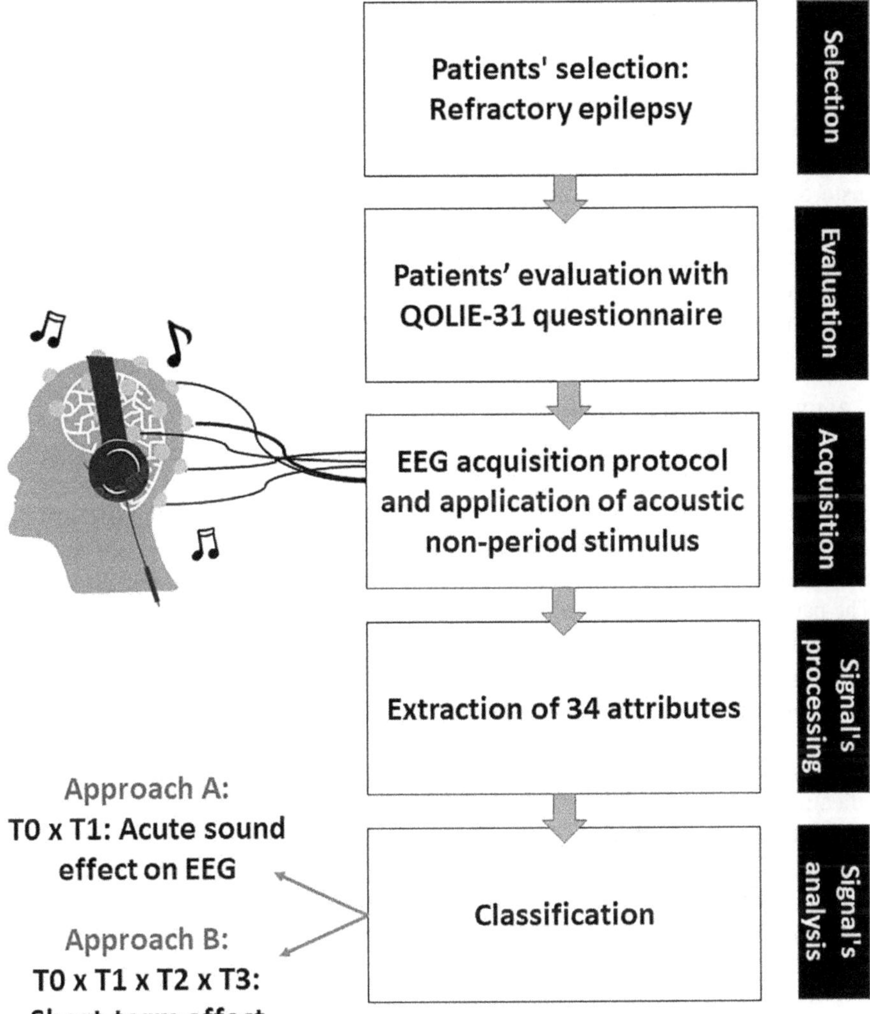

FIGURE 6.1   Proposed method: This study focuses on the development of an EEG database, with signals from refractory epilepsy patients before and after the application of an acoustic non-period stimulation. These signals will be analyzed with machine learning techniques. For this, we will perform feature extraction, test some classifiers in the differentiation of these signals, and discuss the sound effects in these patients.

extraction of 34 attributes and the use of classical classifiers such as Decision trees and Support vector machines (SVMs) to differentiate these signals and analyze if they have a meaningful contrast. These classifications will be evaluated by six metrics: accuracy, kappa statistic, sensitivity, specificity, F-score, and AUC. Figure 6.1 below summarizes the objectives of this work.

6.3.4 Database

6.3.4.1 Aperiodic Binaural Acoustic Stimulation (ABAS) Development

Inspired by these several well-succeeded studies based on binaural beats, our laboratory developed the ABAS. It was developed on Matlab software and later exported to Audacity 2.0. The audio was recorded in WAV format, aiming to reproduce it without distortion in notebooks and cell phones.

The ABAS consists of a 400 Hz baseband soundtrack, randomly interrupted by pulses. These pulses are rapid events of 50 μs, 420 Hz frequency, and 20% higher amplitude when compared to the baseband. Each second of sound always had four pulses but with different interpulse intervals. Finally, the sound applied to each ear was identical to the other one, except for the pulse locations.

6.3.4.2 Selection of Subjects

The participants were recruited from the Outpatient Clinic of Neurology of Hospital das Clínicas de Pernambuco (HC/UFPE). The sample consisted of 16 patients, of both sexes. Among these 16 patients, two were excluded as they could not finish the exam routine. Of the 14 remaining patients, 10 patients did not present epileptiform discharges at any time of the examination, and 04 patients presented discharges. The patients were then divided into two groups: Group 1 (G1), composed of patients with epileptiform discharges ($n = 04$); and Group 2 (G2), patients who did not present discharges ($n = 10$).

As an inclusion criterion, participants who had a clinical diagnosis of epilepsy were over 18 years of age, and who were refractory to drug treatment were considered. The criteria for refractory epilepsy were defined according to the ILAE classification (Kwan, Arzimanoglou, Berg, Brodie, Allen Hauser, Mathern, Moshé, Perucca, Wiebe, and French, 2010). Participants who failed to complete any of the exam protocols and were not available for the evaluations were excluded from the survey. The study was conducted in compliance with the guidelines of Resolution 466/2012 of the National Health Council and the Declaration of Helsinki of 1964 and approved by the Ethics Committee of the Health Sciences Center of Federal University of Pernambuco, CAAE number 79271517.2.0000.5208, Recife, Brazil. All participants signed the Informed Consent Term (ICT) prior to the start of the research. Patients were informed of the goals and procedures, as well as the risks and benefits, and could discontinue the assessments at any time, without the need for further explanation.

6.3.4.3 Questionnaire

The patients were invited to answer the questionnaires of evaluation (semi-structured interview, Quality of Life 31—QOLIE-31). The QOLIE-31 is a specific questionnaire for people with epilepsy. It consists of 31 questions, distributed into seven domains about perception of seizures (five items), and QoL considering the disease scenario, emotional, cognitive and memory aspects, energy, fatigue, perception about the effects of medication, and social limitations. The questions were slowly read to the patients, and responses were recorded as per the Likert scale. Each question is given a number ranging from 01 to 06 and this numbering is assigned a value, which is as per the table of scores of correction of the QOLIE-31 (Silva, Marques, Alonso, Azevedo, Westphal-Guitti, Caboclo, Sakamoto, and Yacubian, 2006). The final score ranges from 0 to 100 points. Higher scores reflect better quality of life, whereas lower scores reflect worse quality of life.

6.3.4.4 EEG Acquisition Equipment

For the acquisition of the electroencephalographic data, the NEURON-SPECTRUM-4/EP digital EEG was used at the sampling rate of 500 Hz, and high-pass filter of 0.1 Hz. Participants were comfortably accommodated on stretchers, for placement of the electrodes. In this process, the ears and forehead were sanitized with an abrasive solution before placement of the electrodes to reduce impurities and oiliness of the skin. Twenty-one channels were used, of which 02 were reference channels and 19 channels were positioned according to the 10–20 system. Then, at each electrode site, conductive gel was used to improve the conductivity of the electrical signal, which was checked by inspecting the impedance between each electrode and referenced to be less than 0.5 kΩ.

6.3.4.5 Data Acquisition Protocol

After the preparation and positioning of the electrodes, the activation protocol was performed. This protocol aims to increase the sensitivity to the examination, as well as to detect specific alterations that can be provoked by the activation tests. The protocol is routinely performed in the HC-PE neurology sector and is attended by nurses and physicians. The protocol consists of events such as hyperventilation, photic stimulation, and assessments during sleep. In order to perform the EEG and as part of the activation protocol, it was also requested that the patient had a sleep deprivation of four hours the night before the EEG recording. During the time of hyperventilation, the patient is asked to breathe deeply (forced and rapid breathing) on a regular basis for three minutes, thereafter receiving photic stimulation. This stimulation is performed with a lamp that produces flashes with frequencies ranging from 0.5 to 20 Hz. The lamp is placed in front of the patient, at a distance of 30 cm from the patient's nose. The frequency (3, 5, 7, 9, 11, 15, 20 Hz) should be triggered in periods of ten seconds (eyes open for five seconds and closed for five seconds) with a time interval of seven seconds. The patient was then asked to sleep for 20 minutes. A schematic describing the whole acquisition protocol is presented below.

6.3.5 Signal Pre-Processing and Feature Extraction

All EEG recordings were processed using rectangular windows of ten seconds each. In addition, two-second overlaps were considered. For this purpose, GNU Octave, a free open-source software was used. Accordingly, feature extraction was performed and 34 attributes were extracted. Table 6.1 shows the complete list of attributes in detail, and also their respective mathematical expressions (Figure 6.2).

TABLE 6.1
List of 34 Extracted Attributes

Attribute	Mathematical Expression	Attribute	
Mean (μ)	$\mu = \dfrac{1}{N}\sum_{n=1}^{N} x_n$	Zero crossings	$\text{ZC} = \sum_{n=1}^{N-1} [\text{SGN}(x_n \times x_{n+1}) \cap \mid x_n - x_{n-1} \geq \text{threshold}]$ $\text{SGN}(x) = \begin{cases} 1, \text{ if } x \geq \text{threshold} \\ 0, \quad \text{otherwise} \end{cases}$
Variance	$\text{var} = \dfrac{1}{N-1}\sum_{n=1}^{N}(x_n - \mu)^2$	Slope sign change	$\text{SSC} = \sum_{n=1}^{N-1} [f(x_n - x_{n-1}) \times (x_n - x_{n+1})]$ $f(x) = \begin{cases} 1, \text{if } x \geq \text{threshold} \\ 0, \quad \text{otherwise} \end{cases}$
Standard deviation (σ)	$\sigma = \dfrac{1}{N-1}\sum_{n=1}^{N} \mid x_n - \mu \mid^2$	Hjorth parameter activity	$\text{Hjorth}_{\text{activity}} = \dfrac{1}{N-1}\sum_{n=1}^{N}(x_n - \mu)^2$
Root mean square	$\text{RMS} = \sqrt{\dfrac{\sum_{n=1}^{N}(x_n)^2}{N}}$	Hjorth parameter mobility	$\text{Hjorth}_{\text{mobility}} = \sqrt{\dfrac{\text{var}\left(\dfrac{dc(t)}{dt}\right)}{\text{var}(x(t))}}$
Average amplitude change	$\text{AAC} = \dfrac{1}{N}\left(\sum_{n=1}^{N}\left\|\dfrac{dx(t)}{dt}\right\|\right)$	Hjorth parameter complexity	$\text{Hjorth}_{\text{complexity}} = \dfrac{\text{Hjorth}_{\text{mobility}}\left(\dfrac{dx(t)}{dt}\right)}{\text{Hjorth}_{\text{mobility}}(x(t))}$
Difference absolute deviation	$\text{DASDV} = \sqrt{\dfrac{1}{N}\sum_{n=1}^{N}\left(\dfrac{dx(t)}{dt}\right)^2}$	Mean frequency	$\text{MNF} = \dfrac{\sum_{j=1}^{M} f_i P_j}{\sum_{j=1}^{M} P_j}$ Where f_i, P_i are the frequencies and power of the spectrum, respectively, and M is the length of the frequencies
Integrated absolute value	$\text{IAV} = \sum_{n=1}^{N} x_n$	Median frequency	$\text{MDF} = \dfrac{1}{2}\sum_{j=1}^{M} P_j$

(Continued)

TABLE 6.1 (*Continued*)
List of 34 Extracted Attributes

Attribute	Mathematical Expression	Attribute	
Logarithm detector	$LOGD = e^{\left(\frac{1}{n}\sum_{n=1}^{N} \log(|x_n|)\right)}$	Mean power	$MNP = \sum_{j=1}^{M} \frac{P_j}{M}$
Simple square integral	$SSI = \sum_{n=1}^{N} x_n^{2}$	Peak frequency	$PKF = \max(P_j)$
Mean absolute value	$MAV = \frac{1}{N}\sum_{n=1}^{N} |x_n|$	Power spectrum ratio	$PSR = \dfrac{PFK}{\sum_{j=1}^{M} P_j}$
Mean logarithm kernel	$MLOGK = \frac{1}{N}\left|\sum_{n=1}^{N} x_n\right|$	Total power	$TP = \sum_{j=1}^{M} P_j$
Skewness (s)	$s = \dfrac{\frac{1}{N}\sum_{n=1}^{N}(x_n - \mu)^{3}}{\sigma^{3}}$	First spectral moment	$SM1 = \sum_{j=1}^{M} f_i P_j$
Kurtosis	$kurt = \dfrac{\frac{1}{N}\sum_{n=1}^{N}(x_n - \mu)^{4}}{\sigma^{4}}$	Second spectral moment	$SM2 = \sum_{j=1}^{M} f_i^{2} P_j$
Maximum amplitude	$MAX = \max(x_n)$	Third spectral moment	$SM3 = \sum_{j=1}^{M} f_i^{3} P_j$
Third moment	$M3 = \left|\frac{1}{N}\sum_{n=1}^{N}(x_n)^{3}\right|$	Variance of central frequency	$VCF = \dfrac{SM2}{TP} - \left(\dfrac{SM1}{TP}\right)^{2}$
Fourth moment	$M4 = \left|\frac{1}{N}\sum_{n=1}^{N}(x_n)^{4}\right|$	Waveform length	$WL = \sum_{n=1}^{N-1} |x_{n+1} - x_n|$
Fifth moment	$M5 = \left|\frac{1}{N}\sum_{n=1}^{N}(x_n)^{5}\right|$	Shannon entropy	$S = \sum_{i} s_i^{2} \log(s_i^{2})$

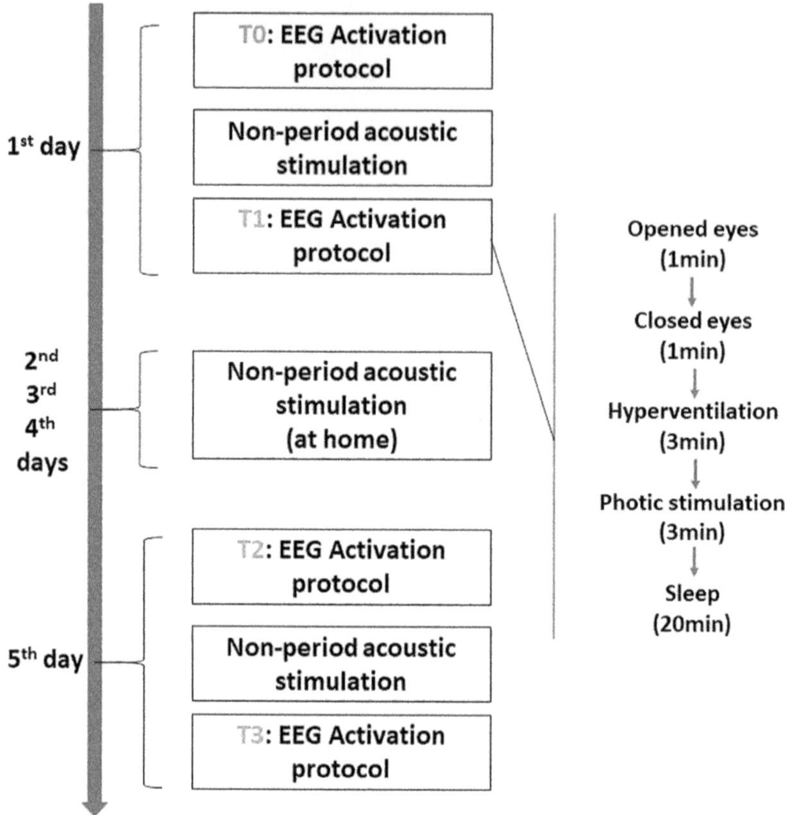

FIGURE 6.2　Image displaying various phases of a process, in sequence (Data acquisition protocol).

6.3.6　CLASSIFICATION

6.3.6.1　Support Vector Machine

SVMs can be used to solve classification or regression problems. The main idea of SVMs is to build a hyperplane as a decision surface to separate the classes in the best possible way (Cortes and Vapnik, 1995). In this way, SVMs perform a nonlinear mapping on the database in a space of high dimension called the feature space. The training process aims to find the optimal hyperplane equation.

The SVM algorithm is well known for its ability to provide good generalization performance. However, this performance may decrease by increasing the complexity of the hyperplane. The type of the machine varies with the type of kernel used to build the optimal hyperplane. Examples of kernels used in the work are the polynomial and radial basis function (RBF) types (Haykin, 2001).

SVMs have been widely used in several medical applications: schizophrenia diagnosis (Espinola, Gomes, Pereira, and Santos, 2020), hepatitis diagnosis (Sartakhti, Zangooei, and Mozafari, 2012), and breast cancer diagnosis (Cordeiro, Santos, and Silva-Filho, 2016, 2017; Cruz, Cruz, and Santos, 2018; de Lima, da Silva-Filho, and dos Santos, 2014; de Lima et al., 2014; de Lima, da Silva-Filho, and dos Santos, 2016; de Vasconcelos, dos Santos, and de Lima, 2018; Ismael and Gomes, 2021; Lima, Azevedo, Cordeiro, Silva-Filho, and Santos, 2015; Pereira, Santana, Lima, and Santos, 2020; Santana, Pereira, Lima, and Santos, 2020; Silva, Santana, Silva Filho, Lima, and Santos, 2020).

6.3.6.2 Decision Trees

Decision trees are a type of supervised machine-learning model that can be used in both classification and regression problems. Decision trees analyze the data through a series of questions related to the attributes. Each question is contained in a node, which branches into child nodes containing the possible answers. The questions then form a hierarchy, forming a tree. The starting point of the tree is the root node which has the highest hierarchical level. The endpoint, on the other hand, is the leaf, a node without children. In this way, the algorithm makes decisions following the structure of the tree. There are several types of Decision trees, which are usually differentiated by the way the method traverses the tree (Kingsford and Salzberg 2008). Random Tree and Random Forest methods are the main ones.

According to Geurts, Ernst, and Wehenkel (2006), a Random Tree algorithm uses a single tree built by a stochastic process. This method considers only a few randomly selected features in each node of the tree.

On the other hand, Random Forests were introduced by Leo Breiman, who was inspired by Amit and Geman. Random Forests consist of a collection of tree predictors, where each tree depends on a group of random variables (Cutler, Cutler, and Stevens 2012). In this way, each tree votes for a class of the problem. In the end, the most voted class is chosen as the prediction of the classifier.

6.3.6.3 Bayesian Networks and Naive Bayes

Bayesian networks are graphical models that represent the variables as nodes. These nodes are connected by arcs, which symbolize the dependence of the variables. In this case, the strength of these variable relationships is determined by a conditional probability. The probability specifies the degree of belief that a node will be in a particular state, given the states of the parent nodes. Thus, the belief is propagated using Bayes Theory, and the probabilities of the nodes are updated (Chen and Pollino 2012). Bayesian networks behave like a linear classifier for a Gaussian distribution. Their behavior is comparable to that of a single-layer perceptron.

There are many applications of Bayesian networks in the medical field: Alzheimer diagnosis (Pinheiro, de Castro, and Pinheiro, 2008; Seixas, Zadrozny, Laks, Conci, and Saade, 2014), psychiatric diseases (Curiac, Vasile, Banias, Volosencu, and Albu, 2009), and breast cancer diagnosis (Cruz-Ramirez, Acosta-Mesa, Carrillo-Calvet, Nava-Fernández, and Barrientos-Martínez, 2007; Kahn Jr, Roberts, Shaffer, and Haddawy, 1997).

6.3.7 Parameter Settings of the Classifiers

The experiments were made by using the following techniques: an SVM with a polynomial kernel of degree (E) 1, 2, and 3 and an RBF kernel with γ of 0.01; Random

Forest with 10, 20, 30, . . ., 100 trees; Random Tree; Naive Bayes; and a Bayesian network. Each configuration was executed 30 times to assess statistical information. An evaluation method was chosen to perform a 10-fold cross-validation, essentially resulting in 90% of instances for training and 10% for validation.

6.3.8 METRICS

We chose six metrics to evaluate the performance of experiments: accuracy, kappa statistic, sensitivity, specificity, F-score, and Area under the ROC Curve (AUC). Accuracy is the probability that the experiment will provide correct results, that is, to correctly classify signals in T0, T1, T2, and T3 classes. In other words, it is the probability of the true positives and true negatives among all the results. The sensitivity metric indicates the rate of a true positive, while specificity is the rate of true negatives. The F-score is calculated from the sensitivity and precision metrics (which are the positive predictions that are actually positive). AUC stands for "Area under the ROC curve". The ROC curve, in turn, is a graph showing the true positive rate vs. the false positive rate. Finally, the Kappa index is a very good measure that can very well handle multi-class problems, as the one proposed here. Accuracy, Sensitivity, specificity, and F-score metrics can be calculated according to Eqs. (6.1)–(6.4) respectively.

$$\text{Accuracy} = \frac{\text{TP} + \text{TN}}{\text{TP} + \text{TN} + \text{FP} + \text{FN}} \tag{6.1}$$

$$\text{Sensitivity} = \frac{\text{TP}}{\text{TP} + \text{FN}} \tag{6.2}$$

$$\text{Specificity} = \frac{\text{TN}}{\text{TN} + \text{FP}} \tag{6.3}$$

$$F \text{ Score} = \frac{2\text{TP}}{2\text{TP} + \text{FP} + \text{FN}} \tag{6.4}$$

where TP is the true positive, TN is the true negative, FP is the false positive, and FN is the false negative.

The κ coefficient (Kappa) is defined as follows:

$$\kappa = \frac{\rho_o - \rho_e}{1 - \rho_e} \tag{6.5}$$

where ρ_o is observed agreement, or accuracy, and ρ_e is the expected agreement, defined as follows:

$$\rho_e = \frac{(\text{TP} + \text{FP})(\text{TP} + \text{FN}) + (\text{FN} + \text{TN})(\text{FP} + \text{TN})}{(\text{TP} + \text{FP} + \text{FN} + \text{TN})^2} \tag{6.6}$$

6.4 RESULTS

This section presents the results obtained for the accuracy of some classifiers used for separating in the classification phase. Figure 6.3 shows the T0 and T1 signals, that is, approach A. Figure 6.4 shows the performance of the same classifiers for separating T0, T1, T2, and T3 signals (approach B). All graphs contain statistical information from the 30 repetitions performed for each configuration. In addition, 10-fold cross-validation was used in all tests.

Furthermore, Tables 6.2 and 6.3 show the results of the mean and standard deviation of all six metrics. Table 6.2 shows the results for approach A, while Table 6.3 shows the results for approach B.

From these results, it is possible to notice that the Random Forest with 100 trees outperformed the other classifiers. It is also worth mentioning that the SVMs with Polykernel with exponent 1 and 2, also presented excellent results, comparable to the Random Forest classifiers, for approach A. In contrast, the Bayesian networks showed the worst results in both approaches.

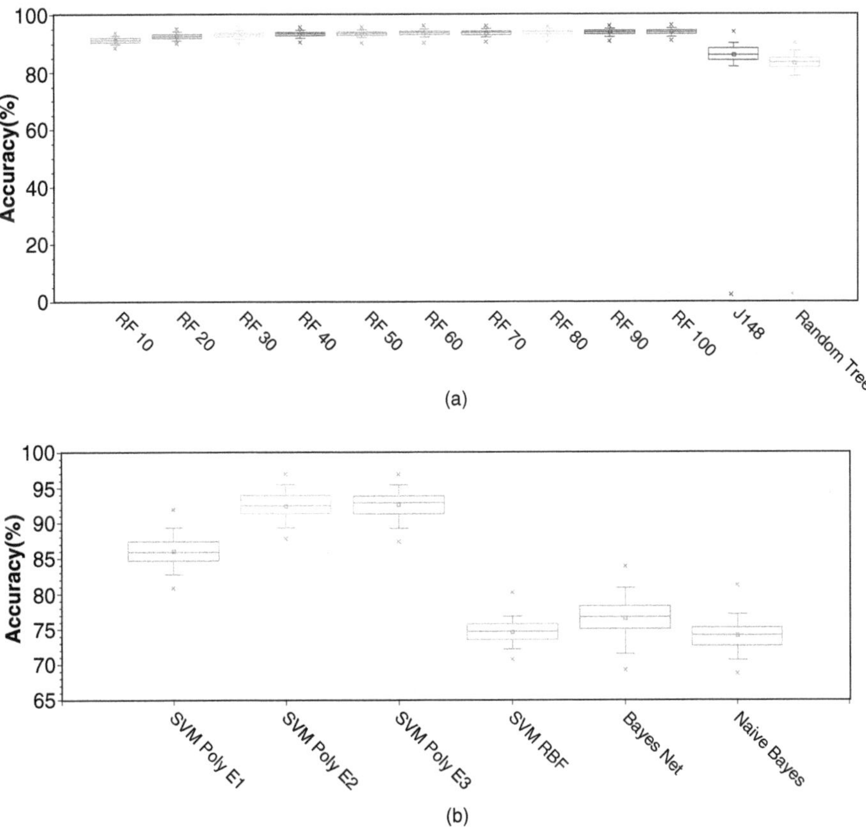

FIGURE 6.3 Classification performance of approach A: Separation of signals before and after the treatment with acoustic stimulus on the first day (T0 and T1), that is, the basal patient's state and immediate state after treatment.

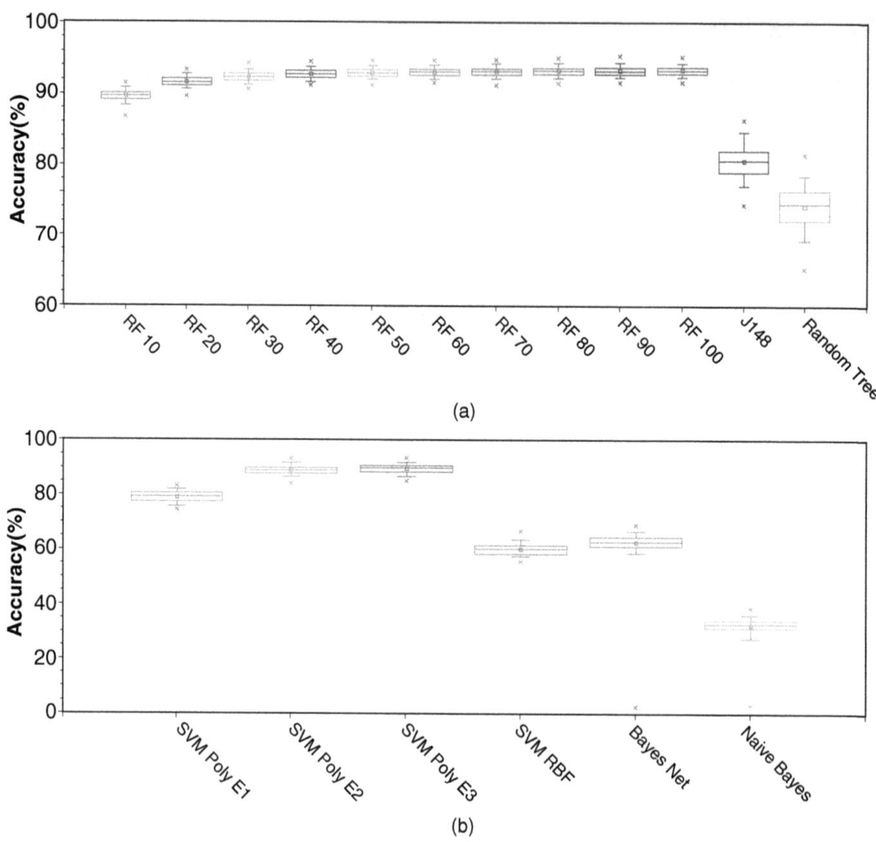

FIGURE 6.4 Classification performance of approach B: Separation of signals before and after the treatment with acoustic stimulus on the first day (T0 and T1) and before and after the treatment on the fifth day (T2 and T3).

6.5 DISCUSSION

In this study, sixteen patients were recruited, of whom 14 met the criteria for inclusion. All of them underwent EEG monitoring during the activation protocol. In addition, they were invited to answer the QOLIE-31 questionnaire. The mean total value of the QOLIE-31 score was 41.95 ± 2.8. In some other studies Beghi, Niero, and Roncolato (2005); Nubukpo, Clement, Houinato, Radji, Grunitzky, Avode, and Preux (2004), who evaluated epileptic patients with this same questionnaire, presented values of a total score between 49.5 and 65.9 points. In another study by Bastos, Laan, Gitaí, Gameleira, and Silva (2009), the researchers evaluated patients with juvenile myoclonic epilepsy, and they found a total score of 62.1. Therefore, we found lower score values than those seen in the literature. However, factors such as regional differences, social and cultural conditions, as well as inclusion criteria of the study sample may be related to this observation. The criterion for the eligibility of this research is patients who are refractory to medication treatment and have no

TABLE 6.2

Classification Performance of Approach A

| | Approach A: T0,T1 | | | | | | | | | | |
| | Accuracy | | Kappa | | Sensitivity | | Specificity | | AUC | | F1 Score | |
Classifier	Mean	Std Dev	Mean	Std Dev	Mean	Std Dev	Mean	Std Dev	Mean	Std Dev	Mean	Std Dev
Random Forest (10 trees)	91.306	1.002	0.784	0.027	0.982	0.006	0.759	0.031	0.971	0.006	0.940	0.007
Random Forest (20 trees)	92.600	0.887	0.817	0.023	0.985	0.005	0.793	0.027	0.981	0.005	0.949	0.006
Random Forest (30 trees)	93.068	0.897	0.829	0.023	0.987	0.005	0.804	0.027	0.984	0.004	0.952	0.006
Random Forest (40 trees)	93.321	0.859	0.836	0.022	0.987	0.005	0.811	0.026	0.986	0.004	0.953	0.006
Random Forest (50 trees)	93.492	0.855	0.840	0.022	0.988	0.005	0.816	0.025	0.987	0.003	0.955	0.006
Random Forest (60 trees)	93.619	0.855	0.843	0.022	0.988	0.005	0.820	0.026	0.987	0.003	0.955	0.006
Random Forest (70 trees)	93.682	0.854	0.845	0.022	0.988	0.005	0.821	0.026	0.988	0.003	0.956	0.006
Random Forest (80 trees)	93.712	0.837	0.846	0.021	0.988	0.005	0.822	0.025	0.988	0.003	0.956	0.006
Random Forest (90 trees)	93.780	0.821	0.847	0.021	0.989	0.005	0.824	0.025	0.988	0.003	0.957	0.006
Random Forest (100 trees)	93.835	0.823	0.849	0.021	0.989	0.005	0.825	0.025	0.989	0.003	0.957	0.006
J48	86.147	2.508	0.673	0.059	0.904	0.027	0.765	0.058	0.843	0.036	0.900	0.018
Random Tree	83.294	2.554	0.605	0.061	0.885	0.028	0.716	0.059	0.800	0.032	0.880	0.019
SVM Polynomial El	86.011	2.082	0.640	0.058	0.968	0.015	0.618	0.062	0.793	0.031	0.906	0.013
SVM Polynomial E2	92.464	1.863	0.821	0.045	0.956	0.018	0.853	0.044	0.905	0.024	0.946	0.013
SVM Polynomial E3	92.646	1.774	0.827	0.042	0.949	0.018	0.875	0.042	0.912	0.023	0.947	0.013
SVM RBF	74.651	1.493	0.233	0.058	0.996	0.006	0.186	0.048	0.591	0.024	0.845	0.008
Bayes Network	76.525	2.731	0.389	0.073	0.909	0.026	0.442	0.062	0.751	0.038	0.843	0.018
Naïve Bayes	74.128	2.019	0.257	0.065	0.959	0.017	0.252	0.053	0.607	0.028	0.837	0.012

TABLE 6.3

Classification Performance of Approach B

Approach A: T0,T1

Classifier	Accuracy		Kappa		Sensitivity		Specificity		AUC		F1 Score	
	Mean	Std Dev	Mean	Std Dev	Mean	Std Dev	Mean	Std Dev	Mean	Std Dev	Mean	Std Dev
Random Forest (10 trees)	89.491	0.753	0.850	0.011	0.964	0.009	0.923	0.008	0.986	0.002	0.920	0.007
Random Forest (20 trees)	91.557	0.681	0.880	0.010	0.973	0.007	0.939	0.008	0.992	0.001	0.937	0.007
Random Forest (30 trees)	92.271	0.651	0.890	0.009	0.977	0.006	0.944	0.007	0.993	0.001	0.943	0.007
Random Forest (40 trees)	92.620	0.622	0.895	0.009	0.979	0.006	0.947	0.007	0.994	0.001	0.946	0.006
Random Forest (50 trees)	92.845	0.606	0.898	0.009	0.979	0.006	0.948	0.007	0.994	0.001	0.947	0.006
Random Forest (60 trees)	92.985	0.618	0.900	0.009	0.980	0.006	0.949	0.007	0.995	0.001	0.948	0.006
Random Forest (70 trees)	93.104	0.618	0.902	0.009	0.981	0.006	0.950	0.007	0.995	0.001	0.949	0.006
Random Forest (80 trees)	93.182	0.629	0.903	0.009	0.981	0.006	0.951	0.007	0.995	0.001	0.950	0.006
Random Forest (90 trees)	93.227	0.629	0.904	0.009	0.981	0.006	0.951	0.007	0.995	0.001	0.950	0.006
Random Forest (100 trees)	93.264	0.610	0.904	0.009	0.981	0.006	0.951	0.007	0.995	0.001	0.951	0.006
J 48	80.506	2.284	0.729	0.032	0.850	0.034	0.915	0.021	0.892	0.020	0.848	0.025
Random Tree	74.169	2.830	0.641	0.039	0.794	0.040	0.889	0.023	0.841	0.024	0.796	0.030
SVM Polynomial El	78.989	1.849	0.698	0.027	0.910	0.025	0.905	0.017	0.931	0.012	0.874	0.019
SVM Polynomial E2	88.907	1.558	0.845	0.022	0.945	0.021	0.939	0.014	0.963	0.009	0.920	0.015
SVM Polynomial E3	89.525	1.532	0.854	0.021	0.936	0.022	0.943	0.014	0.963	0.009	0.918	0.017
SVM RBF	60.109	2.040	0.402	0.032	0.919	0.026	0.627	0.046	0.777	0.021	0.709	0.021
Bayes Network	62.792	2.392	0.466	0.035	0.793	0.035	0.741	0.030	0.845	0.024	0.701	0.026
Naïve Bayes	32.406	2.905	0.077	0.023	0.016	0.010	0.988	0.007	0.684	0.042	0.030	0.020

control over their seizures. This is probably one of the factors that influenced the total lower score in the questionnaire.

As for the domains evaluated by the questionnaire, the highest averages were seen in the emotional aspects (63.33 ± 3.3) and adverse effects of medication (54.38 ± 6.3). Domains such as overall quality of life, sociability, and cognitive aspects presented the lowest mean values, 34.79 ± 4.0, 36.18 ± 7.3, and 37.65 ± 6.4, respectively. This indicates that these are the areas most affected by pharmacoresistant epilepsy.

In addition, it is important to mention that both the ABAS and the whole experimental procedures were well tolerated by patients. They did not wake due to the positioning of the headphones or with the start of the auditory stimulus. No adverse effects and no complex partial convulsions or secondarily generalized seizures occurred associated with the stimulation.

Furthermore, we also investigated whether there were differences in the electrophysiological signals before and after the acoustic stimulation using machine learning techniques. For this, we applied feature extraction (with 34 attributes extracted) and tested multiple classifiers, including classical machine learning methods such as SVMs and Decision trees. These chosen classifiers have low computational cost, which facilitates their introduction into clinical practice. In the following, we experimented with two classification approaches: Approach A, which compares T0 and T1 signals; and approach B, which compares T0, T1, T2, and T3 signals. We achieved good classification performance with both approaches. In the first case, we aimed to analyze if there is an immediate response to the treatment, that is, the acute effect of ABAS. Table 6.2 shows that, overall, Random Forest overcame the other classifiers in all six metrics, with an average accuracy of 93.835 ± 0.823, Kappa index of 0.849 ± 0.021, sensitivity of 0.989 ± 0.005, average specificity of 0.825 ± 0.025, AUC of 0.989 ± 0.003, and average F-score of 0.957 ± 0.006. In the second case, we analyzed the short-term effect of the sound, after five continuous uses of the treatment. Results showed that there is a significant difference between signals, pointing to some neuromodulation. Table 6.3 shows that, overall, Random forest again overcame the other classifiers in all six metrics, with an average accuracy of 93.264 ± 0.610, Kappa index of 0.904 ± 0.009, sensitivity of 0.981 ± 0.006, average specificity of 0.951 ± 0.007, AUC of 0.995 ± 0.001, and average F-score of 0.951 ± 0.006.

Finally, these results provide clues and a theoretical basis for binaural non-periodic sound stimulation effects in epileptic patients. The literature of Quinkert, Schiff, and Pfaff (2010); and Vismer, Forcelli, Skopin, Gale, and Koubeissi (2015) already shows that non-periodic stimulation with an unstructured temporal pattern destabilizes the rhythmic oscillation activity with abnormal patterns within reverberant neural circuits, acting on the ictogenesis and maintenance of epileptiform activity. In addition, we showed in this work that the sound produced clear changes in the patients' electroencephalographic signals. Therefore, this technique appears to be promising and with good applicability. At this time, however, it is not possible to establish if ABAS is abortive or prophylactic, or even if its effect varies with the type of epilepsy. As a bottom-up acoustic stimulation, ABAS may have interfered with the synchronization of brain-stem nuclei involved in auditory neuronal pathways. However, it is also possible that ABAS interfered with higher brain cortical structures. Thereby, further experiments should be performed in the future, considering a larger group of patients and differentiating types of epilepsy.

6.6 CONCLUSION

One-third of patients suffer from refractory epilepsy, which means that medications are not enough to stop seizures. Most of the time, surgery also cannot benefit these patients. In studies with animals, it was observed that non-periodic electrical stimulation can have an anticonvulsant effect. The problem is that this type of stimulus is invasive and dangerous.

A type of stimulation that has been tested in many applications is binaural beats, which can induce alterations in neuronal activity. Thinking about this, we developed a non-period acoustic stimulation as an alternative and incremental therapy.

In order to test the proposed method, we recruited 14 patients with refractory epilepsy. Their electroencephalographic signals were analyzed before and after the application of treatment with ABAS using machine learning. We achieved great results in this pilot study: first, ABAS and the whole experimental procedure were well tolerated by patients, and there were no adverse effects due to the stimulus. Furthermore, we showed that the sound produced clear changes in the patients' electroencephalographic signals, both immediately and in the short term.

In conclusion, these results point to the possibility of applying a non-period acoustic stimulation to attenuate hypersynchronous neuron activity and subsequent crises. In the future, further experiments should be performed with a greater number of volunteers.

ACKNOWLEDGMENTS

The authors are grateful to the Brazilian research agencies CAPES and CNPq, for the partial financial support of this research.

CONFLICT OF INTEREST

All authors declare they have no conflicts of interest.

COMPLIANCE WITH ETHICAL STANDARDS

This study was funded by the Brazilian research agencies CAPES and CNPq.

All procedures performed in studies involving human participants were in accordance with the ethical standards of the institutional and/or national research committee and with the 1964 Helsinki Declaration and its later amendments or comparable ethical standards.

REFERENCES

M. Arrais, J. Modolo, D. Mogul, and F. Wendling. Design of optimal multi-site brain stimulation protocols via neuro-inspired epilepsy models for abatement of interictal discharges. *Journal of Neural Engineering*, 18(1):016024, 2021.

M. C. Bastos, F. V. D. Laan, L. L. G. Gitaí, F. T. Gameleira, and L. H. B. R. D. Silva. Epilepsia mioclônica juvenil: estudo clínico, epidemiológico, terapêutico e da qualidade de vida. *Journal of Epilepsy and Clinical Neurophysiology*, 15(2):65–69, 2009.

E. Beghi, M. Niero, and M. Roncolato. Validity and reliability of the Italian version of the quality-of-life in epilepsy inventory (QOLIE-31). *Seizure*, 14(7):452–458, 2005.

A. T. Berg, S. F. Berkovic, M. J. Brodie, J. Buchhalter, J. H. Cross, W. van Emde Boas, J. Engel, J. French, T. A. Glauser, G. W. Mathern, et al. Revised terminology and concepts for organization of seizures and epilepsies: Report of the ilae commission on classification and terminology, 2005–2009. *Epilepsis*, 51(4):676–685, 2010.

S. H. Chen and C. A. Pollino. Good practice in Bayesian network modelling. *Environmental Modelling & Software*, 37:134–145, 2012.

F. R. Cordeiro, W. P. D. Santos, and A. G. Silva-Filho. A semi-supervised fuzzy growcut algorithm to seg-ment and classify regions of interest of mammographic images. *Expert Systems with Applications*, 65:116–126, 2016.

F. R. Cordeiro, W. P. D. Santos, and A. G. Silva-Filho. Analysis of supervised and semi-supervised growcut applied to segmentation of masses in mammography images. *Computer Methods in Biome-chanics and Biomedical Engineering: Imaging & Visualization*, 5(4):297–315, 2017.

C. Cortes and V. Vapnik. Support-vector networks. *Machine Learning*, 20(3):273–297, 1995.

V. R. Cota, D. de Castro Medeiros, M. R. S. da Páscoa Vilela, M. C. Doretto, and M. F. D. Moraes. Distinct patterns of electrical stimulation of the basolateral amygdala influence pentylenetetrazole seizure outcome. *Epilepsy & Behavior*, 14(1):26–31, 2009.

T. Cruz, T. Cruz, and W. Santos. Detection and classification of lesions in mammographies using neural networks and morphological wavelets. *IEEE Latin America Transactions*, 16(3):926–932, 2018.

N. Cruz-Ramirez, H. G. Acosta-Mesa, H. Carrillo-Calvet, L. A. Nava-Fernández, and R. E. Barrientos-Martínez. Diagnosis of breast cancer using Bayesian networks: A case study. *Computers in Biology and Medicine*, 37(11):1553–1564, 2007.

D.-I. Curiac, G. Vasile, O. Banias, C. Volosencu, and A. Albu. Bayesian network model for diagnosis of psychiatric diseases. In *Proceedings of the ITI 2009 31st International Conference on Information Technology Interfaces,* pages 61–66. IEEE, New York, 2009.

A. Cutler, D. R. Cutler, and J. R. Stevens. Random forests. In *Ensemble Machine Learning*, pages 157–175. Springer, Berlin, 2012.

M. da Silva Junior, R. C. de Freitas, W. P. dos Santos, W. W. A. da Silva, M. C. A. Rodrigues, and E. F. Q. Conde. Exploratory study of the effect of binaural beat stimulation on the EEG activity pattern in resting state using artificial neural networks. *Cognitive Systems Research*, 54:1–20, 2019.

D. de Castro Medeiros, V. R. Cota, M. R. S. da Páscoa Vilela, F. A. G. Mourão, A. R. Massensini, and M. F. D. Moraes. Anatomically dependent anticonvulsant properties of temporally-coded electrical stimulation. *Epilepsy & Behavior*, 23(3):294–297, 2012.

S. M. de Lima, A. G. da Silva-Filho, and W. P. dos Santos. A methodology for classification of lesions in mammographies using zernike moments, ELM and SVM neural networks in a multi-kernel approach. In *2014 IEEE International Conference on Systems, Man, and Cybernetics (SMC),* pages 988–991. IEEE, New York, 2014.

S. M. de Lima, A. G. da Silva-Filho, and W. P. dos Santos. Detection and classification of masses in mammographic images in a multi-kernel approach. *Computer Methods and Programs in Biomedicine*, 134:11–29, 2016.

J. de Vasconcelos, W. dos Santos, and R. de Lima. Analysis of methods of classification of breast thermographic images to determine their viability in the early breast cancer detection. *IEEE Latin America Transactions*, 16(6):1631–1637, 2018.

C. M. Dubé, J. Molet, A. Singh-Taylor, A. Ivy, P. M. Maras, and T. Z. Baram. Hyper-excitability and epilepsy generated by chronic early-life stress. *Neurobiology of Stress*, 2:10–19, 2015.

J. Engel, T. A. Pedley, and J. Aicardi. *Epilepsy: A Comprehensive Textbook*, volume 3. Lippincott Williams & Wilkins, New York, 2008.

C. W. Espinola, J. C. Gomes, J. M. S. Pereira, and W. P. dos Santos. Vocal acoustic analysis and machine learning for the identification of schizophrenia. *Research on Biomedical Engineering*, 2020:1–14, 2020.

R. S. Fisher, W. V. E. Boas, W. Blume, C. Elger, P. Genton, P. Lee, and J. Engel Jr. Epileptic seizures and epilepsy: definitions proposed by the International League against Epilepsy (ILAE) and the International Bureau for Epilepsy (IBE). *Epilepsia*, 46(4):470–472, 2005.

R. S. Fisher, J. H. Cross, J. A. French, N. Higurashi, E. Hirsch, F. E. Jansen, L. Lagae, S. L. Moshé, J. Peltola, E. Roulet Perez, et al. Operational classification of seizure types by the international league against epilepsy: position paper of the ILAE commission for classification and terminology. *Epilepsia*, 58(4):522–530, 2017.

G. Gálvez, M. Recuero, L. Canuet, and F. Del-Pozo. Short-term effects of binaural beats on EEG power, functional connectivity, cognition, gait and anxiety in Parkinson's disease. *International Journal of Neural Systems*, 28(05):1750055, 2018.

P. Geurts, D. Ernst, and L. Wehenkel. Extremely randomized trees. *Machine Learning*, 63(1):3–42, 2006.

V. Gkolias, A. Amaniti, A. Triantafyllou, P. Papakonstantinou, P. Kartsidis, E. Paraskevopoulos, P. D. Bamidis, L. Hadjileontiadis, and D. Kouvelas. Reduced pain and analgesic use after acoustic bin-aural beats therapy in chronic pain-a double-blind randomized control cross-over trial. *European Journal of Pain*, 24(9):1716–1729, 2020.

S. Hauser and S. Josephson. *Neurologia Clínica de Harrison-3*. Amgh Editora, Alegre, Brazil, 2015.

S. Haykin. Neural networks: Principles and practice. *Bookman*, 11:900, 2001.

A. M. Ismael and J. C. Gomes. The efforts of deep learning approaches for breast cancer detection based on x-ray images. In *Biomedical Computing for Breast Cancer Detection and Diagnosis*, pages 290–309. IGI Global, Hershey, PE, 2021.

C. E. Kahn Jr, L. M. Roberts, K. A. Shaffer, and P. Haddawy. Construction of a Bayesian network for mammographic diagnosis of breast cancer. *Computers in Biology and Medicine*, 27(1):19–29, 1997.

C. Kingsford and S. L. Salzberg. What are decision trees? *Nature Biotechnology*, 26(9):1011–1013, 2008.

P. Kwan, A. Arzimanoglou, A. T. Berg, M. J. Brodie, W. Allen Hauser, G. Mathern, S. L. Moshé, E. Perucca, S. Wiebe, and J. French. Definition of drug resistant epilepsy: consensus proposal by the ad hoc task force of the ilae commission on therapeutic strategies. *Epilepsia*, 51(6):1069–1077, 2010.

K. J. Lee, Y. M. Shon, and C. B. Cho. Long-term outcome of anterior thalamic nucleus stimulation for intractable epilepsy. *Stereotactic and Functional Neurosurgery*, 90(6):379–385, 2012.

S. Lima, W. Azevedo, F. Cordeiro, A. Silva-Filho, and W. Santos. Feature extraction employing fuzzy-morphological decomposition for detection and classification of mass on mammograms. In *Conference proceedings: Annual International Conference of the IEEE Engineering in Medicine and Biology Society. IEEE Engineering in Medicine and Biology Society. Annual Conference,* volume 2015, pages 801–804, IEEE, New York, 2015.

B. A. Malow, R. Kushwaha, X. Lin, K. J. Morton, and M. S. Aldrich. Relationship of interictal epilep-tiform discharges to sleep depth in partial epilepsy. *Electroencephalography and Clinical Neuro-Physiology*, 102(1):20–26, 1997.

E. Niedermeyer, W. Froescher, and R. Fisher. Epileptic seizure disorders. *Journal of Neurology*, 232(1):1–12, 1985.

P. Nubukpo, J. Clement, D. Houinato, A. Radji, E. Grunitzky, G. Avode, and P. Preux. Psychosocial issues in people with epilepsy in Togo and Benin (West Africa) II: quality of life measured using the QOLIE-31 scale. *Epilepsy & Behavior*, 5(5):728–734, 2004.

F. J. Perales, L. Riera, S. Ramis, and A. Guerrero. Evaluation of a VR system for pain management using binaural acoustic stimulation. *Multimedia Tools and Applications*, 78(23):32869–32890, 2019.

J. M. S. Pereira, M. A. Santana, R. C. F. Lima, and W. P. Santos. Lesion detection in breast thermography using machine learning algorithms without previous segmentation. In W. P. dos Santos, M. A. de Santana, and W. W. A. da Silva, editors, *Understanding a Cancer Diagnosis*, 1st edition, pages 81–94. Nova Science, New York, 2020.

H. D. O. Perez, G. Dumas, and A. Lehmann. Binaural beats through the auditory pathway: from brainstem to connectivity patterns. *Eneuro*, 7(2):232, 2020.

P. R. Pinheiro, A. K. A. de Castro, and M. C. D. Pinheiro. A multicriteria model applied in the diagnosis of Alzheimer's disease: A Bayesian network. In *2008 11th IEEE International Conference on Computational Science and Engineering,* pages 15–22. IEEE, New York, 2008.

A. W. Quinkert, N. D. Schiff, and D. W. Pfaff. Temporal patterning of pulses during deep brain stimulation affects central nervous system arousal. *Behavioural Brain Research*, 214(2):377–385, 2010.

M. A. Santana, J. M. S. Pereira, R. C. F. Lima, and W. P. Santos. Breast lesions classification in frontal thermographic images using intelligent systems and moments of haralick and zernike. In W. P. dos Santos, M. A. de Santana, and W. W. A. da Silva, editors, *Understanding a Cancer Diagnosis*, 1st edition, pages 65–80. Nova Science, New York, 2020.

J. S. Sartakhti, M. H. Zangooei, and K. Mozafari. Hepatitis disease diagnosis using a novel hybrid method based on support vector machine and simulated annealing (SVM-SA). *Computer Methods and Programs in Biomedicine*, 108(2):570–579, 2012.

F. L. Seixas, B. Zadrozny, J. Laks, A. Conci, and D. C. M. Saade. A Bayesian network decision model for supporting the diagnosis of dementia, Alzheimer's disease and mild cognitive impairment. *Computers in Biology and Medicine*, 51:140–158, 2014.

S. D. Shorvon, F. Andermann, and R. Guerrini. *The Causes of Epilepsy: Common and Uncommon Causes in Adults and Children*. Cambridge University Press, Cambridge, 2011.

S. Shorvon, R. Guerrini, E. Trinka, and S. Schachter. *The Causes of Epilepsy: Diagnosis and Investigation*. Cambridge University Press, Cambridge, 2019.

T. I. d. Silva, C. M. Marques, N. B. Alonso, A. M. Azevedo, A. C. Westphal-Guitti, L. O. S. F. Caboclo, A. C. Sakamoto, and E. M. T. Yacubian. Tradução e adaptação cultural do quality of life in epilepsy (QOLIE-31). *Journal of Epilepsy and Clinical Neurophysiology*, 12(2):107–110, 2006.

W. W. A. Silva, M. A. Santana, A. G. Silva Filho, S. M. L. Lima, and W. P. Santos. Morphological extreme learning machines applied to the detection and classification of mammary lesions. In T. K. Gandhi, S. Bhattacharyya, S. De, D. Konar, and S. Dey, editors, *Advanced Machine Vision Paradigms for Medical Image Analysis*, pages 55–95. Elsevier, London, 2020.

S. Sisodiya, W.-R. Lin, B. Harding, M. Squier, and M. Thom. Drug resistance in epilepsy: expression of drug resistance proteins in common causes of refractory epilepsy. *Brain*, 125(1):22–31, 2002.

M. Sundaram, R. Sadler, G. Young, and N. Pillay. EEG in epilepsy: current perspectives. *Canadian Journal of Neurological Sciences*, 26(4):255–262, 1999.

K. Tóth, K. T. Hofer, Á. Kandrács, L. Entz, A. Bagó, L. Eross, Z. Jordán, G. Nagy, A. Sólyom, D. Fabó, et al. Hyperexcitability of the network contributes to synchronization processes in the human epileptic neocortex. *The Journal of Physiology*, 596(2):317–342, 2018.

M. S. Vismer, P. A. Forcelli, M. D. Skopin, K. Gale, and M. Z. Koubeissi. The piriform, perirhinal, and entorhinal cortex in seizure generation. *Frontiers in Neural Circuits*, 9:27, 2015.

J. G. Webster. *Medical Instrumentation: Application and Design*. John Wiley & Sons, Hoboken, NJ, 2009.

7 Artifacts Removal in Electroencephalogram (EEG) Signals

Jammisetty Yedukondalu, M Krishna Chaitanya, and Lakhan Dev Sharma

7.1 INTRODUCTION

Functional near-infrared spectroscopy (fNIRS), electroencephalography (EEG), and some non-invasive methods have cutting-edge cognitive science, cognitive psychology, and neuroscience research. Spectroscopy (fNIRS), magnetoencephalography (EMG), and other technologies are also important [1]. One technique for measuring brain activity is EEG, which records impulses from multiple scalp electrodes [2]. The health of the patient [3] is also important, as is the diagnosis and identification of various brain diseases [4]. In contrast, EEG has a high degree of precision but is often distorted by outside noise, leading to a variety of distortions [5]. The source of artifacts is not only measurement instruments but also human subjects, with the former causing issues such as high electrode impedance, line noise, and faulty electrodes [6]. Physiological artifacts including muscular activity, eye blinks, eye movements, and heart activity that occur in EEG signals are only a few examples [7]. The physiological signals, like EEG and electrocardiogram (ECG), were putrefied utilizing sliding mode singular spectrum analysis into reconstructed components, which aid in extracting the prejudiced topographies [8].

In real-world applications like brain-computer interfaces (BCIs), such physiological aberrations may interfere with cerebral impulses and be mistaken for regular occurrences [9]. Furthermore, artifacts may mimic the cognitive or pathologic movement, skewing visual clarification and analysis in medical studies such as Alzheimer's disease and sleep disorders [10] and so on. As a result, identifying and removing artifacts is the most essential preprocessing step before being used, whether in clinical diagnosis or in practical applications. Strategies that have been improved by refining current algorithms, integrating other methods, or automating the removal process may be divided into two groups: either using a reference channel to estimate artifactual signals or splitting the EEG signal into new realms. Examples of alternative strategies are regression [11], the Wavelet Transform algorithm, hybrid approaches [13], Empirical-mode Decomposition (EMD), and Blind Source Separation (BSS) [12]. A circulant Singular System Analysis (SSA) followed by a four-stage cascaded Savitzky-Golay filter is used to remove baseline wandering

DOI: 10.1201/9781003252092-9

and power line interfaces in the ECG signal while preserving its morphological characteristics [14]. A similar technique can be extended to the EEG signals for the elimination of artifacts. Bayesian-optimized K-Nearest Neighbor (BO-KNN) and EEG signals have been proven to be effective methods for characterizing mental strain [15]. Entropy-centered topographies were extracted from an EEG signal decayed by means of a stationary wavelet transform [16].

In spite of the significant investigation on artifact identification and elimination of EEG signals, no one ideal solution for all forms of artifacts has been identified. In view of this problem, we aim to conduct a complete assessment of the primary approaches for removing artifacts from EEG that have been presented in the literature. First, we'll go over the features of EEG signals and the many sorts of artifacts that can be found. Then we go through the most commonly used removal strategies, as well as their benefits and cons. Finally, a comparison study based on specific requirements is provided.

7.2   BACK GROUND

7.2.1   EEG CHARACTERISTICS

EEG is a record of impulsive electrical action in the brain that allows voltage changes in brain activity to be detected [17]. EEG signals have a frequency that varies from 0.01 to 100 Hz, which may be split into five frequency groups as shown in Table 7.1.

7.2.2   ARTIFACT TYPES

When collecting EEG data from recording equipment, signal artifacts are more noticeable [18]. Unwanted signals called artifacts are due to noise in the environment, experimental errors, and physiological artifacts. Furthermore, external elements such as the environment and experiment error are classed as non-physiological artifacts, whereas physiological artifacts (for example: heartbeat, muscular activity, and eye blink) are classified as physiological artifacts [19]. The experimental error may be readily decreased with proper process and forethought. Physiological artifacts, on the other hand, are more difficult to eliminate since they require specific algorithms [20]. Figure 7.1 depicts the artifacts in EEG signals.

TABLE 7.1
Basic Brain Waves and Their Frequency Range

Name of the Band	Frequency (Hz)	Description
Gamma	30–80	Concentration, problem solving
Beta	13–30	Active mind, busy
Alpha	8–13	Reflective, restful
Theta	4–13	Drowsiness
Delta	1–4	Sleep, dreaming

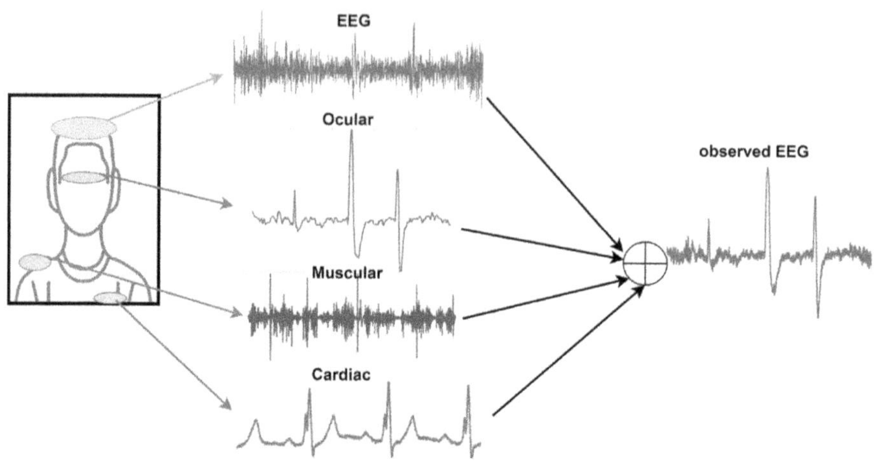

FIGURE 7.1 Physiological artifacts in EEG signals.

7.2.2.1 Physiological Artifacts

Ocular artifacts: Ocular artifacts are an important source of artifacts in EEG recordings [21]. Ocular artifacts are generated by the movement and blinking of the eye, and they can extend across the scalp and be picked up by EEG activity. Artifacts caused by the movement of the eye, in particular, are caused by changes in the retina's alignment. Eye blink artifacts are induced by ocular conductance owing to contact changes between the cornea and the eyelid, as well as the shifting of the cornea dipole with the movement of the eyelid. Furthermore, due to the effect of volume conduction, both ocular artifacts are present. Such ocular signals have the potential for the electrooculogram to be recorded (EOG). EOG signals have a much larger amplitude than EEG [22], and their frequency is similar to that of EEG signals. As a result, once we eliminate EOG artifacts, bidirectional interference will produce a removal error.

Muscle artifacts: Muscle activity contamination of EEG data is a well-known and difficult problem that can occur in a variety of muscle groups [23]. These artifacts can be created by any muscular contraction and stretching in close proximity to signal recording locations, the patient talking, sniffing, swallowing [19], and so on. In principle, muscle artifacts evaluated by EMG have a large frequency range of 0–200 Hz. Independent Components Analysis (ICA)[24] may be a good way to reduce EMG contamination.

Cardiac artifacts: When an electrode is placed on or close to a blood vessel [23], cardiac artifacts can occur owing to the heart's expansion and contraction. Pulse artifacts, with a frequency of roughly 1.2 Hz, can appear in the EEG as a comparable waveform, making them difficult to eliminate. An ECG is a kind of cardiac activity that measures the electrical signal produced by the heart [25].

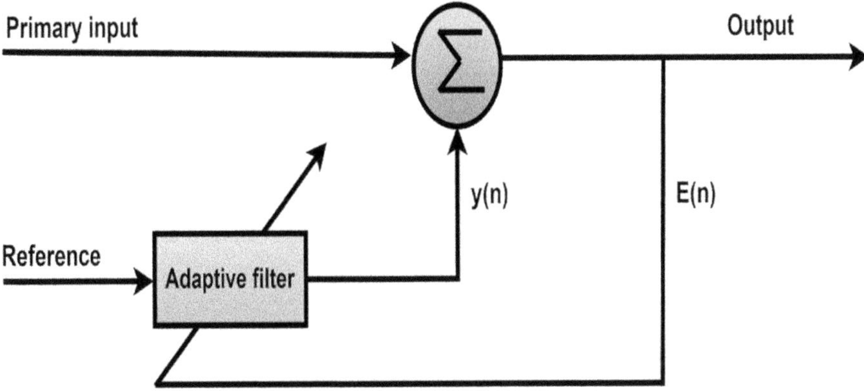

FIGURE 7.2   Adaptive noise canceller.

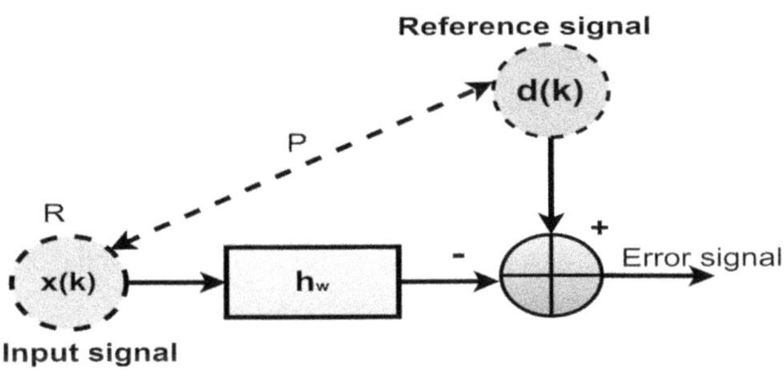

FIGURE 7.3   Basic flow diagram of artifacts elimination from EEG signals.

7.2.2.2 Non-Physiological Artifacts

Instrument artifacts are non-physiological artifacts caused by electrode misalignment and cable movement. With proper process and forethought, these artifacts may be erased. A simple filter, with its identifiable frequency spectrum, may easily reduce such artifacts from ambient sources. Even though white noise has a wide frequency range, a high-frequency filter may still eliminate the bulk of artifacts [12,26]. Provides relevant literature for dealing with volume conduct artifacts (Figure 7.2).

7.3 ARTIFACT REMOVAL TECHNIQUES

A basic flow diagram of artifact removal is shown in Figure 7.3 as well as artifact removal methods are discussed in this section.

7.3.1 REGRESSION TECHNIQUES

Regression is a simple and commonly employed technique for reducing artifacts from EEG data. Regression techniques rely on removing artifact signals from EEG recordings. It is based on the assumption that the EEG and ocular artifacts (OAs) are linearly uncorrelated. Due to the fact that EEG and EOG both involve brain activity, identifying the reference artifact signals may be exceedingly challenging [27]. Here, Eq. (7.1) displays the basic mathematical analysis.

$$EEG_r(n) = EEG_s(n) + \gamma EOG(n); \text{ with } n = 1, 2, \ldots \quad (7.1)$$

Here, the real EEG signals are referred to as EEG_s, the recorded EEG signals are referred to as EEG_r, and the proportion of EOG signals is referred to as γ.

7.3.2　FILTERING METHODS

The elimination of EEG artifacts involves the use of a variety of filtering methods, namely Kalman filtering, adaptive filtering (AF), and Wiener filtering (WF), each of them was employed using a different optimization theory. Two frequently used filtering techniques are briefly illustrated in the following sections.

7.3.2.1　Adaptive Filtering (AF)

The required EEG signals are unfortunately being interfered with by ECG, EMG, and EOG artifact frequencies. AF eliminates significant data and frequency band overlap [28]. However, there are two specific drawbacks to this: (i) Reference noise signals must be used to minimize the noise content in the original signals, and (ii) It's possible that utilizing the reference noise won't affect the useful information in the original signals.

7.3.2.2　Wiener Filtering (WF)

In order to design a linear time-invariant filter and lower the mean square error between the pure EEG records and the appraised signal, the genuine EEG data are estimated using the linear statistical filtering method known as Wiener filtering. Determining the power spectral densities of the calculated and artifact signals is the only way to calculate the linear filter because statistics are unknown [29]. Figure 7.4 depicts the WF block diagram.

7.3.3　BLIND SOURCE SEPARATION (BSS)

The basic aim of BSS is to identify sources among a variety of signals [30]. Some of the BSS algorithms are covered in the sections that follow.

7.3.3.1　Principal Component Analysis (PCA)

One easy way to eliminate artifacts utilizing the orthogonality principle is through the use of principal component analysis (PCA), a BSS approach [31]. PCA is a technique for multivariate data analysis that requires reducing the total correlated variables from a huge number to a manageable set of uncorrelated variables. A PCA is described as a "linear projection that turns multivariate data into a set of components known as principle components (PCs)" [32]. The singular value decomposition (SVD) technique is used to compute PCs. From the covariance matrix (C), eigenvalues for SVD are calculated. The most significant eigenvalues are correlated with maximum variance, while the least significant eigenvalues are correlated with the

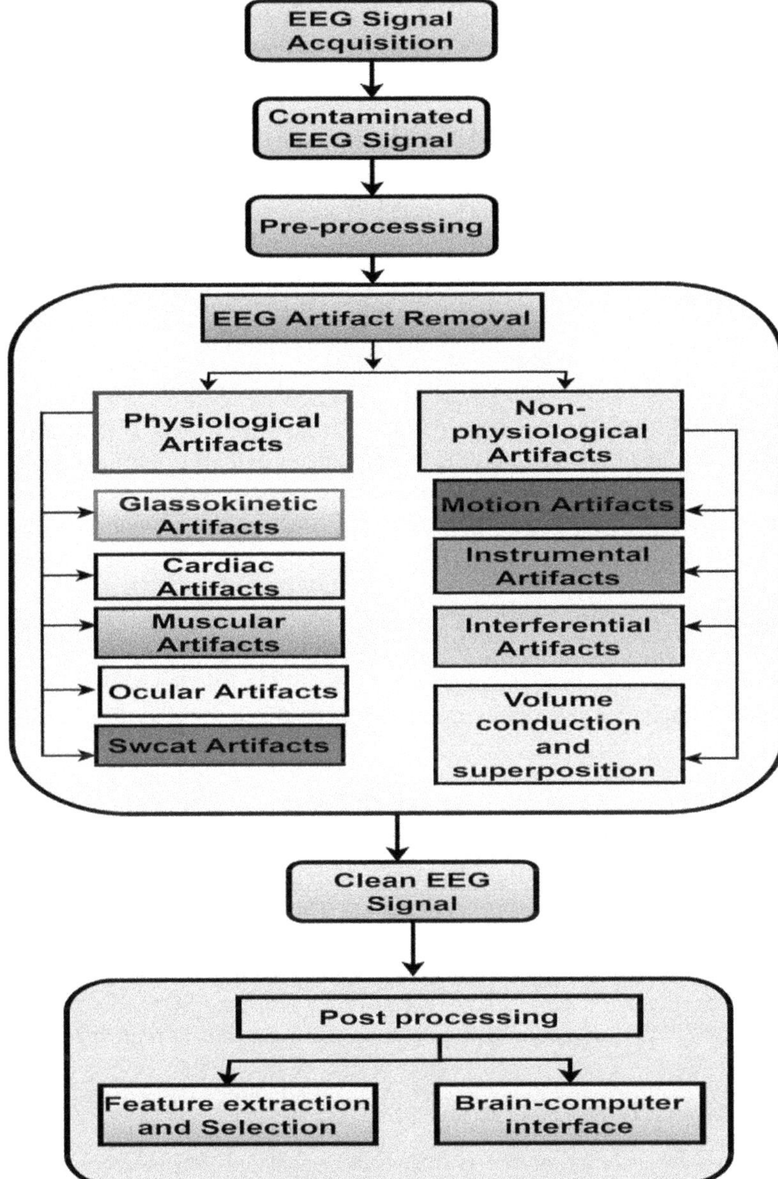

FIGURE 7.4   Wiener filter basic block diagram.

lowest variance. Assuming the unique EEG signal (EEG_{or}) and artifacts like EMG and EOG are combined with the recorded EEG signals (EEG_{re}), Eq. (7.2) is derived.

$$EEG_{re} = EEG_{or} + a\,EOG + b\,EMG \qquad (7.2)$$

Here a, b are real constants. The orthogonality requirement is not ever upheld being the nonlinearity between the electrical signals of brain neurons due to eye blinks and

EMs related to original EEG data [33]. In comparison to the regression approach and filtering techniques, PCA performs better. Other artifacts cannot be eliminated, but PCA may remove OAs.

7.3.3.2 Independent Component Analysis (ICA)

A potent BSS technique for removing artifacts from EEG recordings is ICA. The main presumption of this technique is that the measured EEG signals are a linear combination of underlying independent sources [33]. Assuming that the underlying sources $V(l)$ are N and that the recorded EEG signals $S(l)$ utilize N channels; Eq. (7.3) is derived.

$$S(l) = MV(l) \tag{7.3}$$

Where $S(l) = [S_1(l), S_2(l), \ldots, S_N(l)]^T$ and $V(l) = [V_1(l), V_2(l), \ldots, V_N(l)]^T$. The transpose operator is denoted by T and the time index operator by l. M is putting together the unidentified matrix. The purpose of ICA is to retrieve V from S deprived of knowing M and V. To achieve Eq. (7.4) in this case, a distinct un-mixing matrix K must be identified.

$$Z(l) = KV(l) \tag{7.4}$$

Z is the estimated value of V. If and only if $K = M-1$, Z is exactly identical to V. ICA's main drawback is that it requires many channels to acquire data from artifactual sources.

7.3.3.3 Canonical Correlation Analysis (CCA)

In 1936, Hotelling suggested CCA. The coordinate system may also be important if there is a significant linear affiliation among both groups of multidimensional variables. Although it might not be apparent, this correlation connection might be looking for two linear transformations. After each set of parameters is changed, the coordinates are maximally correlated. Compared to ICA, which relies on higher-order statistics (HOS), this approach utilizes second-order statistics (SOS). Because muscle artifacts don't have a stereotypical topography, CCA can simply remove them [34].

7.3.4 Wavelet Transform (WT)

WT uses a wavelet function that is scaled and translated [35] to decompose EEG signals in the time domain.

$$\varphi_{a,b}(n) = \frac{1}{\sqrt{a}}\varphi(\frac{n-b}{a} \tag{7.5}$$

where a and b are real numbers and $N = 1, 2, 3, \ldots, N$. Because the wavelets resembled OAs, Discrete Wavelet Transform (DWT) removes OAs [36]. The goal of the exceptional and non-redundant DWT transform technique is to clean up the artifacts from the time-domain EEG signals. To get estimated and precise coefficients for this investigation, the signal is distributed among a number of high-pass and low-pass filters [35]. Up till the target frequency is attained, the procedure is iteratively repeated. When this is accomplished, the output is up-sampled, and thereafter a factor of 2 down-sampling was employed to obtain the restored signal.

7.3.5 Empirical Mode Decomposition (EMD)

The EMD decomposes the EEG signals into a few oscillatory processes known as intrinsic mode functions (IMFs) [37]. Two requirements must be met by the generated IMFs:

1. The total number of outliers and zero-crossings within the dataset must be equal or deviate by no more than one.
2. The local maxima, which must always be zero, determines the average value of the enclosure at any given position.

It is a data-driven approach; unlike WT, the putrefaction is not carried out by means of bass utilities that have been predefined. The methods for performing EMD are as follows:

1. Determine all of the local peaks and minima for the provided EEG signal, $x(t)$.
2. Compute the topmost envelope $u(t)$ and bottom envelope $l(t)$ by interpolating between the maxima and minima.
3. To obtain the first IMF, compute the mean m1 of upper and lower envelopes and remove it from the signal.

Based on information about amplitude and frequency, EMD breaks down the signals. Due to their overlap at higher frequencies, the EMG artifacts and the EEG signals cannot be separated, but these particular EMG artifacts can be eradicated by employing various extensively used current artifact exclusion procedures.

7.3.6 Singular Spectrum Analysis (SSA)

For removing artifacts among the multi-channel and single-channel EEG recordings, SSA is a potent decomposition technique. Multi-channel data is mostly used using the BSS approach. The SSA technique is essentially split into two parts, with each step being further broken down into two stages [38].

1. SVD and Time delay embedding are the two decomposition methods.
2. Two reconstruction techniques include grouping and diagonal averaging.

When compared to BSS techniques, the SSA technique can better remove muscular artifacts. Artifacts may be further eliminated by combining the SSA with additional BSS techniques.

7.3.7 HYBRID METHODS

In addition to the algorithms mentioned above, there are still many other effective and innovative techniques. The following are some important hybrid techniques.

7.3.7.1 Discrete Wavelet Transforms – Adaptive Filtering Method (DWT-AFM)

An allusion signal is needed to eradicate the noise in EEG data using ICA. DWT can be used to overcome this issue. By using low-frequency wavelet coefficients to filter out OAs, the reference EOG signal may be produced from the provided data [39]. In contrast to ICA, improved artifact removal does not also need a huge quantity of information. The drawback of DWT is that it is unable to eliminate artifacts efficiently if their spectrum overlaps with that of the original EEG signals [35]. Adaptive noise canceller (ANC) is another name for the AFM. This issue may be fixed using the ANC. The disadvantage of the ANC is that, in order to remove artifacts, it needs a reference signal. Problems with spectrum overlap and reference signals can both be resolved by combining DWT with ANC [40]. The reference EOG signal produced by DWT is utilized as an input reference to the ANC in the OA elimination process. When employing this hybrid approach, artifacts are removed more effectively than when employing DWT and ANC alone.

7.3.7.2 Discrete Wavelet Transform – Blind Source Separation (DWT-BSS)

One of the amalgam techniques to more efficiently eliminate artifacts is the DWT-BSS. Multi-channel data may often be used with the BSS approach. The drawbacks of both strategies have been covered in earlier sections. It is possible to combine the benefits of both strategies in order to get over these drawbacks. One of these techniques can be utilized as the first technique based on single-channel and multi-channel. For the single-channel technique, the wavelet coefficients are applied to BSS (ICA or CCA) after the time series signal is first decomposed using DWT [41]. The first technique for multi-channel data can be DWT or BSS, and the output signal is then fed into the second technique to remove artifacts. If ICA and CCA are first employed, the time domain signal is split into ICs and CCs. These coefficients are further divided by DWT to more effectively remove artifacts from the EEG data.

7.3.7.3 Empirical Mode Decomposition – Blind Source Separation (EMD-BSS)

Different techniques such as DWT, EMD, SSA, etc., should be utilized for ambulatory or single-channel data processing. A hybrid model that combines many techniques can improve performance in terms of artifact removal. DWT uses specified mother wavelets to decompose the data. DWT is insufficient for stochastic data that is nonlinear and non-stationary, such as EEG signals. EMD is a data-driven approach that may also be used channel-wise to decompose into IMFs for multi-channel data [42].

7.3.7.4 Singular Spectrum Analysis –Adaptive Noise Canceller (SSA-ANC)

One of the fusion approaches for removing artifacts among multi-channel as well as single-channel EEG recordings is SSA-ANC. It may be used with portable devices when multi-channel data gathering is not feasible due to the nature of ICA and CCA as multi-channel data approaches. In an amalgam technique like SSA-ANC, the allusion signal for removal of EOG artifacts using ANC is provided by SSA, similar to how DWT uses eigenvalues. The EOG reference signal is created using the last low-frequency components of the DWT [43]. The lower eigenvalues that are created when using SVD on the trajectory matrix are also used to generate the reference signal in SSA [44]. Since ANC receives the input reference EOG signal, which is produced from the output of SSA, the artifact removal performance is better than using SSA or ANC alone.

7.3.7.5 Singular Spectrum Analysis –Blind Source Separation (SSA-BSS)

OAs and muscular artifacts are removed from the recorded EEG signals using SOS and HOS within the effective BSS techniques of ICA and CCA [45]. BSS techniques are multi-channel, and each one has benefits and drawbacks of its own. To eliminate artifacts from EEG signals, BSS techniques are integrated with SSA in a hybrid manner. The single or multi-channel data of EEG is decayed using SSA, and the decayed data is then additionally treated by BSS techniques for eliminating artifacts.

7.4 EEG ARTIFACT DATASETS

The previously reviewed study employed a variety of datasets, including manual datasets, Mendeley, Git-hub databases, BCI-IV databases, etc. Table 7.2 summarizes the various open-source dataset types used in the works under consideration.

TABLE 7.2

EEG Artifacts Open-Source Datasets

Dataset	Type of Artifact	Nature	Dataset Link
A semi-simulated EEG/EOG dataset for the comparison of EOG artifact rejection techniques [46]	Ocular	Simulated	https://data.mendeley.com/datasets/wb6yvr725d/4
EEG eye artifact dataset [39]	Ocular	Real	https://osf.io/2qgrd/
EEG dataset contaminated with artifact/noise	Ocular, Head/Jaw Movement	Real	https://github.com/inabiyouni/EEG_dataset_for_artifact-noise_detection
The TUH EEG Artifact Corpus (TUAR) [47]	5 Types	Real	https://isip.piconepress.com/projects/tuh_eeg/
DATA SET 2A [48]	Eye Artifacts	Real	http://www.bbci.de/competition/iv/#dataset2a

7.5 PERFORMANCE COMPARISON OF CURRENT TECHNIQUES

Table 7.3 provides a tabular analysis of the literature and techniques. The artifacts cannot all be eliminated by separate methods. According to the requirements of the reference channel, procedures are categorized. Online automated process applications, whether single or multi-channel, require prior knowledge to optimize performance and eliminate artifacts. Both physiological and non-physiological artifacts can be removed using various techniques. Regression techniques are fundamental for eliminating artifacts but call for multi-channel data and reference channels. Filtering techniques work by initially calculating artifactual elements and removing them from the original, contaminated EEG signals. However, when subtracting, some of the original EEG signals are also lost. The majority of researchers only allow typical artifacts to be removed using ICA [49]. Since muscle artifacts are not typical, ICA cannot effectively eliminate them. Although CCA can solve this issue, doing so increases simulation time and computing costs, making CCA unsuitable for use in online applications. When only a single or few channels of data are available for ambulatory analysis, multi-channel data processing techniques like ICA and CCA cannot be applied.

When only a rare channel or a single channel of data is accessible for ambulatory analysis, multi-channel data processing techniques like ICA and CCA cannot be applied. SSA and EMD algorithms can be used in single and multi-channel applications, though EMD has the disadvantages of mode mixing and aliasing. The SSA approach only eliminates one kind of artifact. If the reference channel is present, regression techniques may be used intuitively [7]. Even though ICA and CCA are multi-channel approaches, Ensemble EMD (EEMD)-ICA eliminates EOG

TABLE 7.3

Comparison of the Artificial Approaches Mentioned in the Survey

References	Method	Channel	Automatic	Reference Electrode Required
[40]	Regression	Multi	Yes	Yes
[28]	AF	Both	Yes	Yes
[27]	ICA	Multi	Yes	No
[50]	CCA	Multi	Yes	No
[35]	DWT	Both	No	No
[36]	EMD	Both	No	No
[51]	SSA	Both	Yes	No
[12]	DWT-AFM	Both	Yes	No
[52]	DWT-BSS	Both	No	No
[49]	EMD-BSS	Both	No	No
[53]	SSA-ANC	Both	Yes	No
[53]	SSA-BSS	Both	No	No
[54]	CiSSA-DWT	Both	Yes	No

artifacts while EEMD-CCA eradicates EMG artifacts from a single channel [53]. The single-channel data is decomposed into several IMFs by EEMD. For additional processing to get rid of artifacts, these IMFs can be used with ICA or CCA. Because EEMD is a data-driven approach, it successfully reduces artifacts compared to WT-ICA. A few channel techniques employ fast multivariate EMD (FMEMD)-CCA to eliminate muscle artifacts more quickly [21]. It was suggested to automatically eliminate OAs using WT-ICA in conjunction with SVM. Regression and filtering approaches can't get rid of ECG artifacts; hence the recursive least square (RLS) notch filter method is suggested [55]. By using a hybrid approach, all of the aforementioned techniques efficiently eliminate artifacts.

7.6 CHALLENGES

7.6.1 ALGORITHM SPECIFIC CHALLENGES

Necessity of reference channel: An additional reference channel requires controlling its placement and noise. Although the ECG and EMG sensors can detect muscular activity, muscle movements cause very dynamic artifacts. To cover these dynamics, EMG sensors must be put at several sites, which is impractical. Thus, WTs and BSS algorithms should be used to remove EMG and ECG artifacts. Since gel paste is applied to the skin before fixing EOG and EMG electrodes, adding an additional reference channel may cause discomfort to study participants. Reference channel-dependent approaches require robust/correct reference signal recording. A reference channel breakdown or loose connection might disrupt preprocessing.

Neuronal activity may also be recorded via the Fp1 and Fp2 EOG reference channels in addition to EOG. EOG-based ocular artifact reduction techniques are plagued by bidirectional contamination error. These techniques erroneously assume that the EEG and EOG signals are uncorrelated when in reality, they are not. Cross-contamination amid EEG and EOG data can result in issues with artifact removal. EOG signals might have recorded neural activity, thus getting rid of them may also involve getting rid of neuronal data.

Multi versus single-channel EEG data application: Multi-channel data contains more information than single-channel data, although single-channel EEG devices have recently seen an increase in popularity because of their greater convenience and portability. Applications like driver sleepiness monitoring or home healthcare applications typically utilize a single EEG electrode, in contrast to applications like clinical diagnostics, prosthetics, wheelchair control, etc. that typically involve EEG signals from many EEG channels. Researchers are forced to employ single-channel EEG artifact reduction techniques in these circumstances.

Proficiency of operator: A good EEG artifact removal tool should be simple to operate and require the operator to have a thorough understanding of how the algorithms function. Operator proficiency determines the efficiency of manual or semiautomatic methods. Expert EEG analysts may improve ICA-based semiautomatic algorithms. Manually discovering poor ICs involves subject expertise and visualization employing topographic maps, power spectrums, and time-domain features to find artifacts. ICA-based semiautomatic procedures can be improved by an experienced operator.

Calibration requirements: Calibration is the first step in several EEG artifact reduction algorithms when adjusting parameters or thresholds. In order to estimate a noise source's contribution to the EEG channels, regression-based techniques generate artifact propagation coefficients. The physiological artifacts in the EEG data are eliminated by these calibration parameters. Threshold calibration is necessary for several automated wavelet analysis-based artifact reduction techniques.

Real-time constraints: The quality of life for people with movement disabilities may be improved by EEG applications like neurofeedback and BCIs. For these applications, precise real-time control is necessary. Results of BCI categorization may be impacted by EEG signal artifacts with amplitudes comparable to or greater than brain activity. As a result, controlling a wheelchair or prosthetic arm may not be convenient. So, it is important to take into account precise real-time artifact removal methods.

Various optimal algorithms for different types of artifacts: The best EEG artifact reduction method must be able to handle various artifacts. Nonetheless, applying a single technique to all EEG artifact forms is difficult. In the past, a certain kind of artifact was eliminated using algorithms. In recent years, the focus of research has switched to artifact removal algorithms that can eliminate any kind of artifact.

7.6.2 GENERAL CHALLENGES

Choosing the evaluation criteria: Comparing the effectiveness of various EEG artifact removal algorithms is of significant difficulty because of the absence of appropriate validation methods. Validation can often be done in one of two ways. EEG data is used initially. It is challenging to quantify a noisy or pure EEG signal from a composite EEG signal. SNR, MSE, and other such objective evaluation metrics are challenging to quantify. Therefore, the most common technique is still the visual evaluation of artifact removal algorithms using real EEG data. This assessment is neither scalable nor impartial. There is no universally accepted method for applying objective assessment criteria to real EEG data, and eye inspection is still the primary method for evaluating the effectiveness of artifact removal algorithms. Second, employ synthetic EEG data. This method estimates noise from the contaminated signal the pure EEG signals are known. SNR, MSE, etc. can be calculated. Simulated data cannot accurately depict raw EEG signals. Researchers often use simulated datasets that usually deal with one form of artifact, making it difficult to compare algorithms for numerous types.

Deficiency of open-source EEG artifact datasets: The lack of an EEG artifact dataset that is widely accepted is a challenge for researchers developing artifact removal techniques. Researchers use artifact-free, single-artifact simulated datasets that don't accurately represent EEG signals. Others may gather data in carefully controlled experimental settings, but they can only visually review it. It is challenging to compare algorithms between studies because most researchers don't open-source their artifact databases, which is related to reproducibility. If you're interested in a particular dataset, contact authors who claim to be able to provide the data.

Nonexistence of open-source executions: Progress on EEG artifact reduction is limited by a lack of open-source implementations. The development of computer vision algorithms is sped up by open-source and pre-trained object classification, detection, and segmentation techniques. By using this technique, researchers can avoid changing codes and concentrate on solving their problems. Unfortunately, code implementations are not shared within the EEG community. The majority of EEG analysis programs and tools contain ICA and other widely used methods. One must start from scratch if one wants to research lesser-known artifact removal methods. Even worse, it takes more time and coding to integrate a custom algorithm into an EEG processing pipeline using the current libraries and toolboxes than it does to actually fix the issue.

Nonexistence of hardware-optimized executions: The difficulty for researchers is to create EEG-based prototypes without using hardware-optimization techniques. When developing a product, academic researchers typically write a code to demonstrate a notion. Because it takes more effort to optimize the code for real-world deployment, successful prototypes are rarely put into production. The code's commercial viability depends on it being optimized for low-cost hardware. While academia lacks adequate oversight and training, industry-based embedded systems developers create algorithms that are hardware-optimized. Sometimes the gap between the software and hardware prevents academic prototypes from being commercialized. Hardware must be optimized by EEG experts.

Exceptional encounters of machine learning created procedures: In the field of EEG signal processing, there has recently been a lot of study done on applications of machine learning, particularly deep learning. However, the improved performance comes at an additional processing cost and necessitates vast amounts of training data, which isn't always available, particularly when discussing brain signals. To address concerns with data scarcity, it is necessary to investigate transfer learning and data augmentation strategies for EEG signals in more detail.

Shortage of benchmarks/competitions: Large open-source datasets, which were frequently used in competitions, were one of the key factors of the rapid development in the field of computer vision. Therefore, whenever a new model is suggested, researchers compare their findings using test sets of well-known datasets, which makes it simple to assess their suggested approaches. Unfortunately, there isn't agreement among EEG experts on a single benchmark dataset for artifact removal, which makes it challenging to compare various models.

Reproducibility issues: Promoting uniform data storage practices can help create the homogeneity required for reproducibility. The lack of agreement on a single data-storage format, as well as the fact that different libraries and EEG headset suppliers output data in different formats, all add to the difficulty. Therefore, using a library or framework that is not part of the manufacturer's resource pool is challenging. If these resources are accessible and open-sourced, valuable research time can be saved.

7.7   CONCLUSION

Electrodes are used to record EEG signals from the scalp, which are produced by the brain. This time-domain EEG data is contaminated by various physiological and non-physiological artifacts. Numerous techniques are covered in this research from the works of numerous authors. However, no single technique can effectively and precisely remove the artifacts. In this study, the benefits and drawbacks of each strategy are explored. Artifactual reference signals are necessary for the elimination of regression algorithms, artifacts, and filtering procedures. BSS techniques efficiently eliminate the artifacts, but they need a lot of multi-channel data and are computationally challenging. The removal of artifacts is not as effective as it might be using the single-channel and multi-channel DWT, EMD, and SSA approaches. Efficiency is increased compared to using just one approach by combining many or using the hybrid method. In this regard, researchers are working to identify the best method for reducing EEG signal artifacts. Future artifact removal approaches will be combined with current developments, such as machine learning, artificial intelligence (AI), and optimization techniques, to create a single system that will be more accurate and efficient.

REFERENCES

1. Frederik, V.; Luca, F.; Esin, K.; Jitkomut, S.; Pedro, A.V.; Daniele, M. Critical comments on EEG sensor space dynamical connectivity analysis. *Brain Topography* 2016, 32, 1–12.
2. Henry, J.C. Electroencephalography: Basic principles, clinical applications, and related fields. *Neurology* 2006, 67, 2092.
3. Hirsch, L.J.; Brenner, R.P. *Atlas of EEG in Critical Care*; John Wiley and Sons: Hoboken, NJ, 2010; Volume 30, pp. 187–216, ISBN 9780470746707.
4. Nunez, P.L.; Srinivasan, R. *Electric Fields of the Brain: The Neurophysics of EEG*, 2nd ed.; Oxford University Press: New York, USA, 2005; pp. 154–169, ISBN 9780195050387.
5. Radüntz, T.; Scouten, J.; Hochmuth, O.; Meffert, B. Automated EEG artifact elimination by applying machine learning algorithms to ICA-based features. *Journal of Neural Engineering* 2017, 14, 8–15.
6. Ge, S.; Yang, Q.; Wang, R.; Lin, P.; Gao, J.; Leng, Y.; Yang, Y.; Wang, H. A brain-computer interface based on a few-channel EEG-fNIRS bimodal system. *IEEE Access* 2017, 5, 208–218.
7. Fatourechi, F.; Bashashati, A.; Ward, R.K.; Birch, G.E. EMG and EOG artifacts in brain computer interface systems: A survey. *Clinical Neurophysiology* 2007, 118, 480–494.
8. Sharma, L.D.; Bhattacharyya, A. A computerized approach for automatic human emotion recognition using sliding mode singular spectrum analysis. *IEEE Sensors Journal* 2021, 21(23), 26931–26940.
9. NaeemMannan, M.; Ahmad, K.M.; Shinil, K.; Myung, Y.J. Effect of EOG signal filtering on the removal of ocular artifacts and EEG-based brain-computer interface: A comprehensive study. *Complexity* 2018, 2018, 18–36.

10. Tamburro, G.; Fiedler, P.; Stone, D.; Haueisen, J.; Comani, S. A new ICA-based fingerprint method for the automatic removal of physiological artifacts from EEG recordings. *PeerJ* 2018, 6, e4380.

11. Husseen, A.H.; Emmanuel, J.; Sun, L.; Emmanuel, I. Complexity measures for quantifying changes in electroencephalogram in Alzheimer's disease. *Complexity* 2018, 2018, 1–12.

12. Sweeney, K.T.; Ward, T.E.; McLoone, S.F. Artifact removal in physiological signals practices and possibilities. *IEEE Transactions on Information Technology* 2012, 16, 488–500.

13. James, C.J.; Hesse, C.W. Independent component analysis for biomedical signals. *Physiological Measurement* 2005, 26, 15–39.

14. Chaitanya, M.K.; Sharma, L.D. Electrocardiogram signal filtering using circulant singular spectrum analysis and cascaded Savitzky-Golay filter. *Biomedical Signal Processing and Control* 2022, 75, 103583.

15. Sharma, L.D., Chhabra, H., Chauhan, U., Saraswat, R.K., Sunkaria, R.K. Mental arithmetic task load recognition using EEG signal and Bayesian optimized K-nearest neighbor. *International Journal of Information Technology* 2021, 13(6), 2363–2369.

16. Sharma, L.D., Bohat, V.K., Habib, M., Ala', M.A.Z., Faris, H., Aljarah, I. Evolutionary inspired approach for mental stress detection using EEG signal. *Expert Systems with Applications* 2022, 197, 116634.

17. Niedermeyer, E.; Lopes da Silva, F.H. *Electroencephalography: Basic Principles, Clinical Applications, and Related Fields*, 5th ed.; Raven Press: New York, USA, 2005; pp. 654–660, ISBN 978–0781789424.

18. Jebelli, H.; Hwang, S.; Lee, S. EEG-based workers' stress recognition at construction sites. *Automation in Construction* 2018, 93, 315–324.

19. Urigüen, J.A.; Garciazapirain, B. EEG artifact removal—State-of-the-art and guidelines. *Journal of Neural Engineering* 2015,12, 031001.

20. Islam, M.K.; Rastegarnia, A.; Yang, Z. Methods for artifact detection and removal from scalp EEG: A review. *Clinical Neurophysiology* 2016, 46, 287–385.

21. Mcmenamin, B.W.; Shackman, A.J.; Greischar, L.L.; Davidson, R.J. Electromyogenic artifacts and electroencephalographic inferences revisited. *Neuroimage* 2011, 54, 4–9.

22. Garrick, L.W.; Robert, E.K.; Anita, M.; Jeffrey, F.C.; Nathan, A.F. Automatic correction of ocular artifacts in the EEG: A comparison of regression-based and component-based methods. *International Journal of Psychophysiology* 2004,53, 105–119.

23. Goncharova, I.I.; Mcfarland, D.J.; Vaughan, T.M.; Wolpaw, J.R. EMG contamination of EEG: Spectral and topographical characteristics. *Clinical Neurophysiology* 2003, 114, 1580–1593.

24. Chen, X.; Liu, A.; Chiang, J.; Wang, Z.J.; Mckeown, M.J.; Ward, R.K. Removing muscle artifacts from EEG data: Multichannel or single-channel techniques? *IEEE Sensors Journal* 2016, 16, 1986–1997.

25. Lee, K.J.; Park, C.; Lee, B. Elimination of ECG Artifacts from a Single-Channel EEG Using Sparse Derivative Method. In *Proceedings of the 2015 IEEE International Conference on Systems,* Man, and Cybernetics, Kowloon, China, 9–12 October 2015.

26. Qin, Y.; Xu, P.; Yao, D. A comparative study of different references for EEG default mode network: The use of the infinity reference. *Clinical Neurophysiology* 2010, 121, 1981–1991.

27. Abdullah, A.K.; Zhang, C.Z.; Abdullah, A.A.A.; Lian, S. Automatic extraction system for common artifacts in EEG signals based on evolutionary stone's BSS algorithm. *Mathematical Problems in Engineering* 2014, 2014, 324750.

28. Zhang, A.; Li, W. Adaptive Noise Cancellation for Removing Cardiac and Respiratory Artifacts from EEG Recordings. In *5th World Congress on Intelligent Control and Automation,* Hangzhou, China, pp. 15–19, June 2004.

29. Izzetoglu, M.; Devaraj, A.; Bunce, S.; Onaral, B. Motion artifact cancellation in NIR spectroscopy using Wiener filtering. *IEEE Transactions on Biomedical Engineering* 2005, 52, 934–938.

30. Mijović, B.; De Vos, M.; Gligorijević, I.; Taelman, J.; Van Huffel, S. Source separation from single-channel recordings by combining empirical-mode decomposition and independent component analysis. *IEEE Transactions on Biomedical Engineering* 2010, 57(9), 2188–2196.

31. Jiang, X.; Bian, G.B.; Tian, Z. Removal of artifacts from EEG signals: A review. *Sensors* 2019, 19(5), 987.

32. Roy, V.; Shukla, S. A survey on artifacts detection techniques for electro-encephalography (EEG) signals. *International Journal of Multimedia and Ubiquitous Engineering* 2015, 10(3), 425–442.

33. Wang, G.; Teng, C.; Li, K.; Zhang, Z.; Yan, X. The removal of EOG artifacts from EEG signals using independent component analysis and multivariate empirical mode decomposition. *IEEE Journal of Biomedical and Health Informatics* 2016, 20(5), 1301–1308.

34. De Clercq, W.; Vergult, A.; Vanrumste, B.; Van Paesschen, W.; Van Huffel, S. Canonical correlation analysis applied to remove muscle artifacts from the electroencephalogram. *IEEE Transactions on Biomedical Engineering* 2006, 53(12), 2583–2587.

35. Khatun, S.; Mahajan, R.; Morshed, B.I. Comparative study of wavelet-based unsupervised ocular artifact removal techniques for single channel EEG data. *IEEE Journal of Translational Engineering in Health and Medicine* 2016, 4, 2000108.

36. Yang, B.; Zhang, T.; Zhang, Y.; Liu, W.; Wang, J.; Duan, K. Removal of electrooculogram artifacts from electroencephalogram using canonical correlation analysis with ensemble empirical mode decomposition. *Cognitive Computation* 2017, 9(5), 626–633.

37. Karatoprak, E.; Seker, S. An improved empirical mode decomposition method using variable window median filter for early fault detection in electric motors. *Mathematical Problems in Engineering* 2019, 2019, 8015295.

38. Xu, S.; Hu, H.; Ji, L.; Wang, P. Embedding dimension selection for adaptive singular spectrum analysis of EEG signal. *Sensors* 2018, 18(3), 697.

39. Reinmar, K.; Andreea, S.; Catarina, D.; Andreas, S.; Valeria, M.; Gernot, M.-P. *EEG EEG Eye Artifact Dataset*, 2020, https://doi.org/10.17605/OSF.IO/2QGRD, https://osf.io/2qgrd/

40. Chen, Y.; Zhao, Q.; Hu, B.; Li, J.; Jiang, H.; Lin, W. et al., A method of removing ocular artifacts from EEG using discrete wavelet transform and kalman filtering. In *IEEE International Conference on Bioinformatics and Biomedicine,* Shenzhen, pp. 15–18, December 2016.

41. Raghavendra, B.S.; Dutt, D.N. Wavelet enhanced CCA for minimization of ocular and muscle artifacts in EEG. *World Academy of Science, Engineering, and Technology* 2011, 5(9), 419–424.

42. Chen, X.; Xu, X.; Liu, A.; Mckeown, M.J.; Wang, Z.J. The use of multivariate EMD and CCA for denoising muscle artifacts from few-channel EEG recordings. *IEEE Transactions on Instrumentation and Measurement* 2018, 67(2) 359–370.

43. Peng, H.; Hu, B.; Shi, Q.; Ratcliffe, M.; Zhao, Q.; Qi, Y. et al. Removal of ocular artifacts in EEG: An improved approach combining DWT and ANC for portable applications. *IEEE Journal of Biomedical and Health Informatics* 2013, 17(3), 600–607.

44. Maddirala, A.K.; Shaik, R.A. Removal of EOG artifacts from single channel EEG signals using combined singular spectrum analysis and adaptive noise canceler. *IEEE Sensors Journal* 2019, 16(23), 8279–8287.

45. Zou, L.; Chen, X.; Dang, G.; Guo, Y.; Wang, Z.J. Removing muscle artifacts from EEG data via underdetermined joint blind source separation: A simulation study. *IEEE Transactions on Circuits and Systems II: Express Briefs* 2020, 67(1), 187–191.

46. Klados, M. A semi-simulated EEG/EOG dataset for the comparison of EOG artifact rejection techniques. *Data Brief* 2019, 8, 1004–1006. https://doi.org/10.17632/WB6YVR725D.4

47. Hamid, A.; Gagliano, K.; Rahman, S.; Tulin, N.; Tchiong, V.; Obeid, I.; Picone, J. The temple university artifact corpus: An annotated corpus of EEG artifacts. In *IEEE Signal Processing in Medicine and Biology Symposium (SPMB),* Philadelphia, PA, USA, (n.d.). https://par.nsf.gov/biblio/10199675

48. Tangermann, M.; Müller, K.R.; Aertsen, A.; Birbaumer, N.; Braun, C.; Brunner, C.; Leeb, R.; Mehring, C.; Miller, K.J.; Mueller-Putz, G.; Nolte, G. Review of the BCI competition IV. *Frontiers in Neuroscience* 2012, 6, 55.

49. Mahajan, R.; Morshed, B.I. Unsupervised eye blink artifact denoising of EEG data with modified multiscale sample entropy, kurtosis, and wavelet-ICA. *IEEE Journal of Biomedical and Health Informatics* 2015, 19(1), 158–165.

50. Mannan, M.M.N.; Kamran, M.A.; Jeong, M.Y. Identification and removal of physiological artifacts from electroencephalogram signals: A review. *IEEE Access* 2018, 6, 30630–30652.

51. Liu, Q.; Liu, A.; Zhang, X.; Chen, X.; Qian, R.; Chen, X. Removal of EMG artifacts from multichannel EEG signals using combined singular spectrum analysis and canonical correlation analysis. *Journal of Healthcare Engineering* 2019, 2019, 4159676.

52. Chavez, M.; Grosselin, F.; Bussalb, A.; Fallani, F.D.V.; Navarro-Sune, X. Surrogate-based artifact removal from single-channel EEG. *IEEE Transactions on Neural Systems and Rehabilitation Engineering* 2018, 26(3), 540–550.

53. Acharjee, P.P.; Phlypo, R.; Wu, L.; Calhoun, V.D.; Adalı, T. Independent vector analysis for gradient artifact removal in concurrent EEG-fMRI data. *IEEE Transactions on Biomedical Engineering* 2015, 62(7), 1750–1758.

54. Yedukondalu, J.; Sharma, L.D. Circulant singular spectrum analysis and discrete wavelet transform for automated removal of EOG artifacts from EEG signals. *Sensors* 2023, 23(3), 1235.

55. Dai, C.; Wang, J.; Xie, J.; Li, W.; Gong, Y.; Li, Y. Removal of ECG artifacts from EEG using an effective recursive least square notch filter. *IEEE Access* 2019, 7, 158872–158880.

8 Multi-Channel and Multi-Label Decision-Making System (MCL-DMS) for Sleep Stage and Sleep Disorder Recognition from EEG Signals

Yi-Hsuan Cheng, Margaret Lech,
and Richardt H. Wilkinson

8.1 INTRODUCTION

Sleep is an essential part of our human life; it spans about one-third of our lifetime. Insufficient sleep affects a person's mental and physical health and may lead to many other undesirable consequences. To give some examples, insufficient sleep decreases the ability to regulate body temperature, weakens the immune system, increases blood pressure, creates difficulty in controlling blood sugar levels, reduces the efficiency of the digestive system, and increases the risk of cardiovascular disease. Sleep disorders can exacerbate fatigue, anxiety, and depression. A lousy sleep leads to poor memory and lack of concentration which can increase the risk of accidents (Walker 2018). It is therefore essential to develop means of accurate assessment of sleep quality. This type of assessment is often referred to as sleep scoring. At present, sleep scoring is conducted manually by highly qualified experts making a visual inspection of lengthy time waveforms recorded overnight by multiple EEG electrodes. In addition to EEG, other related signals such as electrocardiograms (ECG), electromyograms (EMG), or body movements can also be inspected to support the diagnosis. The marking process follows sleep-scoring standards outlined by the American Academy of Sleep Medicine (Berry et al. 2013) or the Rechtschaffen and Kales standard (Kales and Rechtschaffen 1968). Since a typical recording time of EEG is eight hours, the process is expensive, tedious, and time-consuming. The sleep experts have to undergo years of training to spot multiple correlated factors contributing

DOI: 10.1201/9781003252092-10

to specific types of sleep disorders. The observations are described by giving score labels to selected time intervals of the recordings. For example, W is typically used as a label for the wake, S1–S4 for sleep stages, and R for rapid eye movement (REM) states. Some of the most often encountered sleep disorders are labeled as insomnia, bruxism, narcolepsy, nocturnal frontal lobe epilepsy (NFLE), periodic leg movement (PLM), REM behavioral disorder, and sleep-disordered breathing (SDB). To ensure high-quality, accurate labeling, at least two experts independently score the same recordings, and a third person checks the scoring for consistency. Despite these measures, the process is still prone to human error. EEGs are routinely used to monitor brain activities, analyze sleep stages, and diagnose sleep disorders. The EEG data collection procedure is conducted during overnight polysomnography (PSG) (Biswal et al. 2017; Acharya et al. 2018). It uses an array of sensors placed on different parts of the patient's head. Due to the recent developments in machine learning (ML), automatic EEG analysis and sleep scoring have attracted attention of researchers. A steadily growing body of research offers different ML approaches to sleep scoring. For easier cross-validation and comparison, sleep studies tend to validate the proposed methods using the same datasets of EEG recordings.

This study contributes by introducing a new automatic scoring system annotating the EEG sleep data with sleep stage and sleep disorder labels. The system eliminates the need for arbitrary decision-making schemes and compensates for the training data imbalance. The information fusion between sleep stage and sleep disorder enhances the classification accuracy. We validate the proposed MCL-DMS against baseline approaches using a dataset from the Sleep Disorders Center of the Ospedale Maggiore of Parma, Italy [cyclic alternating pattern (CAP)] (Terzano et al. 2001).

8.2 RELATED WORKS

Traditional sleep scoring techniques rely on the costly and time-consuming manual evaluation of PSGs. However, recent ML advancements offer the possibility of automating this process. The research progressively improves the automatic scoring process starting from the relatively simple single-modality and single-label diagnosis and gradually progressing toward the ultimate but, at the same time, more challenging multi-modal and multi-label scoring.

The current body of work is dominated by sleep stage recognition techniques from EEG, ECG, and other related signals in a single-modality approach. Many of these studies detect sleep stages in healthy subjects to eliminate confounding factors and simplify the process. For example, Kim et al. (2017) used the heart rate variability (HRV) recordings from the CAP database to classify three sleep stages in healthy individuals (wake, light sleep, and deep sleep). The classification was based on the noise-reduced fractal properties of the HRV that were found to be indicative of the sleep stage. A sensitivity of 77% and specificity of 73% were reported for the three sleep-stage categories and 72% accuracy in distinguishing between deep and light sleep. In another example, Sharma et al. (2018) applied EEG recordings of healthy people from the Sleep EDF database to detect six sleep stages [wake W, four sleep levels (from light sleep to deep sleep) S1, S2, S3, and S4, and rapid eye movement R]. A traditional processing framework was applied where features extracted from the EEG waveforms were used to train the support vector machine (SVM) model. The features included log energy, signal fractal dimension, and sample entropy. An average accuracy of 91.5% was reported. Timplalexis et al. (2019) also used the Sleep EDF database to classify five sleep stages of healthy people. However, in this study, a mixture of time and frequency domain features was used to train the ensemble of bagged trees (EBT) classifier. An average accuracy approaching 89% was reported.

From the detection of sleep stages in healthy individuals, the research progressed toward the detection of sleep stages in both healthy people and people suffering from sleep disorders. For example, Tripathi et al. (2020) investigated the detection of six sleep stages from EEG recordings of four groups of individuals (healthy, bruxism, insomnia, sleep-disordered breathing, and REM behavior disorder). The recordings were sourced from the CAP database (Terzano et al. 2001). Entropy features calculated within separate spectral bands of the wavelet transform were used to train a hybrid learning classifier. The classifier applied class-specific residuals and distances from nearest neighbors to categorize sleep stages in a pairwise binary manner. The results reveal accuracies of 91.77%, 88.14%, 80.13%, and 73.88% for the automated categorization of wake vs. sleep, wake vs. REM vs. non-REM, wake vs. light sleep vs. deep sleep vs. REM sleep, and wake vs. S1-sleep vs. S2-sleep vs. S3-sleep vs. REM sleep schemes, respectively. No disorder-specific observations were reported. Sharma et al. (2021) used the EEG data of individuals representing eight sleep ailment categories (healthy, insomnia, bruxism, narcolepsy, NFLE, PLM disorder, REM behavior disorder, and sleep-disordered breathing) to detect six sleep stages. The data source was the CAP database (Terzano et al. 2001). Statistical norm features were used to train an ensemble of the EBT classifier. The highest average accuracy achieved was 85.3%.

Alongside sleep-stage detection methods, several studies investigated the related problem of sleep disorder diagnosis. In this case, instead of labels denoting sleep stages, the training data were marked with the type of sleep ailment. Sharma et al. (2021) analyzed ECG signals from the CAP database to distinguish between two categories of sleep i.e., healthy and insomnia. The statistical norm features extracted from wavelet transform sub-bands were applied to train two sleep disorder recognition classifiers, K-nearest neighbor (KNN) and SVM.

The SVM provided the highest accuracy of 97.87% when using features from the REM sleep stage only. Widasari et al. (2020) used ECG signals from the CAP database to detect four categories of sleep disorders (healthy, insomnia, sleep-disordered breathing, and REM behavior disorder). Spectral and speech quality features extracted from ECG recordings were applied to train the ensemble of the EBT classifiers. The experimental results led to 84.01% sensitivity, 94.17% specificity, and 86.27% accuracy. It was also shown that the proposed method could efficiently classify sleep disorders using the 30-second intervals of ECG data. Sharma et al. (2021) used EEG signals from the CAP database (Terzano et al. 2001) to detect sleep disorders. Time-domain statistical features known as Hjorth parameters were used in two different ways. The first method used the EBT classifier to detect four categories (healthy, insomnia, sleep-disordered breathing, and REM behavior disorder). The accuracy achieved was 96.5%. The second method applied the EBT and boosted trees to detect six categories (healthy, narcolepsy, NFLE, PLM disorder,

REM behavior disorder, and sleep-disordered breathing). The average accuracy, in this case, was 91.3%. A multi-modal approach combining Hjorth features from two modalities [electrooculogram (EOG) and EMG] was recently investigated by Sharma et al. (2022). The Hjorth features were applied to train an EBT model leading to 94.3% accuracy in detecting six categories (healthy, insomnia, narcolepsy, NFLE, PLM disorder, and REM behavior disorder).

While the single-modality, single-label scoring of sleep data is well advanced, very few examples of efficient multi-modal and multi-label studies exist. Therefore, in this study, we would like to address this gap and propose a new multi-label sleep stage and sleep disorder classification system from a single modality represented by EEG data.

8.3 METHODOLOGY

8.3.1 STRUCTURE OF THE NN SYSTEM

The proposed MCL-DMS approach shown in Figure 8.1 was designed to identify the sleep stage and the sleep disorder from the same data sample of the EEG signal simultaneously. It consists of two levels of classification. The first level includes two groups of five single-label classification channels, one group identifying the sleep stage and the other group the sleep disorder. Each channel has its own separate convolutional neural network (CNN) classifier. The five groups correspond to five different sets of EEG electrodes. The classification outcomes (soft probability vectors) given by these two groups of channels are concatenated and passed to two second-stage classifiers structured as fully connected shallow NNs. One of the networks is trained to identify the sleep stage, and the other is trained to identify the sleep disorder. This way, sleep stage and sleep disorder are identified twice. The difference is that during the first stage of classification, each CNN makes its decision based on the physical EEG data having only one label representing either sleep stage or sleep disorder. In contrast, each of the second-stage NNs makes the decision using a combined sleep stage and sleep disorder information in the form of concatenated metadata (probability vectors). The shallow NNs make the final diagnostic decision by arbitrating between decisions made by two first-level assessors. The first-level assessors work with limited single-label information; therefore, their decisions may not always be correct. The second-level assessors can compensate for these limitations by working with two-label information. For example, certain sleep disorders may be associated with specific sleep stages; therefore, knowing the sleep stage could enhance the accuracy of disorder detection.

8.3.2 PRE-PROCESSING

8.3.2.1 EEG Time Waveforms

The EEG recordings represented time waveforms collected from electrodes placed on patients' heads, as shown in Figure 8.2 (Klem et al. 1999). The sampling frequency was 512 Hz, providing a signal bandwidth of 256 Hz. We have normalized the amplitudes of all recordings to the range of ±1. For the classification of the sleep stage, time waveforms recorded from five electrodes, C, F, O, P, and T (Table 8.1) were used. Whereas to classify sleep disorders, time waveforms from three electrodes,

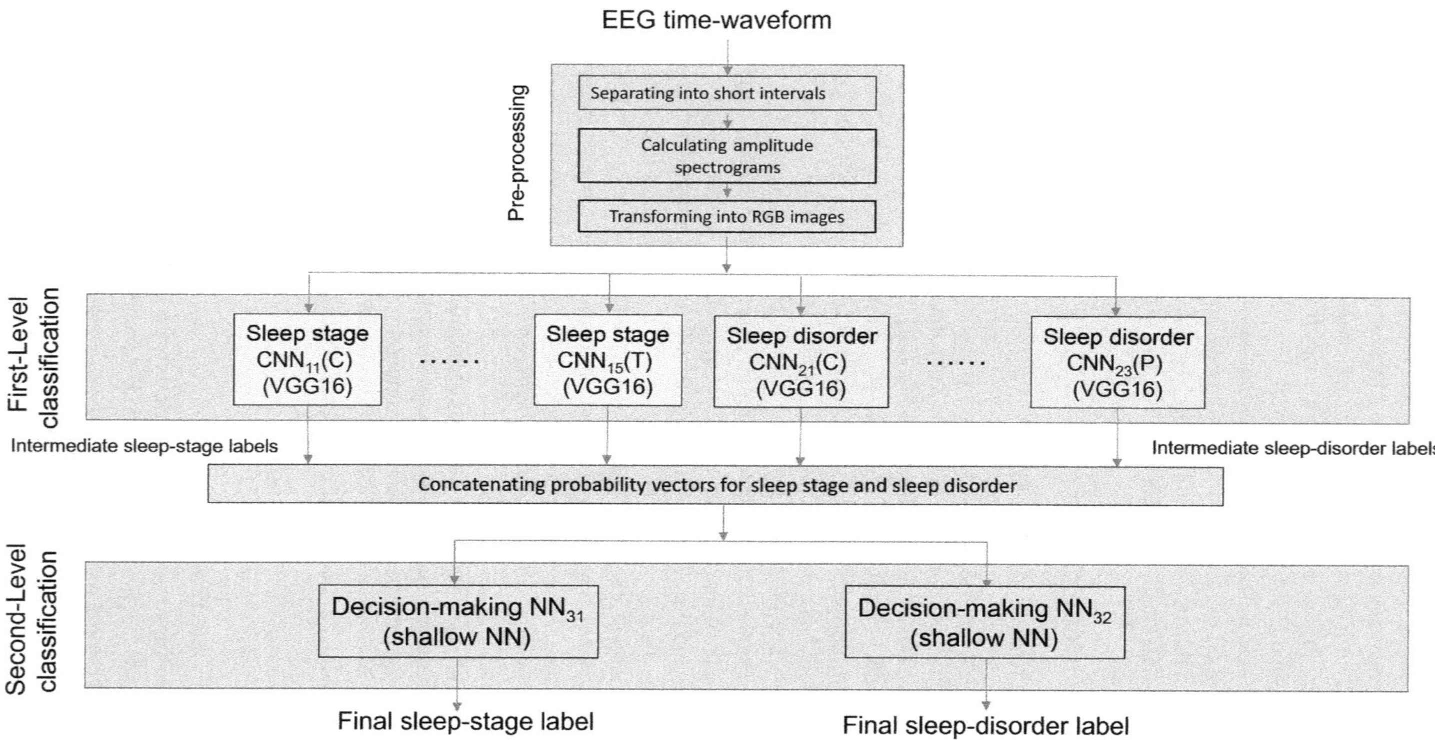

FIGURE 8.1   Diagram showing the proposed MCL-DMS for sleep stage and sleep disorder classification from EEG signals.

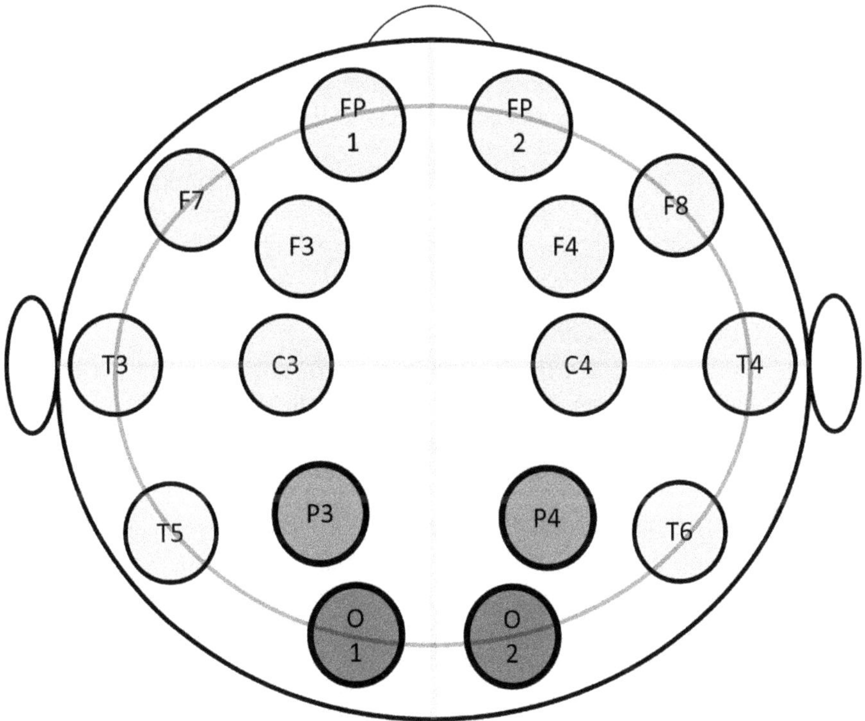

FIGURE 8.2 Positions of EEG electrodes on a person's head according to the 10–20 electrode system described in Ref. [10] (Based on Klem et al. 1999).

TABLE 8.1

Names and Groups of EEG Electrodes Used in Sleep Stage and Sleep Disorder Detection Experiments

Group Name	As per Figure 8.2 (Klem et al. 1999)	Used in Sleep Stage Detection	Used in Sleep Disorder Detection
C	C-R, C-S1, C-S2, C-S3, C-S4, and C-W	Yes	Yes
F	F-R, F-S1, F-S2, F-S3, F-S4, and F-W	Yes	Yes
O	O-R, O-S1, O-S2, O-S3, O-S4, and O-W	Yes	No
P	P-R, P-S1, P-S2, P-S3, P-S4, and P-W	Yes	Yes
T	T-R, T-S1, T-S2, T-S3, T-S4, and T-W	Yes	No

C, F, and P (Table 8.1), were used. Since we aimed to train one of the existing CNN architectures (VGG16) optimized for 2-D image array classification, the EEG waveform recordings were transformed into image representations.

8.3.2.2   Separating into Short Intervals

Raw EEG recordings (time waveforms) collected during about eight hours of sleep were divided into short 10-second intervals. The sleep stage and the sleep disorder labels for each interval were kept the same as those for the recording samples from which these cuttings were made. By applying a one-second stride, there was a 90% overlap between subsequent intervals. With such a significant overlap, we could generate a relatively large number of training data samples required to train deep-learning models. Examples of 10-second intervals of EEG time waveforms for different sleep stages and sleep disorders are presented in Figure 8.3.

8.3.2.3   Calculating Amplitude Spectrograms

For each 10-second interval, a linear amplitude spectrogram was calculated using the short-time Fourier transform. The linear frequency scale was determined experimentally to be most suitable by performing comparison tests with logarithmic frequency scales. The time axis of the spectrograms was also linear.

8.3.2.4   Transforming into RGB Images

The VGG16 architecture was designed to accommodate color input images formatted as three 2D color planes (R, G, and B); it was assumed that the optimal input to such a network should also be given in this format. We have therefore transformed the amplitude spectrogram arrays into color RGB images. The conversion process applied the "Jet" colormap from MathWorks MATLAB (The MathWorks, Inc.). The colormap amplitude range in dB was normalized separately for each group of electrodes by mapping into each group's average minimum and maximum spectral amplitudes calculated across the entire database (Lech et al. 2020). Examples of the resulting spectrogram images for different sleep stages and sleep disorders are shown in Figure 8.3.

8.3.3   First-Level Classification

As shown in Figure 8.1, the first-level classification included two groups of CNN classifiers. The first group was trained to recognize the sleep stage using data provided by five groups of electrodes (C, F, O, P, and T), with each group used to train a separate classifier CNN_{11}–CNN_{15}, respectively. Six sleep stages [wake (W), sleep stages (S1, S2, S3, and S4), and rapid eye movement I] were categorized. The second group was trained to recognize the sleep disorder using data provided by three groups of electrodes (C, F, and P). Each group was used to train a separate classifier CNN_{21}–CNN_{23}. Eight sleep disorders [neutral (N), bruxism (B), insomnia (I), narcolepsy (Na), NFLE (Nf), PLM (P), REM behavior disorder (R), and sleep-disordered breathing (S)] were categorized. The VGG16 CNN model architecture (Qassim et al. 2018; Simonyan and Zisserman 2015) was trained from scratch in all first-level classification channels; no transfer learning was applied. The VGG16 network structure consisted of thirteen 2D convolutional layers and three fully connected layers. The ReLu activation function was used, and the learning rate was set to 0.001.

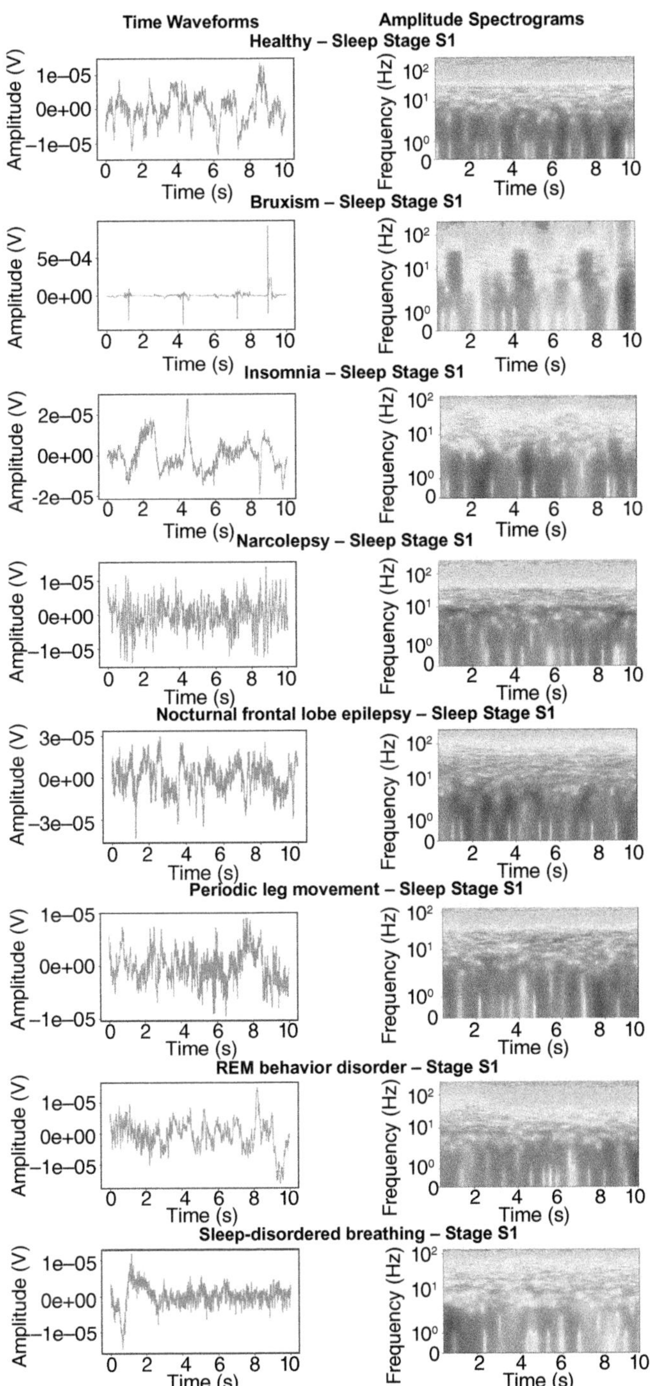

FIGURE 8.3 Examples of EEG time waveforms (10-second intervals) and the correspond-ing spectrograms for the sleep stage S1; healthy sleep; and six sleep disorders: bruxism, insomnia, narcolepsy, NFLE, PLM, REM behavior disorder, and sleep-disordered breathing.

8.3.4   Concatenating Probability Vectors

The probability vectors generated by all the first-level CNNs were concatenated into a single vector P_i providing an input to the second-stage shallow NN classifier. Assuming that N is the total number of training images, $M_1 = 5$ is the number of parallel classification channels (or CNNs) designated to classify the sleep stages; $M_2 = 3$ is the number of parallel first-level classification channels designated to classify the sleep disorder; $C_1 = 6$ is the number of sleep stage categories; and $C_2 = 8$ is the number of sleep disorder categories; for a given image i $(i = 1, \ldots, N)$, we can write the concatenated input vector P_i as

$$P_i = \left\{ \left\{ \mathrm{SP}_{i,j} \right\}_{j=1,\ldots,M_1}, \left\{ \mathrm{DP}_{i,k} \right\}_{k=1,\ldots,M_2} \right\} \tag{8.1}$$

Where SP denotes the probability vectors generated by the five sleep-stage recognition channels (groups of electrodes), and DP corresponds to the probability vectors generated by the three sleep disorder recognition channels. Assuming that sp denotes a scalar probability value of a given sleep stage category, and dp is the scalar probability value of a given sleep disorder category, Eq. (8.1) can be rewritten in a more detailed form as

$$P_i = \left\{ \left\{ \left\{ \mathrm{sp}_{i,j,l} \right\}_{l=1,\ldots C_1} \right\}_{j=1,\ldots,M_1}, \left\{ \left\{ \mathrm{dp}_{i,k,m} \right\}_{m=1,\ldots C_2} \right\}_{k=1,\ldots,M_2} \right\} \tag{8.2}$$

8.3.5   Second-Level Classification

The second-stage decision-making network was a shallow perceptron NN with fully connected layers. It consisted of an input layer and two hidden layers. The size of the input layer was equal to the size of the concatenated probability vectors given by the first-stage classifiers. At the same time, the output layer was equal to the number of categories identified by the NN (i.e., six for the sleep stage classification or eight for the sleep disorder classification). Both hidden layers were of size 128 nodes. The ReLu node activation function was used.

8.3.6   Performance Measures

As measures of the classification performance, we used the average classification accuracy A_C and $F1$ score. The classification accuracy was calculated as

$$A_c = \frac{\mathrm{TP} + \mathrm{TN}}{\mathrm{TP} + \mathrm{TN} + \mathrm{FP} + \mathrm{FN}} \tag{8.3}$$

Where TP, TN, FP, FN represent the numbers of true positive, true negative, false positive, and false negative classification outcomes, respectively. Due to the unbalanced training data across different sleep stages and sleep disorder categories, we have also used the $F1$ score to determine if the model has a margin for improvement. It was given as

$$F1 \text{ score} = \frac{2 * \mathrm{Recall} * \mathrm{Precision}}{\mathrm{Recall} + \mathrm{Precision}} \tag{8.4}$$

where the recall and precision parameters were calculated as

$$\text{Recall} = \frac{\text{TP}}{\text{TP} + \text{FN}} \tag{8.5}$$

$$\text{Precision} = \frac{\text{TP}}{\text{TP} + \text{FP}} \tag{8.6}$$

When the training data contains an imbalanced class representation, high average accuracy across classes can be achieved; however, it is often associated with an uneven distribution of accuracies across individual classes. Highly represented categories achieve higher accuracy, and less represented categories a lower accuracy. This is reflected by low $F1$ scores, which allow us to determine the levels of misclassification. The ultimate goal is to achieve high values of both accuracy and $F1$ scores.

8.4 EXPERIMENTS

8.4.1 DATA DESCRIPTION

The proposed MCL-DMS, and the baseline approaches, were tested using the CAP of the EEG Activity During Sleep database (Terzano et al. 2001) collected at the Sleep Disorders Center of the Ospedale Maggiore of Parma, Italy. It contains EEG and other modality recordings representing normal and pathological sleep conditions. In this study, we have used only the EEG recordings. Table 8.2 shows the six sleep-stage categories, the eight sleep-disorder categories, and the numbers of corresponding spectrogram images used to train models recognizing these categories.

TABLE 8.2

CAP Data Categories and the Numbers of Spectrogram Images Used to Train the Classifiers for the Sleep Stage and Sleep Disorder Detection

Sleep Stage	Number of Images	Sleep Disorder	Number of Images
Wake (W)	218,142	Bruxism (B)	55,978
Stage S1	43,605	Insomnia (I)	193,548
Stage S2	391,109	Normal (N)	325,292
Stage S3	115,127	Narcolepsy (Na)	96,077
Stage S4	147,348	NFLE (Nf)	161,694
Rapid Eye Movement I	194,823	PLM (P)	100,473
Total	1,110,154	REM behavior disorder (REM)	122,388
		Sleep-disordered breathing (S)	54,690
		Total	1,110,140

The CAP database is one of the most popular and frequently used research datasets. The sleep stage and sleep disorder labels allowed us to design a multi-label sleep annotation approach. In addition, the length of the CAP recordings was sufficient to train ML models.

8.4.2 Experiments and Results

8.4.2.1 Experimental Schedule

To generate a comparison baseline for the proposed MCL-DMS, we have conducted experiments using classical single-channel and single-label approaches.

We start with Experiment 1, investigating the performance of a single CNN classifier trained either to detect the sleep stage or the sleep disorder. We compare individual performances of different groups of electrodes.

In Experiment 2, we investigate the first version of the MCL-DMS approach (MCL-DMS1). It comprises two independent sub-systems, one for the sleep stage and one for the sleep disorder. However, each system contains a number of electrode groups (multiple channels); each group with its own CNN and shallow decision-making NN. We compare the NN decision-making with conventional decision-making rules.

Finally, in Experiment 3, we test the performance of the proposed multi-channel and multi-label MCL-DMS2 approach for the simultaneous classification of sleep stage and sleep disorder.

In all experimental scenarios, the training/testing procedures were repeated three times, each time with different mutually exclusive training and testing sets. The results were calculated as average values over the three runs.

8.4.2.2 Experiment 1 – Single-Channel and Single-Label Classification

In this experiment, we create a simple baseline classification scenario where EEG signals from a given group of electrodes are classified by a single VGG16 network. Five groups of electrodes classify the sleep stage, and three other groups of electrodes the sleep disorder (Figure 8.4). Table 8.3 shows the average accuracy and the $F1$ scores achieved.

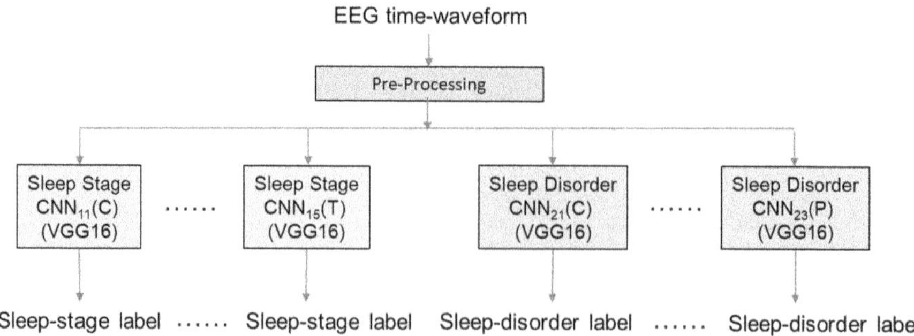

FIGURE 8.4 Experiment 1: Single-channel classification of sleep stages using five channels (groups of electrodes) and sleep disorders using three channels.

TABLE 8.3

Experiment 1: Average Accuracy and *F*1 Scores for Different Channels (Electrode Groups)

Sleep Stage Classification			Sleep Disorder Classification		
Electrode Group (Channel)	Average Accuracy (%)	*F*1 Score	Electrode Group (Channel)	Average Accuracy (%)	*F*1 Score
C	57.27	0.42	C	64.19	0.59
F	55.40	0.43	F	79.05	0.78
O	66.27	0.54	P	74.79	0.75
P	57.46	0.45			
T	55.23	0.43			

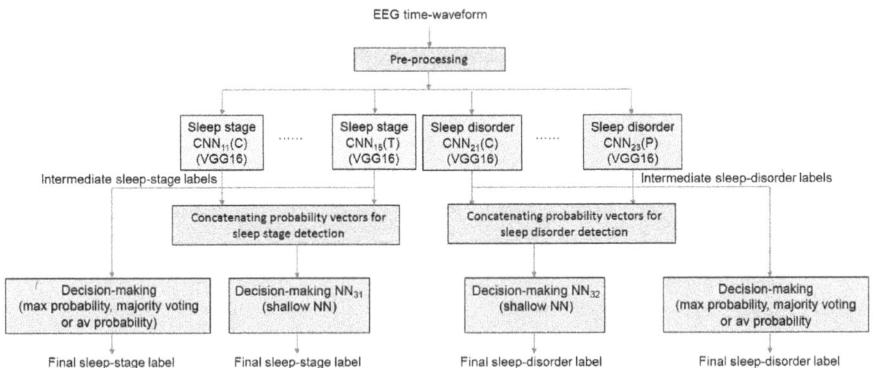

FIGURE 8.5 Experiment 2: Simultaneous multi-channel and multi-label classification of sleep stage and sleep disorder using the first version of the multi-channel decision-making system (MCL-DMS1) with no sleep stage and sleep disorder information fusion.

8.4.2.3 Experiment 2 – Multi-Channel and MCL-DMS1 without Information Fusion between Sleep Stage and Sleep Disorder

In this experiment, we investigate the first version of the multi-channel decision-making system (MCL-DMS1) without information fusion between sleep stage and sleep disorder. It consists of two separate classification branches (Figure 8.5), one for the sleep stage and one for the sleep disorder. Each branch contains groups of electrodes (multiple channels), each group with its own CNN. Classifiers $CNN_{11} - CNN_{15}$ classify the sleep stage and $CNN_{21} - CNN_{23}$ the sleep disorder. Since, in both cases, sleep stage and sleep disorder, the same EEG data are assessed by multiple classifiers, a disagreement between channels (assessors) could occur. For this reason, a decision-making mechanism had to be employed. However, no information fusion between the sleep stage and sleep disorder is applied. To achieve this, all the sleep stage detection CNNs pass their results to a single shallow decision-making NN for the sleep stage recognition (NN_{31}), and all the sleep disorder detection CNNs pass their results to the shallow decision-making NN for the sleep disorder recognition

(NN_{32}). Alternatively, the CNN outcomes can be sent to one of the conventional decision-making units, including maximum probability, majority voting, and average probability. This way, we could test and compare four different decision-making mechanisms. The average accuracy and $F1$ scores achieved by the MCL-DMS1 are presented in Table 8.4.

8.4.2.4 Experiment 3 – Multi-Channel Decision-Making System (MC-DMS2) with Information Fusion between Sleep Stage and Sleep Disorder

This experiment investigates the second version of the multi-channel and MCL-DMS2 with information fusion between sleep stage and sleep disorder. Like in MCL-DMS1, there are two separate classification branches (Figure 8.6), one for the sleep stage and one for the sleep disorder. Each branch contains groups of electrodes (multiple

TABLE 8.4

Experiment 2: Average Accuracy and $F1$ Scores for the MCL-DMS1 Using Different Decision-Making Methods

Sleep Stage Classification			Sleep Disorder Classification		
Decision-Making Method	Average Accuracy (%)	F1 Score		Average Accuracy (%)	F1 Score
Max Probability	78.35	0.63		88.63	0.89
Majority Voting	75.79	0.57		83.77	0.84
Average Probability	42.01	0.34		46.94	0.44
Shallow NN	92.17	0.85		95.08	0.95

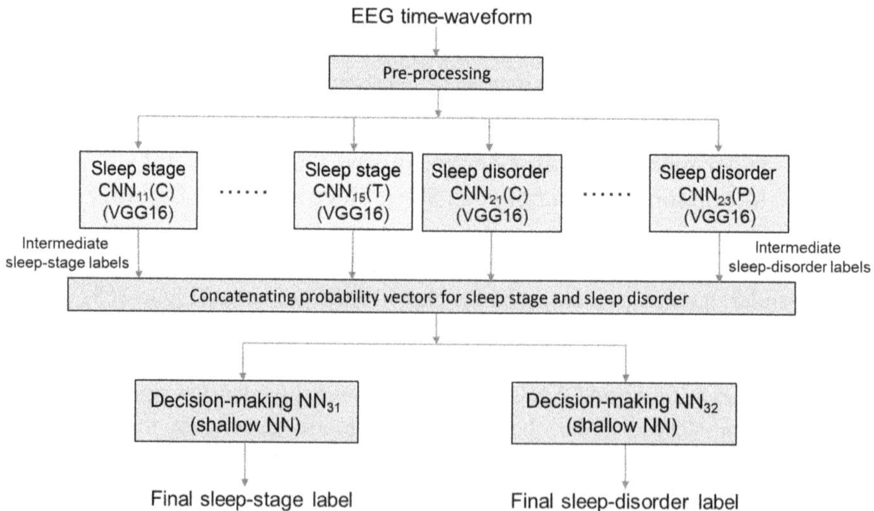

FIGURE 8.6 Experiment 3: Simultaneous multi-channel and multi-label classification of sleep stage and sleep disorder using the second version of the MCL-DMS2 with sleep stage and sleep disorder information fusion.

TABLE 8.5

Experiment 3: Average Accuracy and *F*1 Scores for the MCL-DMS2

Sleep Stage Classification		Sleep Disorder Classification	
Average Accuracy (%)	*F*1 Score	Average Accuracy (%)	*F*1 Score
94.19	0.90	96.02	0.96

channels) with the corresponding CNNs; $CNN_{11} - CNN_{15}$ classify the sleep stage and $CNN_{21} - CNN_{23}$ the sleep disorder. The information from both branches is fused by concatenating the probability vectors and then passing them to the two final decision-making shallow NNs, one for sleep stage recognition (NN_{31}) and one for sleep disorder recognition (NN_{32}). Due to the fusion of information, each NN makes the decision using two labels (sleep stage and sleep disorder) generated by the first-level assessors (CNNs). In contrast, the NNs in the MCL-DMS1 were only getting single-label information from the first-level assessors. The average accuracies and $F1$ scores achieved by the MCL-DMS2 are presented in Table 8.5.

8.4.3 Discussion

Combined outcomes of Experiments 1–3 shown in Figure 8.7 led to several observations regarding the relative performance of the proposed MCL-DMS and the baseline approaches. In the following sections, we have summarized these observations.

8.4.3.1 Comparison between Different Classification Methods

The clear winner showing the best performance for both sleep stage and sleep disorder recognition in terms of accuracy and $F1$ score is the proposed MCL-DMS2. It gives an average accuracy of 94% ($F1$ score 0.90) for the sleep stage and 96% ($F1$ score 0.96) for sleep disorder recognition. It is followed by the MCL-DMS1-NN with 92.2% ($F1$ score 0.85) for the sleep stage and 95% ($F1$ score 0.95) for sleep disorder recognition. The higher $F1$ scores reached by the MCL-DMS1-NN and MCL-DMS2 compared to all other approaches show that the two-level classification with the shallow decision-making NN provides an efficient compensation for the training data imbalance and leads to equally high accuracy across all classes. As expected, the single-channel methods that use only a single CNN classifier (Group C-, F-, O-, P-, and T - CNN for sleep stage and Group C-, F-, and P - CNN for sleep disorder) achieved the lowest performance in terms of the accuracy and $F1$ scores. It indicates that the training data imbalance for the single-channel methods leads to uneven accuracy distribution across classes, with classes with a higher representation having higher accuracy than classes with a lower representation.

8.4.3.2 Comparison between Different Decision-Making Rules in the Multi-Channel and Multi-Label Classification

One of the advantages underlying the MCL-DMS structure's design was the elimination of arbitrary decision-making. Conventional multi-channel decision-making systems use arbitrary rules assuming that, for example, the final decision should be

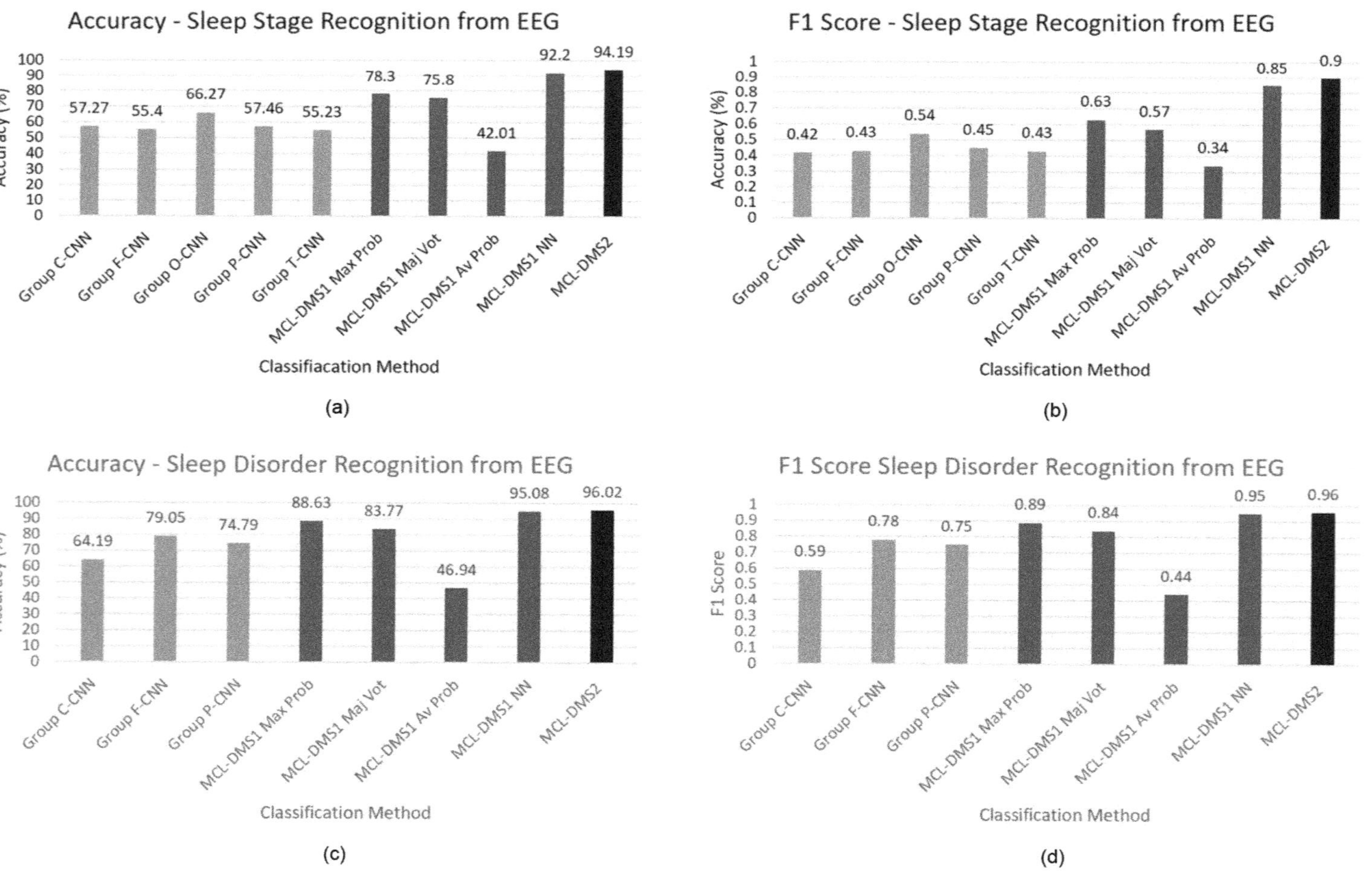

FIGURE 8.7 Average accuracies and F1 scores across different methods for the sleep-stage recognition (a) and (b), and sleep disorder recognition (c) and (d).

derived as an average (maximum or most voted) outcome from multiple assessment channels. Instead of using one of these rules, we have trained shallow NNs to arbitrate between outcomes from multiple assessment channels. Figure 8.7 shows that for both labels (sleep stage and sleep disorders), the shallow decision-making NNs (NN_{31} and NN_{32}) applied within the MCL-DMS1 structure (Figure 8.5) outperformed all three arbitrary rules (majority voting, average probability, and maximum probability). The best-performing arbitrary decision-making rule was maximum probability, followed by majority voting and the least-performing rule was average probability.

8.4.3.3 Comparison between MCL-DMS1 and MCL-DMS2

Both versions of the proposed MCL-DMS (MCL-DMS1 and MCL-DMS2) performed a simultaneous multi-label recognition of sleep stage and sleep disorder. In MCL-DMS1, the final assessor network NN_{31} made the decision based on the learned sleep-stage information only, and the NN_{32} on the learned sleep disorder only. In contrast, in MCL-DMS2, both assessor networks made their decisions using a fusion of sleep stage and sleep disorder information. Figure 8.7 shows that MCL-DMS2 led to about 2% higher accuracy than the MCL-DMS1 while achieving similar $F1$ scores. Certain sleep stages could be affected by specific sleep disorders, and different sleep disorders could be associated with specific sleep stages. Therefore, the fusion of information was a key factor in improving the MCL-DMS2 accuracy over the MCL-DMS1. Since $F1$ was similar in both structures, it appears that the compensation for the training data imbalance is mostly associated with the two-stage classification mechanism, not so much with the fusion of multi-label information. However, the fusion of multi-label information appears to improve diagnostic accuracy.

8.4.3.4 Comparison between Different Groups of Electrodes (Different Channels)

When looking at the baseline single-channel classification methods (Group C, F, O, P, –T - CNN for sleep stage and Group C, F, P- CNN for sleep disorder), it can be observed that some of the groups of EEG electrodes performed better than other. In the case of sleep stage classification (Figure 8.7a and b), group O led to the highest accuracy (66.27%); however, the $F1$ score was relatively low (0.54). Other groups performed with an accuracy slightly above 50% and rather low $F1$ scores of around 0.4. In the case of sleep disorder recognition (Figures 8.7c and d), the highest accuracy of 79% was achieved by electrode F. However, in this case, the $F1$ score was also relatively high (78%), indicating that for the sleep disorder, the training data did not have as large an imbalance as the sleep stage data (see Table 8.2). Group P also performed quite well (accuracy 75%, $F1$ score 0.75), but group C was the lowest performer (accuracy 64%, and $F1$ score 0.59).

8.4.3.5 Comparison with Related Studies

In this section, we present our results in the context of other closely related works. Table 8.6 shows the accuracy of the sleep-stage recognition from EEG signals. Both

TABLE 8.6

A Comparison between Sleep Stage Classification Studies Using EEG Signals

Study	Database	Number of Sleep Categories	Features	Method	Accuracy (%)
Sharma et al. (2018)	Sleep-EDF	6	Log energy, signal fractal dimension, entropy	SVM	91.5%
Timplalexis et al. (2019)	Sleep-EDF	5	Mixture of time and frequency domain features	EBT	88.88%
Tripathi et al. (2020)	CAP	6	Dispersion entropy, bubble entropy	Hybrid learning classifier	71.68%
Sharma, Tiwari and Acharya (2021)	CAP	6	Statistical norm features	EBT	85.1%
This study (2022)	CAP	6	Log spectrograms	MCL-DMS1	92.17%
This study (2022)	CAP	6	Log spectrograms	MCL-DMS2	94.19%

TABLE 8.7

A Comparison between Sleep Disorder Classification Studies Using EEG Signals

Authors	Database	Number of Sleep Categories	Features	Method	Accuracy (%)
Sharma, et al. (2021)	CAP	4	Hjorth parameters	EBT	96.5%
Sharma et al. (2021)	CAP	6	Hjorth parameters	EBT and boosted trees	91.3%
This study (2022)	CAP	8	Log spectrogram	MCL-DMS1	95.08%
This study (2022)	CAP	8	Log spectrogram	MCL-DMS2	96.02%

of the proposed approaches (MCL-DMS1 and MCL-DMS2) outperformed all other studies listed in Table 8.6. Sharma et al. (2018) show a close result to MCL-DMS1; however, a different database (Sleep EDF) was used, making a direct comparison difficult. Table 8.7, on the other hand, shows the accuracy of sleep disorder recognition from EEG signals. Again, both of our approaches outperformed other studies. Although Sharma et al. (2021) show the highest accuracy, it was achieved using four sleep disorder categories making the task less challenging than the six-class recognition used to validate our methods. In addition, it needs to be noted that the related studies listed in Tables 8.6 and 8.7 performed separate training and classification tasks for sleep stage and sleep disorder. Whereas, in this study, we propose a system of classifiers trained to perform both tasks simultaneously.

8.5   CONCLUSION

A new method (MCL-DMS) for simultaneous sleep stage and sleep disorder recognition from EEG signals was proposed and tested. The classification experiments show that a single sample of EEG waveform of 10-second duration can be simultaneously classified to identify the sleep stage (out of six categories) with an average accuracy of 94% and the sleep disorder (out of eight categories) with an average accuracy of 96%. The proposed system of NN classifiers MCL-DMS was shown to outperform baseline approaches using single classifiers. It was shown that a shallow decision-making NN trained to arbitrate between outcomes from different parallel classifiers was more efficient than the conventional maximum probability, majority voting, and average probability methods. It demonstrated that the shallow decision-making network eliminated the need for arbitrary decision-making schemes. A two-stage classification procedure applied by the MCL-DMS was shown to provide an efficient compensation for the training data imbalance. At the same time, the information fusion between sleep stage and sleep disorder was found to be a key factor in improving classification accuracy.

8.6   FUTURE RESEARCH DIRECTIONS

As shown by the current body of work, sleep scoring can be efficiently supported by simultaneous classification of EEG together with other modalities such as ECG, EMG, or EOG. In our future works, we will focus on multi-modal sleep scoring approaches.

ACKNOWLEDGMENT

This research was supported by an Australian Government Research Training Program Scholarship, Engineering Top-up Scholarship, and RMIT Research Stipend. The CAP Sleep database from the Sleep Disorders Center of the Ospedale Maggiore of Parma, Italy, was downloaded via physionet.org.

REFERENCES

Acharya, U.R, S.L. Oh, Y. Hagiwara, J.H. Tan, and H. Adeli. 2018. Deep convolutional neural network for the automated detection and diagnosis of seizure using EEG signals. *Computers in Biology and Medicine*. 100: 270–278. https://doi.org/10.1016/j.compbiomed.2017.09.017

Berry, R.B., R. Brooks, C.E. Gamaldo, S.M. Harding, C.L. Marcus, and B.V. Vaughn. 2013. *The AASM Manual for the Scoring of Sleep and Associated Events: Rules, Terminology and Technical Specifications*. Darien, IL: American Academy of Sleep Medicine.

Biswal, S., J. Kulas, H. Sun, B. Goparaju, M.B. Westover, M.T. Bianchi, and J. Sun. 2017. SLEEPNET: Automated sleep staging system via deep learning. arXiv preprint: https://doi.org/10.48550/arxiv.1707.08262

Kales, A., and A. Rechtschaffen. 1968. *A Manual of Standardized Terminology, Techniques and Scoring System for Sleep Stages of Human Subjects*. Washington, DC: United States Government Printing Office.

Kim, J., J. Lee, and M. Shin. 2017. Sleep stage classification based on noise-reduced fractal property of heart rate variability. *Procedia Computer Science*. 116: 435–440. https://doi.org/10.1016/j.procs.2017.10.026

Klem, G H, H.O. Lüders, H.H. Jasper, and C. Elger. 1999. The ten-twenty electrode system of the international federation. The international federation of clinical neurophysiology. *Electroencephalography and Clinical Neurophysiology. Supplement.* 52: 3–6.

Lech, M., M. Stolar, C. Best, and R. Bolia. 2020. Real-time speech emotion recognition using a pre-trained image classification network: effects of bandwidth reduction and companding. *Frontiers in Computer Science.* 2: 14. https://doi.org/10.3389/fcomp.2020.00014

Qassim, H., A. Verma, and D. Feinzimer. 2018. Compressed residual-VGG16 CNN model for big data places image recognition. In *Proceedings of the 2018 IEEE 8th Annual Computing and Communication Workshop and Conference (CCWC)*, Las Vegas, NV, USA, 8–10 Jan. 2018, 169–175. Piscataway, NJ: IEEE. https://doi.org/10.1109/CCWC.2018.8301729

Sharma, M., D. Goyal, P.V. Achuth, and U.R. Acharya. 2018. An accurate sleep stages classification system using a new class of optimally time-frequency localized three-band wavelet filter bank. *Computers in Biology and Medicine.* 98: 58–75. https://doi.org/10.1016/j.compbiomed.2018.04.025

Sharma, M., J. Tiwari, and U.R. Acharya. 2021. Automatic sleep-stage scoring in healthy and sleep disorder patients using optimal wavelet filter bank technique with EEG signals. *International Journal of Environmental Research and Public Health.* 18(6): 3087. https://doi.org/10.3390/ijerph18063087

Sharma, M., H.S. Dhiman, and U.R. Acharya. 2021. Automatic identification of insomnia using optimal antisymmetric biorthogonal wavelet filter bank with ECG signals. *Computers in Biology and Medicine.* 131: 104246. https://doi.org/10.1016/j.compbiomed.2021.104246

Sharma, M., J. Tiwari, V. Patel, and U.R. Acharya. 2021. Automated identification of sleep disorder types using triplet half-band filter and ensemble machine learning techniques with EEG Signals. *Electronics.* 10 (13): 1531. https://doi.org/10.3390/electronics10131531

Sharma, M., J. Darji, M. Thakrar, and U.R. Acharya. 2022. Automated identification of sleep disorders using wavelet-based features extracted from electrooculogram and electromyogram signals. *Computers in Biology and Medicine.* 143: 105224. https://doi.org/10.1016/j.compbiomed.2022.105224

Simonyan, K. and A. Zisserman. 2015. *Very deep convolutional networks for large-scale image recognition.* https://doi.org/10.48550/arXiv.1409.1556

Terzano, M.G., L. Parrino, A. Sherieri, R. Chervin, S. Chokroverty, C. Guilleminault, M. Hirshkowitz, M. Mahowald, H. Moldofsky, A. Rosa, R. Thomas, and A. Walters. 2001. Atlas, rules, and recording techniques for the scoring of cyclic alternating pattern (CAP) in human sleep. *Sleep Medicine.* 2(6): 537–553. https://doi.org/10.1016/s1389-9457(01)00149-6

The Math Works, Inc. MATLAB. Version 2022a, The Math Works, Inc., 2022. Computer Software. https://www.mathworks.com/.

Timplalexis, C., K. Diamantaras, and I. Chouvarda. 2019. Classification of sleep stages for healthy subjects and patients with minor sleep disorders. In *Proceedings of the 2019 IEEE 19th International Conference on Bioinformatics and Bioengineering (BIBE)*, Athens, Greece, 28–30 October 2019, 344–351. Piscataway, NJ: IEEE. https://doi.org/10.1109/BIBE.2019.00068

Tripathi, R.K., S.K. Ghosh, P. Gajbhiye, and U.R. Acharya. 2020. Development of automated sleep stage classification system using multivariate projection-based fixed boundary empirical wavelet transform and entropy features extracted from multichannel EEG signals. *Entropy.* 22 (10): 1141. https://doi.org/10.3390/e22101141

Walker, M.P. 2018. *Why We Sleep: The New Science of Sleep and Dreams.* London: Penguin Books.

Widasari, E.R., K. Tanno, and H. Tamura. 2020. Automatic sleep disorders classification using ensemble of bagged tree based on sleep quality features. *Electronics.* 9 (3): 512. https://doi.org/10.3390/electronics9030512

Section III

EEG – Signal Classification

9 Analyzing and Decoding Natural Reach and Grasp Action Using Convolutional Neural Network

Abida Nazir, Asim Waris, Shafiq Alam,
Shafaq Mushtaq, Rabia Nazir,
and Imran Khan Niazi

9.1 INTRODUCTION

Reaching and grasping are necessary movements in everyday life. All daily life chores involve various types of hand movements. The majority of hand movements encompass grasping. People with motor disorders lack in functional limbs, but they have retained movement-related cortical potentials (MRCPs), which can be used to transform the intentions of people into computer commands [1,2]. MRCPs reflect the cortical processes involved in the planning and execution of movement; thus, they can be manipulated for the detection and classification of movements [1,3]. There are multiple types of grasping movements, *i.e.*, palmar grasp, spherical grasp, parallel grasp, lateral grasp, cylindrical grasp, and snap grasp, based on the shape of the object to be held and the orientation of the fingers and thumb to grasp the object [1,4–6]. This study focuses on the EEG signal analysis of palmar and lateral grasp movements. The results of neural signal matchup with hand movements can be used for multiple hardware developments for paralyzed and handicapped patients so that they might enjoy a relatively convenient life [7].

In this era of development, an independent lifestyle is gaining the utmost importance. Deficiencies and inadequacies are responded with more and more technical and innovative solutions. Reaching and grasping mark the basis of an independent lifestyle. Patients who have lost the connection path of sensory and motor neurons of arm and hand regions totally depend for a caregiver in order to approach and hold any object. Such a type of dependency is seriously cumbersome and inconvenient. Spinal injury, motor disorder, and paralyzed patients suffer from such type of movement loss [8]. This type of loss can be fixed using a brain-computer interface (BCI). BCI uses brain signals to communicate with hardware devices [9]. These hardware devices are used by paralyzed or disabled patients to reduce their dependency. BCI actually decodes the way in which one plans and executes the movement, giving precise and timely feedback about the user's intentions [2]. This involves decoding the goal of the intended movement and the characteristics of the intended movement, *i.e.*, speed and force [10–13].

A lot of studies address EEG signal exploration. Muller Putz et al. showed that upper limb paralyzed patients have been observed to generate EEG signal patterns by the imagination of hand movements. These patterns can be identified by the power decrease in specific frequency bands that could be classified by BCI. Further, they also highlighted that EEG signals carry information about an object's size, shape, and grasp type [14,15]. Grasp types are encoded over the motor cortex area, while object characteristics activate the fronto-parietal areas [16]. The whole process of grasping is an interplay between neural representations of grasp type and object properties [14].

Schwarz et al. successfully classified palmar, lateral, and pincer grasps from MRCPs. Furthermore, they employed the same technique to discriminate between three grasping actions of bi-manual [17]. They also analyzed neural correlates of goal-directed movement intents vs non-goal-directed movement, and results reflected higher accuracy with goal intention in mind [12]. They also highlighted the importance of central motor areas as the origin of discriminative signals [1,11]. They also investigated hand open, palmar grasp, lateral grasp, pronation, and supination in ten persons with cervical spinal cord injury (SCI) [1].

Baogou Xu et al. studied five different reach and grasp movements, namely, palmar, pinch, twist, push, and plug grasp, and showed the feasibility of decoding multiple reach and grasp movements for natural and relatively intuitive BCI applications [18]. Cristoph Gugher et al. discussed the suitability of different types of BCIs according to the user's needs, environment, and applications.

Most BCIs use gel-based electrodes, while gel-based electrodes are not very much comfortable for daily life use [19]. Studies have shown the use of dry electrodes as a priority by patients as their use is more convenient to users. Therefore, most BCIs use dry electrodes, although their electrodes output and their mounting on the scalp are not very ideal [20]. Studies propose two approaches to dry electrodes. One approach is the use of capacitive sensors, which do not require direct contact with the scalp, thus posing a motion artifact problem. While second approach is the use of micro-electrodes inserted in the first layer of skin through micro needles or bristle sensors, which may be uncomfortable to users [21]. Ofner et al. found discriminative signals originated from central motor areas based on pattern analysis. They also investigated more grasp [22] clinical feasibility studies in individuals having SCIs. Literature studies reflect that EEG pattern analysis is highly informative for devising assistive devices for SCI, paralysis, and motor disorder patients [23]. There is extensive study regarding how EEG correlates with motor movements, but there is still ample room for further exploration of these signals so that they can be manipulated at their best to provide an optimum solution to ease the lives of patients. In this study, we analyzed EEG data using the convolutional neural network (CNN) technique of data classification. This resulted in a classification accuracy of 54.3%.

9.2 MATERIALS AND METHODS

9.2.1 GEL-BASED RECORDINGS

Gel-based electrodes have gel introduced between the electrode and the head scalp. This conductive gel maintains good contact between electrodes and the scalp, but after a few hours, the gel may get dry and new gel must be introduced [20,21,24]. In this study, 15 able-bodied, right-handed subjects were involved for gel-based recordings. The specifications of the subjects involved were as given below.

- Electrode-Type: Gel-based
- Electrodes Positioned Over: Frontal and Parietal
- Electrodes Reference Point: Right Earlobe
- Number of Electrodes: 58 Active
- Number of Participants: 15
- Age: 15–30
- Male: 10
- Female: 5
- Sampling Frequency: 256 Hz

All data is pre-filtered using a Chebyshev filter from 0.01 to 100 Hz. Power noise is reduced using a notch filter. All data is synchronized using the tools for BCI (TOBI) signal server. A force-sensitive resistor, whose resistance changes when mechanical stress, pressure, or force is applied, is used to record movement onset and grasping time point to each object.

9.2.2 WATER-BASED RECORDINGS

Water-based electrodes use water as an interface between electrode and scalp, *i.e.*, may be a sponge filled with water.

- Electrode-Type: Water-based
- Electrodes Positioned Over: Frontal and Parietal
- Electrodes Reference Point: Right Earlobe
- Number of Electrodes: 32 Active
- Number of Participants: 15
- Age: 15–30
- Male: 10
- Female: 5
- Sampling Frequency: 256 Hz

Pre-filtration of data was performed using a 3rd-order anti-aliasing Butterworth filter with a band-pass frequency from DC to 100 Hz. The movement onset and grasping time of each object were recorded using photodiodes. The output of the photodiode was digitized using an amplifier with a sampling frequency of 256 Hz. All data was saved in a computational unit to maintain data fatality.

9.2.3 Dry-Based Recordings

Dry electrodes come in direct contact with the scalp without any gel or water medium. They are either spiky, capacitive, or non-contact type.

- Electrode-Type: Dry Electrode
- Number of Participants: 15
- Male: 10
- Female: 5
- Aged: 15–30
- Electrode Positioned Over: Frontal, Occipital, and Parietal
- Sampling Frequency: 256 Hz

Pre-filtration of data was performed using a 3rd-order anti-aliasing Butterworth filter with a band-pass frequency from DC to 100 Hz. The movement onset and grasping time of each object was recorded using photodiodes. The output of the photodiode was digitized using an amplifier with a sampling frequency of 256 Hz. All the data was saved in a computational unit to maintain data fatality.

9.2.4 EEG Database

In this work, a database by Andreas Schwarz et al. was used. This data base was developed by experiments performed in Graz University of Technology, Austria, and BitBrain Zaragoza, Spain. This database has EEG as well as EOG signals. The initial 58 channels had EEG signals, while the last six channels were dedicated to collecting EOG signals. Schwarz et al. analyzed this database using an LDA classifier. They offered open access to the database for further research and analysis. We explored this database using deep learning techniques of classification. The scope of our study is limited to EEG signals only, and we ignored EOG signals by considering electrodes numbered 1–58.

9.2.5 Experimental Setup

All subjects involved in the experiment were seated in a comfortable position on the chairs in front of the table. Experimental objects, *i.e.*, empty glass and glass with a spoon were placed on the table. Gel-based experiment was performed in a shielded environment, while dry- and water-based electrode experiments were performed in a non-shielded environment. Subjects were directed to stable their right hand on a specific sensorized mean position, which was placed in front of them. In the case of empty glass, they were directed to perform palmar grasp, while in the case of spoon they were asked to perform a lateral grasp. Further, they were instructed to hold the object for 1–2 seconds. After every hold, they placed their hand on the central rest position. A screen was placed in front of them where the number of attempts was counted after every trial. There was 4 second pause before starting a new trial. The total number of trials recorded per condition was 80. Each of the 20 trials was grouped into a run. Three minutes of rest were recorded at the start, after 20 trials, then after 40 trials, and finally in the end of the experiment.

9.2.6 DATA ANALYSIS

Workspace variable analysis of the data reflected the following findings, as tabulated in Table 9.1. Furthermore, the tasks executed, along with the respective duration of tasks performed, were analyzed in order to comprehend the signal database. The results of this analysis are summarized in Table 9.2.

9.2.7 DATA PREPROCESSING

Pre-filtration of data is performed using a Butterworth band-pass filter with a cut-off frequency of 0.3 and 60 Hz. For better feature extraction, data is distributed into multiple windowing. A WOI of [-2 to 3]seconds for each movement trial is defined with movement onset at 0 second. Rest trials have the same duration as the movement trials. Potential artefact contaminated data is filtered out by statistical parameters and filtering techniques. Data having amplitude above 125 µV is considered as abnormal joint probability. Therefore, trials scrutinized for rejection were excluded from further analysis.

TABLE 9.1
Data Analysis

Serial #	Movement Onset	Code
1	Palmar grasp movement onset	503587
2	Lateral grasp movement onset	503588
3	RO	768
4	Vertical eye movement onset	10
5	Horizontal eye movement onset	12
6	Eye blink movement onset	14

TABLE 9.2
Task Types and Respective Duration

Serial #	Task Type	Time (min)
1	Rest recording	3
2	Visual guided paradigm (eye movements)	2
3	Reach and grasp tasks (Run 1,20 trials/condition)	≈ 7
4	Reach and grasp tasks (Run 2,20 trials/condition)	≈ 7
5	Rest recordings	≈ 7
6	Visual guided paradigm (eye movements)	2
7	Reach and grasp tasks (Run 3,20 trials/condition)	≈ 7
8	Reach and grasp tasks (Run 4,20 trials/condition)	≈ 7
9	Rest recording	≈ 7
10	Visual guided paradigm (eye movements)	

9.2.8 POWER SPECTRAL DENSITY AND TIME FREQUENCY ANALYSIS

Power spectral density (PSD) is an analysis of the distribution of power over the whole frequency range. It is used to gain spectral density estimation of data, while time frequency analysis is the characterization and manipulation of signals whose statistics vary in time [24,25]. For PSD calculation, preprocessed data was filtered using a common average reference filter. Further, all trials were epoched from (0–1.5) seconds with reference to movement onset. Welch's method of overlapping was used to calculate PSD. One-second window was developed for PSD calculation with 25% overlap.

PSD average per condition and a confidence interval were calculated using non-parametric t-percentile bootstrap statistics (alpha = 0.05). In order to gain the grand-average PSD, the average over the participant specific mean and its respective confidence interval were calculated. Time frequency analysis was studied using event-related synchronization maps in range from 2 to 40 Hz. Each movement condition using a specific reference interval of [-2-1]seconds was analyzed.

Figure 9.1 (left) represents the filtered signal of both movements. The black wavy line represents the filtered signal of palmar grasp movement onset, while the brown wavy line represents filtered lateral grasp movement onset signal. The right graph represents the PSD of the filtered signal reaching phase with an interval (0–1.5) seconds. Figure 9.1 (lower) spectrogram represents the frequency distribution of the signal during the movement execution phase.

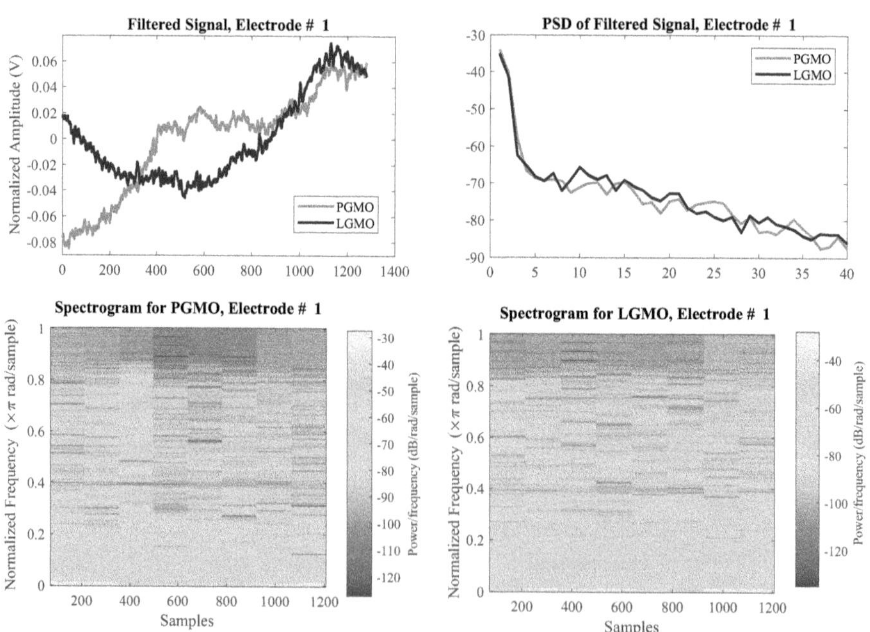

FIGURE 9.1   PSD of filtered signal.

9.2.9 Movement-Related Cortical Potentials

All preprocessed EEG signals were resampled to 16 Hz to reduce computational load, and then a common average reference (CAR) filter was applied. Then filtering was done by using a Butterworth low pass filter with a cut-off frequency of 3 Hz. For reasonable conclusion extraction, all study data was normalized. All rest trials and movement recordings were epoched to the WOI [-2–3], and time- and condition-specific averages were calculated. Further, a 95% confidence interval was calculated for every condition using non-parametric t-percentile bootstrap statistics.

We calculated the MRCPs of 4 random channels of gel-based electrodes of subject number 6.

- Fcz = Channel # 13
- C1 = Channel # 25
- Cz = Channel # 26
- C2 = Channel # 27

In the case of water-based electrodes, the following channels are used for MRCP calculations.

- Fcz = Channel # 2
- C1 = Channel # 5
- Cz = Channel # 6
- C2 = Channel # 7

In the case of dry-based electrodes, the following channels are used for the calculation of potentials.

- Fcz = Channel # 10
- C1 = Channel # 16
- Cz = Channel # 17
- C2 = Channel # 18

9.2.10 Multiclass Classification

The classification approach used is central neural network analysis. All preprocessed EEG signals are resampled to 16 Hz to reduce computational load, and then a CAR filter is applied. Further a 4th-order zero-phase Butterworth low pass filter having a cut-off frequency of 3 Hz is applied. All preprocessed trials of the experiment, *i.e.*, movement as well as rest conditions, were divided in a calibration set, which consisted of the first 90% of all recorded trials per conditions (TPC) designated as the training set and the remaining 10% of all recorded TPC considered as the test set [26,27].

The train set is the set of data that is used to train and make the model learn the patterns or hidden features in the data. In each epoch, the same training data is fed to the neural network repeatedly, and the model continues to learn the features of the data. On the basis of these learned features, it further classifies the validation as well as the test data. In order to get better classification accuracy, the training set should have a diversified set of inputs so that the model is trained in all scenarios and can predict any unseen data sample that may appear in the future. The validation set is a set of data separate from the training set that is used to validate our model performance during training, while the test set is a separate set of data used to test the model after completing the training.

Using an unseen test dataset, after multiple iterations, an optimum test accuracy of around 54.2% was achieved, which is fairly above the adjusted chance level accuracy of 49.06%. The signal, which is to be classified is given to the input layer, and after multiple layer mapping iterations, the output is the classified label, which is computed using extracted features from the image signal. Individual neurons in the previous layer are connected to the neurons in the subsequent layer; this correlation is called the receptive field. Features extraction from the input signal image is done using a receptive field. The exact location of a feature is of importance until its detection. Thus, the convolution layer is accompanied by the pooling layer. The major benefit of the pooling technique is that it reduces trainable parameters. There are multiple pooling techniques, like max-pooling and average pooling. Max-pooling is a more efficient technique as it reduces map size very significantly [27–29].

A fully connected layer is like a fully connected network in conventional models. The first phase output is fed into the fully connected layer, and then the dot product of the input vector and weight vector is performed in order to get the final output. For every time point within WOI, a CNN is trained to get classifications with optimum accuracy. It is worthy to mention that the classifier classifies the data into three classes, *i.e.*, palmar grasp, lateral grasp, and rest onset (RO); thus, it is not a binary classification but a multiclass. The occurrences of palmar and lateral are theoretically equal (80), and RO occurrences were only 3 of 3 minutes each. Each occurrence of rest is then converted into 80 windows of 5 second each.

9.3 RESULTS

9.3.1 GEL-BASED RECORDINGS

Figure 9.2 represents the MRCPs for the grand average for the palmar and lateral grasp conditions for gel-type of electrodes. A negative deflection can be observed around time ($t = 0$ s), which starts almost one second before the movement onset. This is actually MRCP. This is also highlighted by a vertical dotted line. A gray wavy line inside shaded regions represents the average of palmar and lateral grasp movement potentials, while a thick shaded region represents a 95% confidence interval. The time interval (0–1.5 seconds) marks the reach and grasp phases; therefore, around 1.5 seconds, there is a prominent positive peak. After that, the graph gradually descends down, which represents the hold and release phases.

Figure 9.3 shows the result of multiclass single trial decoding. The grand average classification accuracy obtained with gel-based electrodes is 58.5%. Bar graphs show that the minimum classification accuracy with gel-based electrodes is that of subject # 3, which is 50%, while the maximum accuracy of 70% is achieved by subject # 4. All subjects attained test accuracy higher than chance level 49.7.

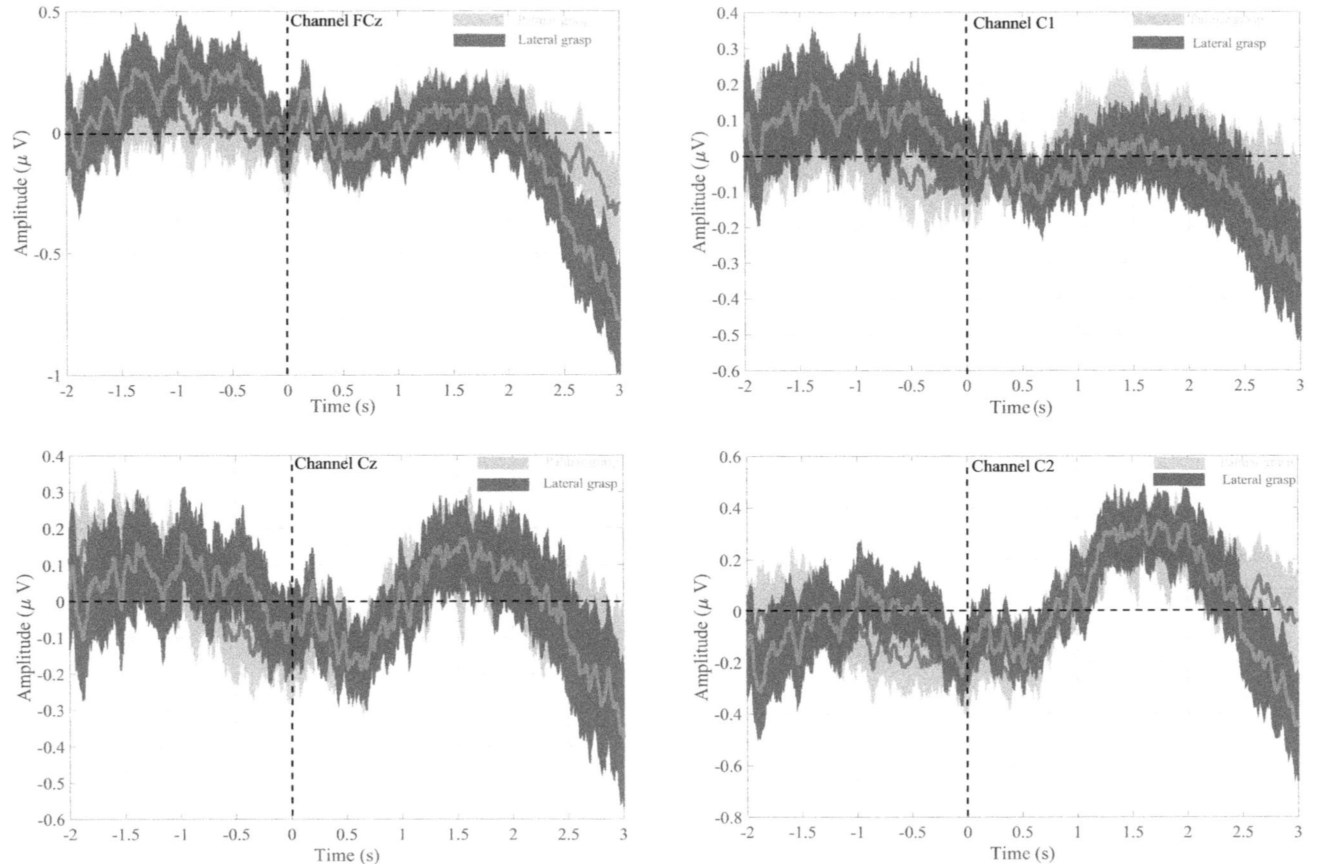

FIGURE 9.2   MRCPs of gel-based recordings.

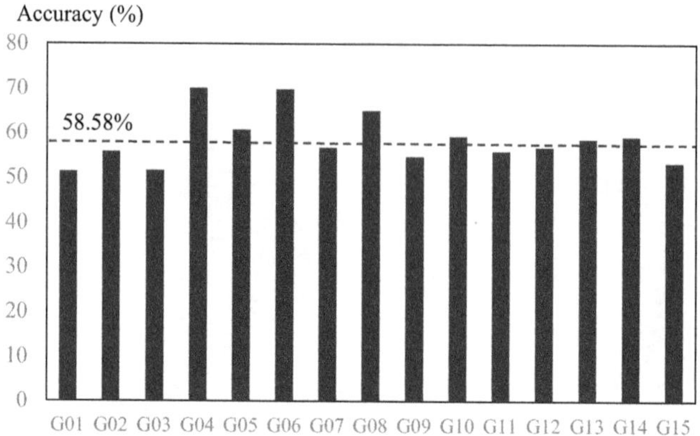

FIGURE 9.3　% Accuracy of all subjects with gel-based electrodes.

FIGURE 9.4　Best confusion matrix of gel-based electrodes.

Figure 9.4 represents the best confusion matrix obtained in gel-based data. As it can be noticed in col.1 that 59 times the classifier identifies lateral grasp as lateral grasp, while 25 times the classifier recognizes lateral grasp as palmar grasp. This results in a 72.8% true positive rate for LG. While col.2 depicts that 37 times target class and output class matches and 25 times palmar grasp is falsely recognized as lateral grasp, which results in a 47.4% true positive rate for palmar grasp. In the same way, col.3 depicts that RO is 72 times recognized as RO, 7 times as PG, and 2 times as LG. This results in an 88.9% true positive rate for RO and the overall best classification accuracy achieved by any subject in the case of gel-based electrodes reaches up to 70%.

9.3.2 Water-Based Recordings

Figure 9.5 shows the MRCPs of water-based electrodes for channels C1, Cz, Fcz, and C2. One second before the movement onset, negative turning starts and reaches its maximum around the movement onset ($t = 0$). Around (1–1.5 seconds), there is a prominent positive peak after that potential returns back to baseline.

Figure 9.6 summarizes subject-specific accuracies while using water-based electrodes for recordings. Average accuracy with water-based electrodes reaches up to 52.6%. Subject # 7 recording data is best classified with an accuracy of 56.3%, while subject # 15 recording reaches to a minimum accuracy of around 48%. Overall test accuracy when using water-based electrodes approaches 52.6%. All subjects achieved test accuracies higher than chance level 49.7, except subject # 15, which was 48%.

Figure 9.7 represents the best confusion matrix achieved while classifying water-based recordings.

Light grey boxes represent correctly classified occurrences. 47 times lateral grasp is classified as lateral, while 49 times palmar grasp is truly classified as palmar. RO is 48 times recognized as true. This results in a RO true positive rate of 59.3%, a PG true positive rate of 52.1%, and a LG true positive rate of 58%, and overall 56.3% of the best classification accuracy is achieved by subject #7. The dark gray column (rightmost) represents true positive (light grey) and false negative (mid-grey) percentages of classified categories, whereas the bottom row represents true positive (light grey) and false negative (mid-grey) percentages with reference to TPC.

9.3.3 Dry-Based Recordings

Figure 9.8 summarizes the MRCP of dry-based electrode recordings of randomly chosen four channels of palmar and lateral grasp movements. All these figures show a prominent negative dip of potential around (0 seconds) time scale; this is actually MRCP. This is also highlighted by a vertical dotted line. A gray wavy line inside shaded regions represents the average of palmar and lateral grasp movement potentials, while a thick shaded region represents a 95% confidence interval. The time interval (0–1.5 seconds) marks the reach and grasp phases; therefore, around 1.5 seconds, there is a prominent positive peak. After that, the graph gradually descends down, which represents the release and return to the base position phase.

Figure 9.9 summarizes results of multiclass single trial decoding. All subject-specific accuracies are shown in bar graph, while horizontal dotted line represents overall average accuracy while using dry-based electrodes for recordings. Subject # 12 data achieved best test classification accuracy of around 55.3%, while subject # 9 recording achieved a minimum test accuracy of 47.9%. Overall accuracy when using dry-based electrodes approaches 51.7%.

Figure 9.10 represents the best confusion matrix achieved. As it can be observed in matrix col.1, the target class and output class match 45 times, while 38 times lateral grasp is recognized as palmar grasp and 6 times as RO. Col.2 depicts that 24 times the palmar grasp is recognized as a palmar grasp, while 38 times, it is recognized as lateral grasp. Col.3 shows RO is 67 times classified as RO, 8 times as palmar grasp, and 6 times as lateral. Rightmost gray col. represents the true positive (light grey) and false negative (mid-grey) classifications of classifiers. The bottom row summarizes the

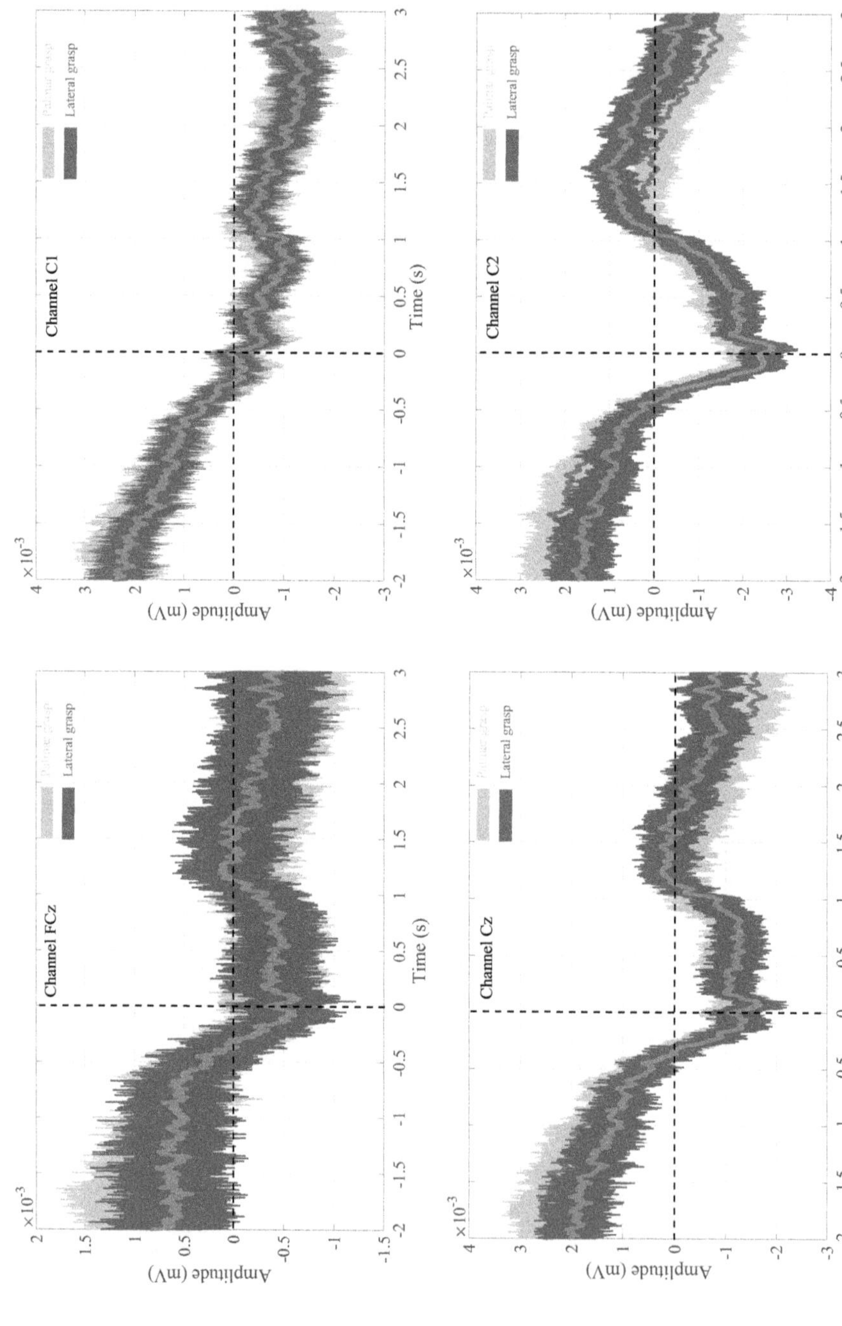

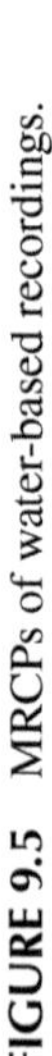

FIGURE 9.5 MRCPs of water-based recordings.

Accuracy (%)
60
50
40
30
20
10
0
52.62%
V01 V02 V03 V04 V05 V06 V07 V08 V09 V10 V11 V12 V13 V14 V15

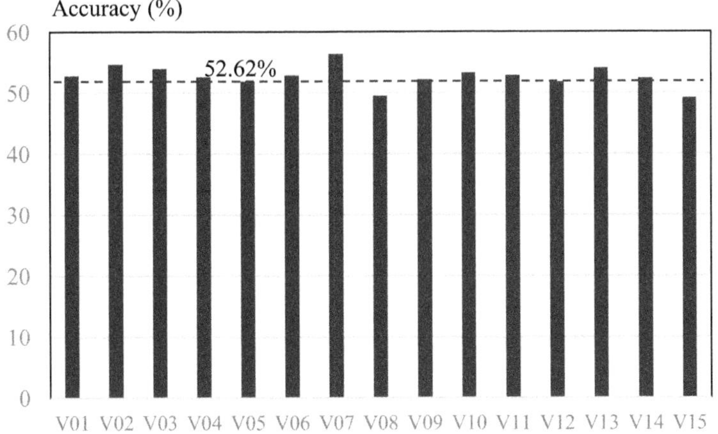

FIGURE 9.6 % Accuracy of all subjects with water-based electrodes.

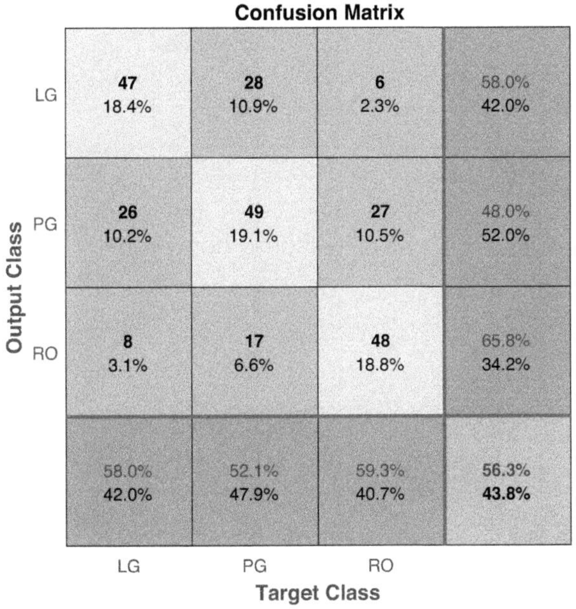

Confusion Matrix
Output Class
LG
PG
RO
47
18.4%
28
10.9%
6
2.3%
58.0%
42.0%
26
10.2%
49
19.1%
27
10.5%
48.0%
52.0%
8
3.1%
17
6.6%
48
18.8%
65.8%
34.2%
58.0%
42.0%
52.1%
47.9%
59.3%
40.7%
56.3%
43.8%
LG
PG
RO
Target Class

FIGURE 9.7 Best confusion matrix of water-based electrode.

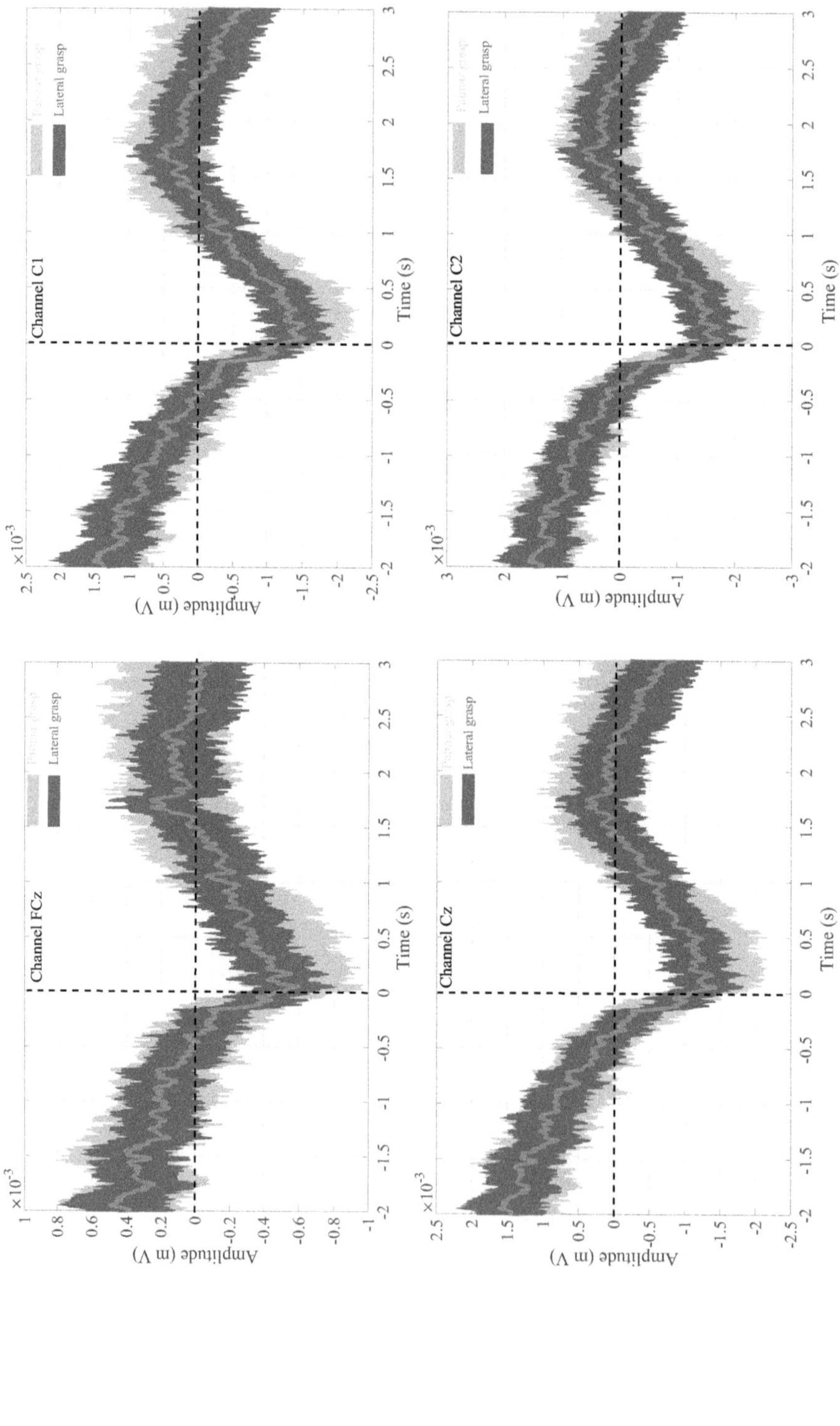

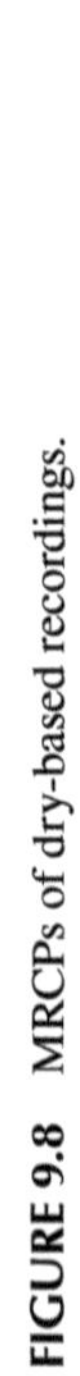

FIGURE 9.8 MRCPs of dry-based recordings.

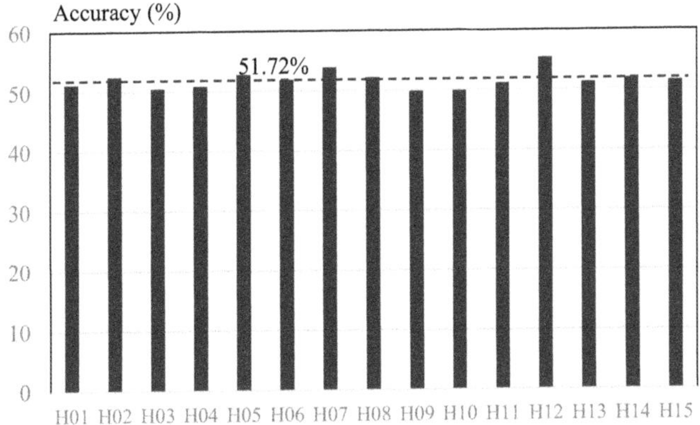

FIGURE 9.9   % Accuracy of all subjects with dry-based electrodes.

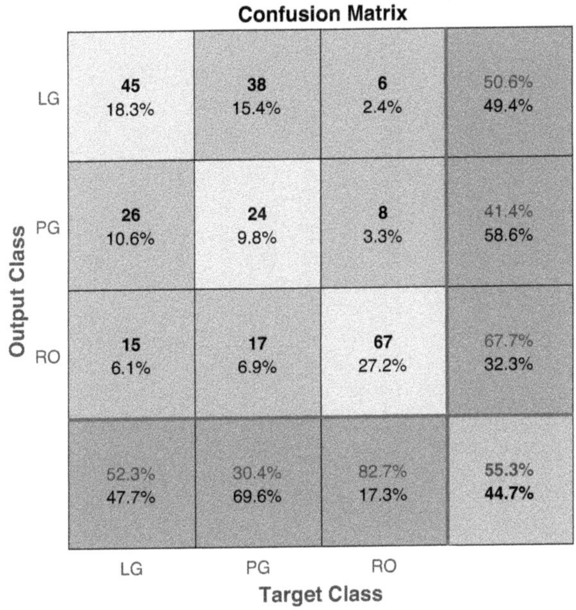

Confusion Matrix

FIGURE 9.10   Best confusion matrix of dry-based electrode.

true positive (light grey) and false negative (mid-grey) classifications with reference to the actual number of occurrences in trials.

9.3.4 BEHAVIORAL ANALYSIS

Figure 9.11 summarizes subject-specific behavioral analysis for all types of electrodes and motions. We noticed the reaction time of every trial for all conditions and individuals. Movement onset time is considered a reference point, and signals of all trials are averaged to conclude a time window for reach, grasp/hold, and release [14,18]. Figure 9.11 represents the behavioral analysis of all subjects. As it can be seen in the graphs, reach and

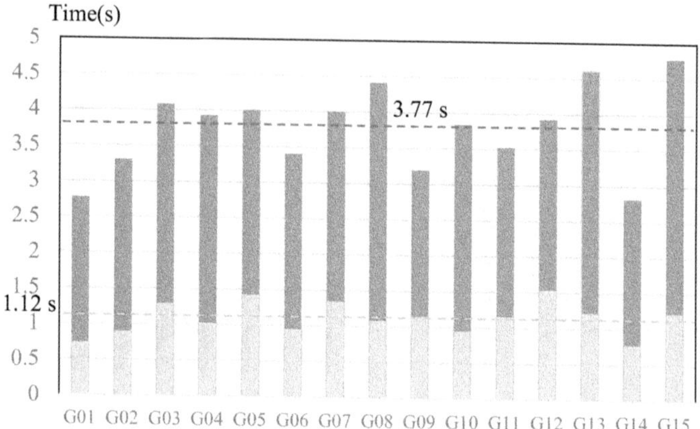

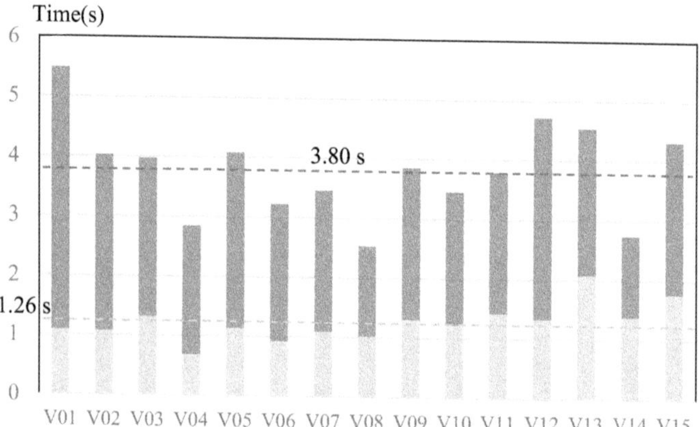

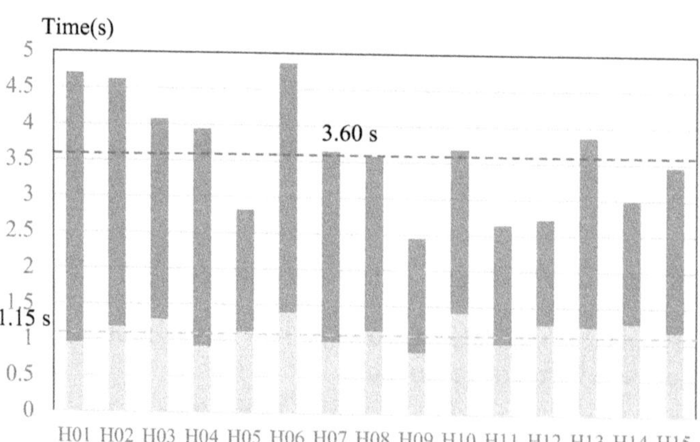

FIGURE 9.11 Subject-specific time involved in palmar and lateral grasps for all electrode-types.

Sub Figure (a1) Gel-based palmar grasp. Sub Figure (a2) Gel-based lateral grasp. Sub Figure (b1) Water-based palmar grasp. Sub Figure (b2) Water-based lateral grasp. Sub Figure (c1) Dry-based palmar grasp Sub Figure (c2) Dry-based lateral grasp.

(*Continued*)

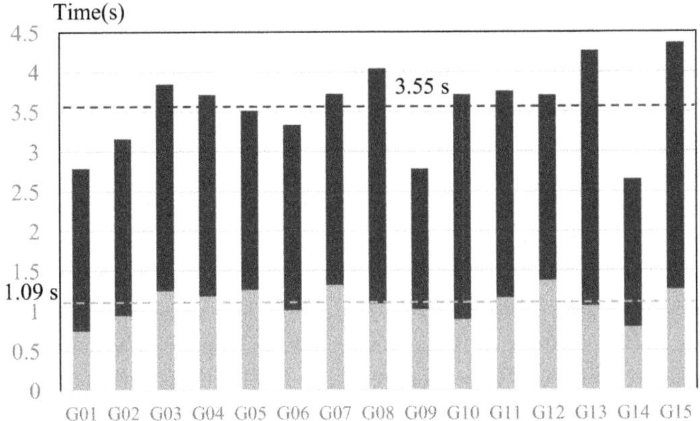

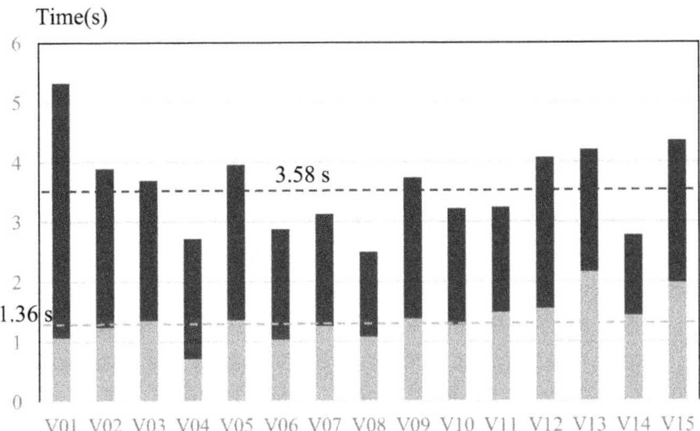

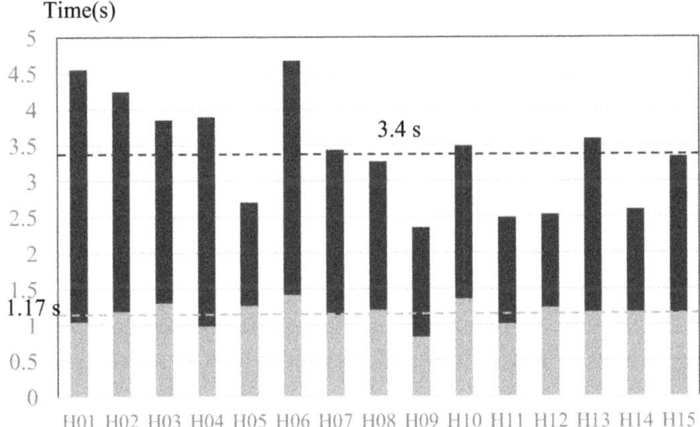

FIGURE 9.11 (*Continued*)	Subject-specific time involved in palmar and lateral grasps for all electrode-types.

Sub Figure (a1) Gel-based palmar grasp. Sub Figure (a2) Gel-based lateral grasp. Sub Figure (b1) Water-based palmar grasp. Sub Figure (b2) Water-based lateral grasp. Sub Figure (c1) Dry-based palmar grasp Sub Figure (c2) Dry-based lateral grasp.

grasp actions are represented by a lightly shaded region. It lasts from (0–1.1seconds/1.36 seconds). The first horizontal dotted line represents the mean over all subjects for specific electrodes and grasp types. A convincing similarity is observed for reach and grasp as well as for the release and hold phases. The dark shaded region represents the hold and release phases. The second horizontal dotted line represents the mean of the hold and release phases. As it can be observed in the graphs, the time taken in the case of palmar grasp (grey graphs) is relatively higher than the lateral grasp (black graphs).

In this research, we analyzed and classified types of movement, i.e., palmar grasp, lateral grasp, and RO. Data is classified on the basis of MRCPs. Most discriminative information lies between (1–1.5 seconds). Overall test accuracy reached 54.2%. Data also contain EOG signals, but in our study, we only considered EEG signals. The number of electrodes used in the experimental study was not equal, *i.e.*, 58 electrodes for gel-type, 32 electrodes for water-type, and 11 dry-type electrodes. Therefore, it can't be inferred directly which type of electrodes are best suited for EEG recording for the best classification.

9.4   DISCUSSION

The results of this study confirmed that EEG correlates of reach and grasp action can be decoded up to a reasonable classification accuracy. We used a multiclass classification approach, which incorporated both movement and rest conditions. MRCPs of all types of electrodes were drawn, and a pictorial analysis represented that a negative dip just around ($t=0$ second) marks the onset of MRCP. After that, the graph ascends, which represents movement and the hold phase. There is a great similarity between MRCPs achieved as a result of deep learning algorithms and the reference study.

Overall classification accuracy calculated on unseen test data resulted in 54.2% classification accuracy, with gel-based recording yielding 58.5%, water-based 52.6%, and dry-based 51.7%. The adjusted chance level for this study was 49.7%, with an interval alpha$=0.05$. If we compare it with the reference study, accuracy decreased by around 5.8%, but it followed the same trend as in the case of gel-based headsets, whose achieved accuracy was 62.3%, followed by water-based 61.3% and dry-based headset 56.4%. An unexpected decrease in accuracy can be attributed to multiple technical factors and certain unknowns and assumptions made. The theoretical study and practical dataset do not match at every bit. Theoretically, there are 80 TPC, but when we analyzed the data, multiple subjects performed under and over trials. This intersubject variation resulted in a decrease of classification accuracy. Further, a direct comparison between types of electrodes and classification accuracy cannot be linearly drawn as the number of channels is variable, *i.e.*, gel$=58$, water$=32$, and dry$=11$. If the number of channels is equal, then we can conclude, in comparison to the accuracy achieved, which type of electrodes is best for recording neural signals.

9.5   STUDY LIMITATION AND FUTURE WORK

In this study, we investigated whether neural correlates recorded through three different types of electrodes can be decoded into natural reach and grasp actions. As the number of EEG and EOG channels is not equal, it cannot be considered that the preprocessing of data is uniform. Further, it is also noticed that experiments with water- and dry-based electrodes are performed in BitBrain Spain, while gel-based electrode experiment is performed in Graz University, Austria, which can contribute to a variable experimental environment and therefore non uniformity of data recorded and thus results. It is also mentioned in the reference study that the object position between gel-based and water-based studies is not exactly replicated, and therefore it is a deviation from the theoretical study. In addition, we also analyzed the fact that the number of TPC is theoretically equal to 80, but in depth analysis of the data reflected that many subjects deviated from the theoretical number and performed a variable number of trials, which contributed to reduced classification accuracy. Moreover, the number of electrodes used with all three types is not equal (gel=58, water=32, and dry=11); therefore, a clear and definite classification accuracy trend regarding electrode-type cannot be concluded. Therefore, as a part of further research, an experiment could be performed with an equal number of electrodes in the same environment so that a clear and convincing result could be achieved, which may direct the use of the best electrodes to record neural signals for limb rehabilitation.

9.6 CONCLUSION

This study proves that EEG and natural reach and grasp movements are easily decodeable. MRCPs and associated action relationship and their best identification and classification can be used to develop assistive rehabilitative devices, which can transform the lives of paralysis, SCI patients, and amputees. Three types of electrodes were used in this study, as the number of electrodes is not exactly equal; therefore, we cannot make a direct comparison between electrode-types and classification accuracy. However, the low number of dry electrodes resulted in lower classification accuracy.

REFERENCES

1. P. Ofner, A. Schwarz, J. Pereira, D. Wyss, R. W. Burger, & G. R. Müller-Putz, "Attempted arm and hand movements can be decoded from low-frequency EEG from persons with spinal cord injury", *Scientific Reports* (2019), 9, 7134.
2. J. Meng, S. Zhang, A. Bekyo, J. Olsoe, B. Baxter, & B. He, "Non-invasive electroencephalogram based control of a robotic arm for reach and grasp tasks", *Journal of Big Data* (2016), 6, 38565.
3. J.-H. Cho, J.-H. Jeong, D.-J. Kim, & S.-W. Lee, "A novel approach to classify natural grasp actions by estimating muscle activity patterns from EEG signals", *Human-Computer Interaction arXiv:2002.00556v1* (2020), 4, 4.
4. M. D. Luciw, E. Jarocka, & B. B. Edin, "Multi-channel EEG recordings during 3,936 grasp and lift trials with varying weight and friction", *Scientific Data* (2014), 1, 140047.
5. A. Schwarz, O. Patrick, P. Joana, I. S. Andreea, & G. R. M¨uller-Putz, "Decoding natural reach-and-grasp actions from human EEG", *Journal of Neural Engineering* (2017), 15, 016005.
6. B. Xu, L. Deng, D. Zhang, M. Xue, H. Li, H. Zeng, & A. Song, "Electroencephalogram source imaging and brain network based natural grasps decoding", *Journal of Big Data* (2021), 15, 797990.
7. A. Ubeda, J. M. Azofin, R. Chavarriaga, & J. R. Millán, "Classification of upper limb center-out reaching tasks by means of EEG-based continuous decoding techniques", *Journal of Neuro Engineering and Rehabilitation* (2017), 14, 9.

8. E. Pirondini, M. Coscia, J. Minguillon, J. R. Millan, D. Van De Ville & S. Micera, "EEG topographies provide subject-specific correlates of motor control", *Scientific Reports* (2017), 7, 13229.

9. M. S. AL-Quraishi, I. Elamvazuthi, S. A. Daud, S. Parasuraman, & A. Borboni, "EEG-based control for upper and lower limb exoskeletons and prostheses: a systematic review", *Sensors* (2018), 18, 3342.

10. P. Ofner, & G. R. Müller-Putz, "Decoding of velocities and positions of 3D arm movement from EEG", *IEEE Engineering in Medicine and Biology Society* (2012), 14, 6406–6409.

11. M. Jochumsen, C. Rovsing, H. Rovsing, I. K. Niazi, K. Dremstrup, & E. N. Kamavuako, "Classification of hand grasp kinetics and types using movement related cortical potentials and EEG rhythms", *Computational Intelligence and Neuroscience* (2017), 2017, 7470864.

12. J. Pereira, P. Ofner, A. Schwarz, A. I. Sburlea, & G. R. Müller-Putz, "EEG neural correlates of goal-directed movement intention", *Sensors* (2017), 31, 4329.

13. J.-H. Cho, J.-H. Jeong, K.-H. Shim, & S.-W. Lee, "Classification of various grasping tasks based on temporal segmentation method using EEG and EMG signals", In *8th Graz Brain-Computer Interface Conference,* Graz University of Technology, Austria (2019).

14. A. I. Sburleaa, M. Wilding, G. R. Müller-Putz, "Disentangling human grasping type from the object's intrinsic properties using low-frequency EEG signals", *Neuroimage: Reports* (2021), 1, 100012.

15. H. A. Agashe, A. Y. Paek, Y. Zhang, & J. L. Contreras-Vidal, "Global cortical activity predicts shape of hand during grasping", *Frontiers in Neuroscience* (2015), 9, 121.

16. M. M. Ramadhan, S. K. Wijaya, & P. Prajitno, "Classification of EEG signals from motor imagery of hand grasp movement based on neural network approach", In *2019 IEEE International Conference on Signals and Systems (ICSigSys),* Bandung, Indonesia (2019).

17. A. Schwarz, J. Pereira, R. Kobler, & G. R. Muller-Putz, "Unimanual and bimanual reach-and-grasp actions can be decoded from human EEG", *IEEE Transactions on Biomedical Engineering* (2020), 67, 1684–1695.

18. B. Xu, D. Zhang, Y. Wang, L. Deng, X. Wang, C. Wu, & A. Song, "Decoding different reach-and-grasp movements using noninvasive electroencephalogram", *Journal of Neural Engineering* (2017), 15, 684547.

19. J. Pereira, A. Ioana Sburlea, & G. R. Müller-Putz, "EEG patterns of self-paced movement imaginations towards externally-cued and internally selected targets", *Scientific Reports* (2018), 67, 13394.

20. V. Mihajlovíc, G. Garcia-Molina, & J. Peuscher, "Dry and water-based EEG electrodes in SSVEP-based BCI applications", *Biomedical Engineering Systems and Technologies* (2012), 357, 23–40.

21. C. Guger, G. Krausz, B. Z. Allison, & G. Edlinger, "Comparison of dry and gel based electrodes for P300 brain–computer interfaces", *Frontiers in Neuroscience* (2012), 6, 60.

22. G. R. Muller-Putz, R. Rupp, P. Ofner, J. Pereira, A. Pinegger, A. Schwarz, M. Zube, U. Eck, B. Hessing, & M. Schneiders, "Applying intuitive EEG-controlled grasp neuroprostheses in individuals with spinal cord injury: Preliminary results from the More Grasp clinical feasibility study", *Sensors* (2017), 2017, 5949–5955.

23. P. Ofner, A. Schwarz, J. Pereira, & G. R. Müller-Putz, "Upper limb movements can be decoded from the time-domain of low-frequency EEG", *Frontiers in Neuroscience* (2017), 12, e0182578.

24. S. Leach, K. Chung, L. Tüshaus, R. Huber, & W. Karlen, "A protocol for comparing dry and wet EEG electrodes during sleep", *Frontiers in Neuroscience* (2020), 14, 586.

25. A. Schwarz, C. Escolano, L. Montesano, & G. R. Müller-Putz, "Analyzing and decoding natural reach-and-grasp actions using gel, water and dry EEG systems", *Frontiers in Neuroscience* (2020), 14, 849.
26. Y. Gaol, B. Gaol, Q. Chen, J. Liu, & Y. Zhang, "Deep convolutional neural network-based epileptic electroencephalogram (EEG) signal classification", *Frontiers in Neurology* (2020), 14, 375.
27. C. Zhong, X. Bai, & B. Dong, "Understanding the convolutional neural networks with gradient descent and back propagation", *Journal of Physics: Conference Series* (2018), 1004(1), 012028.
28. R. Yamashita, M. Nishio, R. K. G. Do & K. Togashi, "Convolutional neural networks: an overview and application in radiology", *Insights Imaging* (2018), 9, 611–629.
29. L. Alzubaidi, J. Zhang, A. J. Humaidi, A. Al-Dujaili, Y. Duan, O. Al-Shamma, J. Santamaría, M. A. Fadhel, M. Al-Amidie & L. Farhan, "Review of deep learning: concepts, CNN architectures, challenges, applications, future direction", *Journal of Big Data* (2021), 8(1), 53.

10 Classification of Motor Imagery EEG Signals Based on Sparse Representations of Empirical Mode Decomposition Features

José Antonio Alves de Menezes,
Juliana Carneiro Gomes, Vitor de Carvalho Hazin,
Júlio César Sousa Dantas,
Marcelo Cairrão Araújo Rodrigues,
Pedro Luís Gurgel Nogueira, and
Wellington Pinheiro dos Santos

10.1 INTRODUCTION

10.1.1 CONTEXT AND MOTIVATION

The brain-computer interface (BCI) has enabled control or communication with various devices through brain sensors (Wolpaw and Wolpaw, 2012), and opens space for the most varied applications, such as touch-free text input systems, controls for wheelchairs, cursors, prostheses, exoskeletons, and virtual reality systems (Sreeja and Samanta et al., 2020). The electroencephalogram (EEG) plays an important role in several types of brain applications and is popular for being non-invasive. In addition to its common use in disease diagnosis, sleep assessment, and neurofeedback, the EEG has also been widely used in BCI applications (Fouad, Amin, El-Bendary, and Hassanien, 2015), especially using motor imagery (MI-BCI), which consists in limb movement imagination. In this sense, we seek to identify and classify MI in order to have a set of brain commands that will compose the interface. However, the nature of the brain signal picked up by the EEG is non-stationary and poses challenges. The signals are so diverse and time-varying that the usefulness of pattern recognition computational models is limited to the time close to the signal collection.

DOI: 10.1201/9781003252092-13

Furthermore, a long recording time is required to achieve good performance for these models, which, in practice, can make the user reluctant to use them (Jiao, Zhang, Chen, Yin, Jin, Wang, and Cichocki, 2018).

Classifications based on sparse representations of some EEG attribute (SRC) (Ameri, Pouyan, and Abolghasemi, 2016; Shin, Lee, Lee, and Lee, 2012) are increasingly useful to obtain good performance from untrained patterns (Betthauser, Hunt, Osborn, Masters, Lé-vay, Kaliki, and Thakor, 2017). This way, allowing a smaller volume of data to be necessary in the training process of a classification model. Jiao et al. (2018); Meng, Yin, She, Gao, Kong, and Luo (2021); and Sreeja et al. (2020) seek to improve this approach by focusing on optimizing and learning dictionaries for sparse representation. Miao, Wang, and Liu (2017); Xu, Sun, Jiang, Chen, He, and Xie (2020); and Zhang, Nam, Zhou, Jin, Wang, and Cichocki (2018), in turn, choose to focus on improving the attributes that will be represented.

Empirical mode decomposition (EMD) (Alam and Samanta, 2017a) is characterized as a good method to contribute to the generation of attributes extracted from non-stationary signals. Thus, several works use it in the BCI based on Motor Imagery (Bashar and Bhuiyan, 2016; Chen and You, 2017; Davies and James, 2014; Saha and Ali, 2016). This method presents itself as an option to be combined with SRC, which has not yet been explored.

We propose to evaluate the use of sparse representation classification (SRC) attributes derived from EMD in order to verify the hypothesis that this combination is promising in the classification of MI in a multiclass problem. We compare the SRC model with a conventional model (MLP). We also evaluated a hybrid approach for the classification of sparse representations with MLP (RSMLP). For both approaches, we use attributes derived from EMD. However, we also extract these attributes directly from the conventional frequency bands, bypassing the application of EMD, in order to arrive at a second comparison. To overcome the difficulty imposed by the base size limitation, we used data augmentation. Attribute selection methods were used to select the most significant ones, specifically random forest (RForest) and particle swarm optimization (PSO).

The structure of the subsequent sections is organized as follows: in Section 10.1.2, we comment on works related to MI-BCI and particularly related to SRC and EMD techniques; in Section 10.2, we present the used materials, methods, and theoretical concepts necessary for a good understanding of this work; and in Sections 10.3 and 10.4, we show the results and discussion. Finally, our conclusions and future work are described in Section 10.5.

10.1.2 Related Works

10.1.2.1 Motor Imagery-Based BCI

Several works have proposed methods aiming to improve MI classification. Zhang, Robinson, Lee, and Guan (2021) experimented with different techniques to adjust CNNs, for instance. In this study, they tested a subject-independent categorization to overcome the small amount of EEG signals per participant. The main idea of the work is to train the network with data from different subjects. Then, using the data from the chosen subject, the pre-trained model is altered and adjusted. With that in mind, the researchers tested a variety of network adaptation mechanisms: classifier optimization, adaptation of convolutional layers, and multiple proportions of training (the number of layers retrained with the data of the patient). In order to test the proposed method, they used EEG signals from 54 healthy participants who imagined right- and left-hand movements. Spatial and temporal filters with max-pooling, three convolutional blocks, and a fully connected layer with Softmax were employed in the CNN. Finally, the study found that, when compared to standard methods (with subject-specific training), the proposed method had 32.50% greater accuracy. In addition, the best results were achieved with the adaptation of three of the four convolutional layers, as well as the Softmax layer. This means that only the first layer was properly trained with data from other patients.

As in the previous work, Zhu, Li, Yao, Zhang, and Xu (2019) also proposed a subject-independent training approach. The author's idea was to train BCIs with data from numerous participants and transfer the learning to classify a new subject. Thus, the authors modified the classic CSP method and applied a band-pass filter. With this, they designed a structure with greater discriminative ability called a separate channel convolutional network (SCCN). The methodology was tested on dataset 2b from the BCI Competition IV (2008). Two measures were used to evaluate the results: accuracy and information transfer rate (ITR). The proposed technique had an ITR of 0.83 and an average accuracy of 64%. Unfortunately, simpler classifiers, such as LDA, produced better results (65%).

Amin, Alsulaiman, Muhammad, Mekhtiche, and Hossain (2019) tested another novel technique: the combination of numerous CNN models with varying depths and filters to improve MI categorization results. In this case, the CNN models were based on the AlexNet architecture. The attributes extracted by the various models are then combined and sent into an MLP (MCNN method) or an autoencoder as an input (CCNN method). The authors experimented with four types of CNNs, ranging from one to four convolution blocks and max-pooling, as well as filters with sizes ranging from 10 to 30. The CNN models were trained and tested with two datasets: the High-Gamma Dataset, which is made up of 20 volunteers' EEG signals, and the BCI IV-2a (BCID) dataset. The BCID is made up of EEG data from nine participants who imagined four different sorts of movements: right hand, left hand, foot, and tongue. In terms of training, the study looked at two approaches: subject-specific training and training based on signals from all volunteers. Therefore, based on the BCID, the first approach had an average accuracy of 75.7%. In the second approach, the CCNN outperformed the others, with an average accuracy of 55.34%.

In turn, Dai, Zhou, Huang, and Wang (2020) concentrated on two methods: modifying the CNN's kernel dimensions and data augmentation for each subject. The researchers looked at how kernel size differed between participants and between imaging sessions for the same subject. This analysis found a 10% difference in accuracy with kernel variations. Based on these findings, they presented a CNN with a hybrid convolution scale, named HS-CNN. Further, the paper also presented and tested a new way of data augmentation in which signal windows are recombined in the time and frequency domains. The researchers used two BCIs.

Competition IV databases to validate the method: 2a and 2b. Each dataset is made up of nine healthy people who imagined four and two types of movements, respectively. The proposed method has an average classification accuracy of 87.6%, with improvements of up to 23.25% for dataset 2a and 19.7% for dataset 2b.

In contrast, Zhao, Zhang, Zhu, You, Kuang, and Sun (2019) invested in new methods of representing EEG signals for the classification of MI. Instead of using EEG signals in one dimension, the authors proposed a way to represent them in three dimensions. In this way of representing, the authors sought to keep the spatial distribution information of the electrodes in addition to the temporal information. For feature extraction and classification steps, they also developed a CNN in 3D (multi-branch 3D CNN). The idea with this architecture is to combine multiple CNNs with different receptive fields. Finally, this methodology was tested with data from the BCI Competition IV 2a database, and the multi-branch 3D CNN achieved superior results when compared with small, medium, and large receptive field networks only.

10.1.2.2 EMD and SRC MI-BCI

Recognizing patterns from sparse representations, although it emerged in the field of image classification (Elad, 2010; Wright, Yang, Ganesh, Sastry, and Ma, 2008), is becoming increasingly useful in the classification of biological signals. Wen, Jia, Lian, Zhou, and Lu (2016) review methods of sparse representations of EEG signals for detecting epilepsy.

Betthauser et al. (2017) propose a classification model based on the smallest residual produced in the reconstruction of a sparsely represented sample. The technique is combined with ELM (Ding, Xu, and Nie, 2014; Huang, Zhu, and Siew, 2006; Huang, Wang, and Lan, 2011) to classify myoelectric signals in the control of prostheses. Signals were collected from two amputees, with and without a prosthesis, in addition to eight healthy individuals. The effectiveness of the method was evaluated both offline and online mode. In the first, the subjects perform suggested movements in random positions of their amputated arm, varying the positions in the three dimensions. The classifier is trained, however, using only one position, while the others are used as a test. When the ELM does not sufficiently discriminate, an SRC move is used to resolve the impasse between the doubtful classes. In online mode, subjects perform suggested moves in four untrained positions while receiving real-time feedback using the same classifier combination as in the previous mode. The method was compared with six other classifiers trained with three attribute groups. In all groups of subjects, the proposed method was the one that obtained the lowest error rate with significant performance improvement ($p < 0.001$) for the untrained positions.

This SRC model based on the smallest residual is still little applied in MI-BCI studies. Therefore, it is of interest to this work to evaluate the technique in this new context. The sparse sample is used to reconstruct the original sample, which will be classified according to the class that produced the smallest residue during its reconstruction. A better description of the method can be found in the Subsection 10.2.5.1.

Ameri et al. (2016) and Shin et al. (2012) appear among the first studies exploring SRC in the classification of MI. Since then, sparse representation has been increasingly used in this type of problem. For us, approaches that seek to improve the attributes that will be sparsely represented are interesting to situate the state of the art.

However, these approaches do not classify the samples themselves, but their sparse representations. This differs from the classification by the smallest residue studied in our work (Betthauser et al., 2017). But we find it appropriate to cite the pioneering studies on the combination of sparse representation techniques in the context of MI-BCI.

Miao et al. (2017) propose a classification mechanism for the sparse representations of optimized attributes in space, time, and frequency. The best EEG channels are selected based on relative entropy (spatial optimization); the signals from this subset of channels are decomposed into several overlapping frequency bands (frequency optimization) and time-segmented into overlapping windows (temporal optimization). Attributes based on the CSP are then extracted and the most significant are selected by sparse regression. Finally, a dictionary is generated and optimized to aid in sorting. The approach was evaluated in two databases and obtained an improvement of 21.57% and 14.38% compared to other methods applied in the same databases. In addition to comparison with other methods, the study assesses the impact of dictionary optimization by comparing SRC results with and without dictionary optimization, obtaining a significant improvement of 9.44%.

Zhang et al. (2018) use the same time-frequency attribute optimization method as the previous study (Miao et al., 2017) but use sparse representation as an attribute selector technique to train an SVM classifier (Noble, 2006; Suthaharan, 2016). The approach was evaluated in three databases, where mean accuracies of 88.5%, 83.3%, and 84.3% were obtained, obtaining significant improvement ($p < 0.01$) in relation to the other compared methods.

EMD is another technique that can be used to improve attributes for classifying MI, but it has not yet been combined with the SRC technique. Yusoff, Mahmoud, Malik, and Bahloul, et al. (2018) use EMD to decompose the signal into five components, called intrinsic mode functions (IMF), to extract three attributes. The resulting feature vector is used to train an artificial neural network and obtains good results in discriminating four classes of MI. The technique is compared to discrete wavelet transform (DWT). EMD traits achieve an average accuracy of 90.02%, while DWT traits average an accuracy of 84.77%.

Alazrai, Aburub, Fallouh, and Daoud (2017) have a similar application but extract up to seven attributes from the produced IMFs. The proposed model consists of a three-layer hierarchical SVM classifier, which surpasses the compared model (traditional SVM). Alam and Samanta (2017a) offer an analysis of the applicability of EMD in the identification of MI. In addition to generating attributes, the technique can also be used to remove artifacts (Alam and Samanta, 2017b).

Gaur, Pachori, Wang, and Prasad (2015) use EMD to compose an enhanced EEG signal, considering the average frequency of the MFIs. Three Hjorn parameters plus the absolute power are extracted from the new signal to compose the feature vector. The LDA classifier is then applied in the classification. It was observed that the technique can improve on average 10.5% of classification accuracy.

Park, Looney, Ur Rehman, Ahrabian, and Mandic (2012) evaluate EMD multivariate ex-tension (MEMD) in MI-BCI. Searches for peaks and troughs in n directions (multichannels) of the input signal, improving the location of frequency information. SVM is applied in classification.

We understand that combining the two approaches, EMD and SRC, can help in the classification of MI.

10.2   MATERIALS AND METHODS

10.2.1   DATABASES

Two datasets were used in this work. The first database was provided by the Neurodynamics Research Group of the Federal University of Pernambuco. It consists of 21 EEG signal collections from a single healthy adult male. The collections were performed on alternate days, and each one consists of 60 trials of eight seconds. In each trial, in turn, the MI of the right, left, or feet is performed. EEG data were collected through the g.Hamp amplifier set to a sampling rate of 256 Hz. In addition, 27 active channels were distributed over the premotor, motor, and sensoriomotor cortex. After preparation and placement of the electrodes, the data acquisition protocol was performed as follows (Figure 10.1):

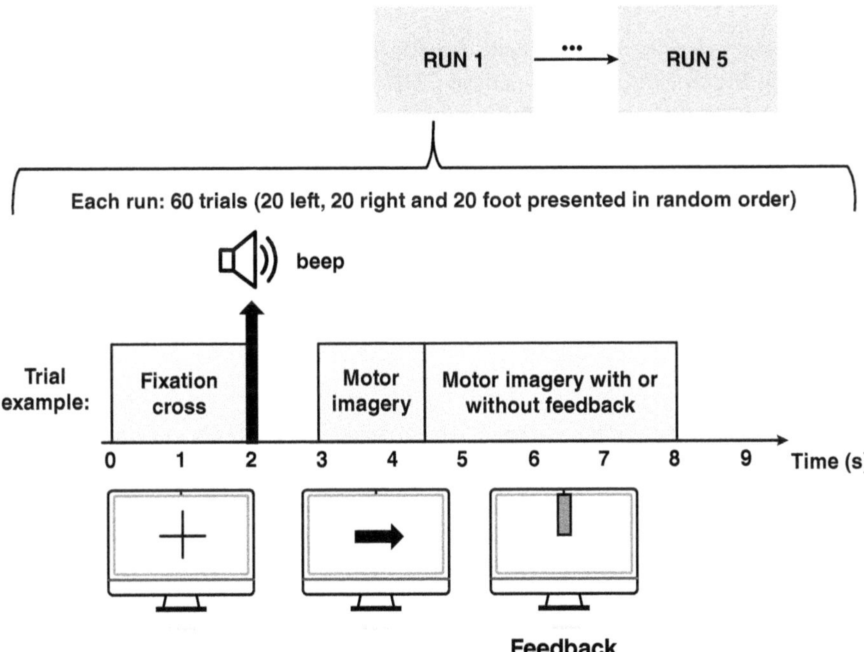

FIGURE 10.1   Database acquisition protocol: the collections were performed in five sessions on alternate days. Each of the sessions is composed of 60 trials of eight seconds, with 20 trials referring to the right hand, 20 to the left hand, and 20 to the foot. At the beginning of each trial, a fixation cross appeared on the screen, followed by a beep, both indicating an impending MI instruction. Then an arrow appeared on the screen, indicating which class should be imagined. Finally, the acquisition of imagination was done both with and without visual feedback.

1. The individual wearing an EEG sits in front of a monitor.
2. In a few moments, a cross appears to alert you of an impending instruction.
3. An arrow will randomly indicate which activity to do in that trial, e.g., an arrow to the right will indicate MI of the right hand, etc.
4. The individual performs the indicated instruction within eight seconds of the trial. It may or may not receive real-time feedback on the quality of its execution.
5. The screen is completely white, and the subject rests for four seconds.
6. The process is repeated until it completes 60 trials.

The second base used was the BCI Competition IV dataset 2b, which is widely used in the classification of MI of the upper limbs. Dataset 2b provides signals from three brain sites: C3, Cz, and C4, organized into several trials labeled with the imagery class. And it is composed of collections of nine subjects. More details about this base can be found in Leeb, Brunner, Müller-Putz, Schlögl, and Pfurtscheller (2008). For each trial, we used the first three seconds of imagery.

10.2.2 Proposed Method

In this work, we propose to evaluate the effectiveness of sparse representations in classifying MI from attributes based on EMD. For this, we use processing, extraction, and selection methods of attributes already related to the manipulation of EEG signals. Figure 10.2 shows how these methods are embedded in our goal flow. Section 10.2.3 brings them up in detail.

10.2.3 Signal Preprocessing and Feature Extraction

The first step of our processing consisted of separating and organizing the trials for each collection. At this stage, the signal could be filtered at 0.5 and 60 Hz and normalized.

EMD was applied to all channels. At least five IMFs were obtained; they approximate the conventional frequency bands (delta, theta, alpha, beta, and gamma) but are more suited to the non-stationary nature of the EEG signal.

However, it was also an option for us to use filtering in the aforementioned conventional frequency bands. These bands are known to carry relevant brain information. Especially alpha and beta bands are related to motor activity.

Once the trial was decomposed or filtered, we segmented it into one second windows and used only the last five seconds to extract features. We can consider that the initial seconds of a trial contain scattered imagery information since the individual was waiting for instructions, so we chose to discard the first three seconds of the trial.

The extracted characteristics were energy, sample entropy, and the absolute power of the segments.

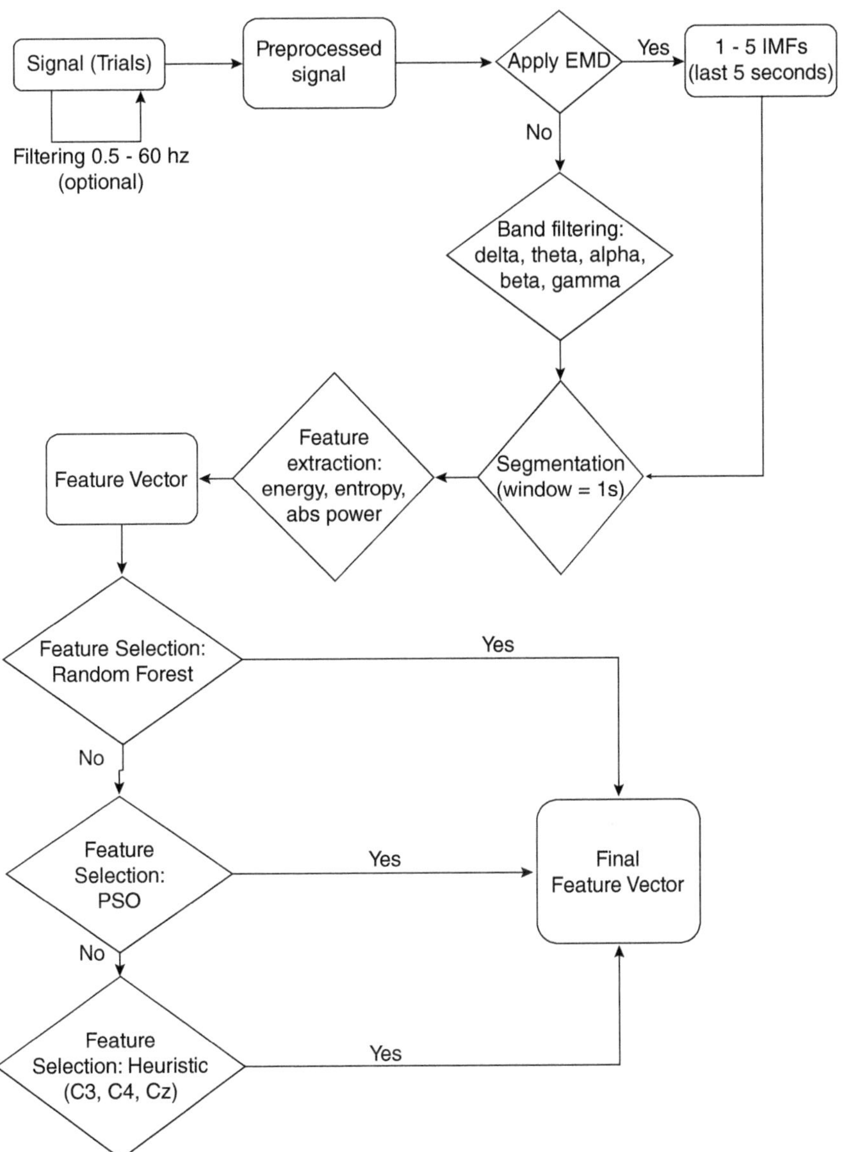

FIGURE 10.2 Trial processing step flow, eight-second window of EEG signal (Section 10.2.1). The flow presents the processing possibilities to obtain the feature vector used in this work. First, the signal is normalized, then you choose to decompose the signal by EMD (setups 1–5, Table 10.1) or into frequency bands (setup6, Table 10.1). Any previous option will generate five signal components, which will be segmented into one second windows. For each segment 3, attributes are extracted (energy, entropy, and absolute power). In dataset 1, the attribute vector will have 2025 attributes in total ($27 \times 5 \times 5 \times 1$). In dataset 2, the attribute vector will have 135 ($3 \times 5 \times 3 \times 3$). This requires the selection of these attributes, which can be done in three ways: using RForest, PSO, or manual. The resulting vector will serve as input for training and validating the classifiers.

10.2.3.1 Empirical Mode Decomposition - EMD

EMD is a self-adaptive method that decomposes the signal without leaving the time domain. It is useful for analyzing non-stationary and non-linear signals, such as brain signals. It consists of breaking the signal into a finite number of IMF (Alam and Samanta, 2017a). For a given signal $x(t)$, it can be decomposed into an IMF $c(t)$ and a residue r(t).

$$x(t) = \sum_{i=1}^{n} c_i(t) + r(t) \tag{10.1}$$

Yusoff et al. (2018) present a good scheme of how the algorithm to obtain the IMF works and can be seen in Figure 10.3.

10.2.4 Feature Selection

In dataset 1, each trial processed carries information from 27 channels, decomposed into 5 IMFs, segmented into five windows of one second, where three functions were calculated for each segment. So our feature vector has a size of $27 \times 5 \times 5 \times 3 = 2025$ attributes. In dataset 2, trials have 3 channels, 5 IMFs, 3 windows of one second, and 3 functions ($3 \times 5 \times 3 \times 3 = 135$ attributes). It is therefore a high number, capable of dispersing the low amount of trials available and making the sorting activity very costly. Then we reduce the vector size using a heuristic approach.

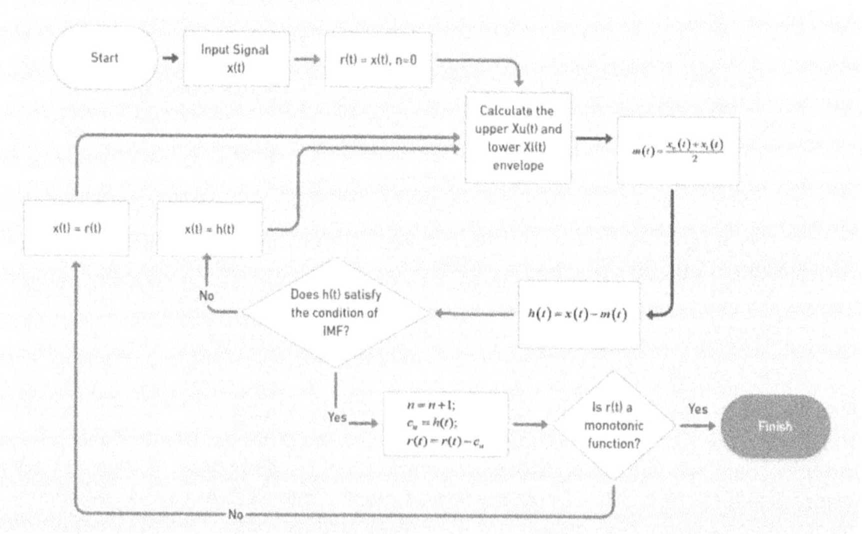

FIGURE 10.3　Flowchart of the empirical mode decomposition algorithm (Yusoff et al., 2018)

It is known by Neuroengineering that certain brain sites are more likely to concentrate MI information. These sites are called C3, C4, and Cz. Both are located close to the central sulcus, in the primary motor cortex and are related to motor activity in the right hand, left hand, and feet, respectively. It should be noted that these are the classes we are trying to identify.

It was also possible to bet which IMFs would be more likely to contain MI. We chose the 3rd and 4th IMFs because of their similarity with beta and alpha bands, commonly related to motor activity (Alazrai et al., 2017; Yusoff et al., 2018).

So, our new vector has $3 \times 2 \times 5 \times 3 = 90$ attributes. We thus mitigate the risk of underfitting signaled by the size of the initial vector and reduce classification costs.

However, it was still of our interest to use computational methods of feature selection, motivated by the notion that we could be missing some important information for the discrimination of the three classes of imagery. Added to the complexity of the brain signal, the interconnection of brain areas does not exhaust the possibility of the information we seek to be reflected in other brain sites.

Two alternatives to heuristic attribute selection are PSO and RForest-aided attribute selection. These methods are explained below.

10.2.4.1 Particle Swarm Optimization - PSO

PSO is a widely established method that works as decision trees, where attributes are ranked according to accuracy. The PSO uses an objective function that seeks to minimally penalize ranking performance, keeping it as high as possible with a reduced number of attributes (Eberhart and Yuhui Shi, 2001; Feng, Ong, Jiang, and Gupta, 2017; Jóhannesson, Bligaard, Ruban, Skriver, Jacobsen, and Nørskov, 2002; Kennedy and Eberhart, 1995; Poli, Kennedy, and Blackwell, 2007; Shi and Eberhart, 1999; van den Bergh and Engelbrecht, 2006; Wang, Yang, Teng, Xia, and Jensen, 2007; and Zhu, Samanta, Li, Rudd, and Frolov, 2018).

The PSO algorithm was inspired by a study of groups of birds looking for a place to build their nests, as well as food. In this case, the movement of the entire pack is based on the overall intelligence of the group. With that in mind, the algorithm initially uses a population of randomly generated particles or individuals, each individual being a candidate for the solution of the fitness function. Each individual is associated with a position vector and a velocity vector. The flock's trajectory is then guided by two sources of information: the position of the best particle in relation to the aptitude function and knowledge of the places previously visited by each particle. In this way, at each iteration of the algorithm, the positions and velocities of the particles are adjusted toward the best global and individual position (Barbosa, Ribeiro, Feitosa, Silva, Rocha, Freitas, Souza, and Santos, 2017; Feitosa, Ribeiro, Barbosa, de Souza, and dos Santos, 2014; Gomes, de Freitas Barbosa, de Santana, de Lima, Calado, Junior, de Almeida Albuquerque, de Souza, de Araujo, Moreno, et al., 2021; Ribeiro, Feitosa, de Souza, and dos Santos, 2014; Sakri, Rashid, and Zain, 2018).

Attribute selection by PSO was implemented in the database using 30 particles and k-NN as an objective function estimator. The individual particle (parameter c_1) and global consciousness were adopted as 0.5. The inertia factor w was 0.9, and the number of neighbors was 30.

10.2.4.2 Random Forest for Attribute Selection

In addition to PSO, we test attribute selection with decision trees, which can be used in classification and regression problems. In particular, RForests are a combination of trees that are built with different samples from the original database. Essentially, each tree is made up of four types of nodes: root, leaf, parent, and child nodes. The starting point is the root and the terminal nodes are the leaves. Thus, using such trees, the algorithm makes a decision after following a hierarchical path that starts at the root node and reaches the leaf node. Thus, after the formation of the forest, a new object that needs to be classified is placed for each of the trees to classify. At the end, each tree casts a vote that indicates its decision on the object's class. The forest then chooses the most voted class for that (Hasan, Nasser, Ahmad, and Molla, 2016) object.

In the case of attribute selection, the measure of importance of each attribute can be calculated according to the reduction of the model's accuracy when the attribute in question is not included in the tree. In other words: decision trees based on less relevant attributes will have a lower ranking performance (Sylvester, Bentzen, Bradbury, Clément, Pearce, Horne, and Beiko, 2018).

In our study, RForests were implemented using 100 trees or iterations.

10.2.5 Classification

The classification activity consisted of estimating which of the three MI classes (right hand, left hand, and foot) a trial belongs to. It is an offline classification of trials (eight-second activities of intense motor imagination). However, it was also part of this study to explore the classification of segments (one second in length). This is a simulation of what would be an online application to identify MI.

Figure 10.4 shows the different approaches to classification used in this study. Assuming that the SRC holds promise for classifying untrained data, it was necessary to compare it with another "common" classifier. We therefore chose the MLP neural network. However, it was also possible to explore the potential of sparse representations in a classifier other than SRC. We then added to our analysis a hybrid approach that used sparse representation but used MLP for classification.

10.2.5.1 Sparse Representation Classification

A sparse representation is a linear combination of a set of vectors, called a dictionary, to obtain a sparse vector, which has a large number of null or near-null values. The dictionary, in turn, is composed of samples from the training base. The classification

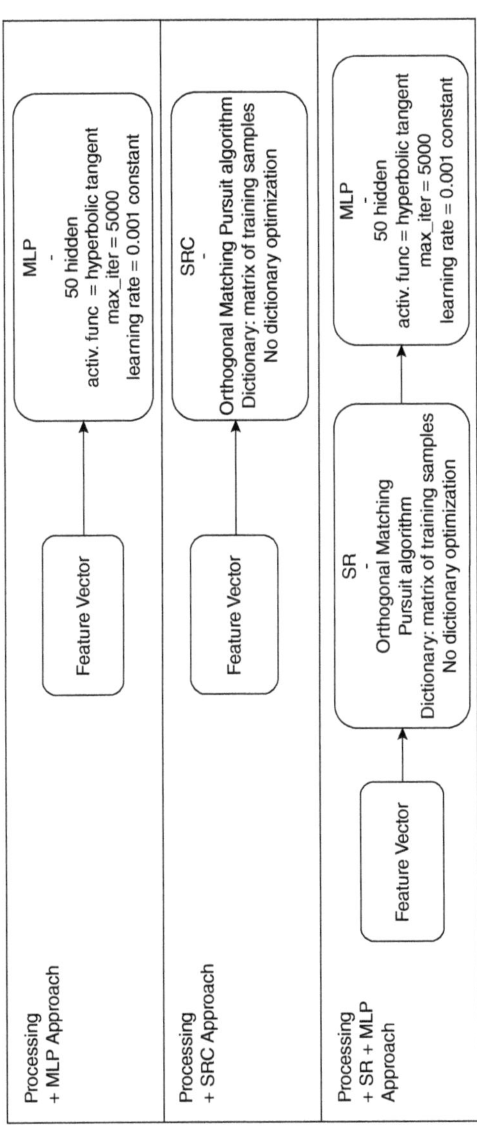

FIGURE 10.4 Classification: three approaches for classifying MI were tested, with a view to future comparison. All three approaches went through the attribute selection step, differing in the type of classifier used. The first approach consisted of classification with MLP; the second approach used the SRC; and the third approach was hybrid, encompassing sparse representation and MLP as a classifier.

of a new sample is done by observing the weights of the linear combinations that most contribute to the construction of the sparse vector. Members of the correct class are expected to contribute more weight.

Let D be a training dictionary, it is an array composed of D_i partitions, with $i = 1, \ldots, n$, where n is the number of classes and D_i is composed of the class's training samples i. A new sample y is reconstructed from a linear combination Dx, where $x = [x_1, x_2, \ldots, x_L]^T$ are the weights associated with each training sample. A sparsity constraint will limit the linear combination to a minimal subset of training samples. This restriction is imposed through the optimization problem.

$$x = \arg\min_{x} \{\frac{1}{2} \| Dx - y \|_2^2 + \lambda \| x \|_1\} \tag{6.2}$$

where $\lambda > 0$ is a sparsity smoothing parameter. Since the transformation will hardly be exact ($Dx = y$) with the sparsity constraint, the residual is then calculated for each class i

$$r_i = \| D_i x_i - y \|_2 \tag{6.3}$$

and the one with the smallest residual is the predicted class for the y sample.

10.2.5.2 Multilayer Perceptron

In 1958, Frank Rosenblatt proposed the perceptron model as the simplest form of an artificial neural network for binary classification. The perceptron consists of a single neuron with synaptic weights and adjustable bias, capable of classifying linearly separable problems (Haykin, 2001).

MLP is a generalization of the Rosenblatt perceptron and consists of several layers: an input layer, one or more hidden layers, and an output layer. Having additional hidden layers allows MLPs to solve more complex problems (Haykin, 2001; Ram-choun, Idrissi, Ghanou, and Ettaouil, 2016).

The training of an MLP is carried out in a supervised manner and aims to adjust the synaptic weights so that the output of the network approaches what is expected. To carry out this adjustment, the most commonly used method is the error retropropagation algorithm, consisting of two phases. In the propagation phase, an output is obtained from an input. Then, in the backpropagation phase, the error is calculated using the obtained and desired outputs. Through the error obtained, it is possible to adjust the weights and iteratively minimize the error (Kumar, Sasank, Praveen, and Rao, 2021).

MLPs have been commonly used in medical applications, such as in the diagnosis of cancer (de Vasconcelos, dos Santos, and de Lima, 2018; Pereira, Santana, Lima, Lima, and Santos, 2020a; Pereira, Santana, Lima, and Santos, 2020b; Pereira, Santana, Silva, Lima, Lima, and Santos, 2020c; Rodrigues, de Santana, Azevedo, Bezerra, Barbosa, de Lima, and dos Santos, 2019; Santana, Pereira, Lima, and Santos, 2020; Santana, Pereira, Silva, Lima, Sousa, Arruda, Lima, Silva, and Santos, 2018), diabetes (Mishra, Tripathy, Mallick, Bhoi, and Barsocchi, 2020), multiple sclerosis (Commowick, Istace, Kain, Laurent, Leray, Simon, Pop, Girard, Ameli, Ferré, et al., 2018), and in the monitoring and diagnosis of COVID-19 (Ahsan, E Alam, Trafalis, and Huebner, 2020; Borghi, Zakordonets, and Teixeira, 2021; Ibrahim, Kamaruddin, Mangshor, and Fadzil, 2020).

10.2.6 Experiments Settings

The scheme shown in Figure 10.2 enabled a series of options for signal processing that served as a parallel input for the classifiers, as shown in Figure 10.4. We started with a heuristic approach first and then made variations, combining other processing options as they proved promising. Table 10.1 lists the combinations chosen in this work. The 10-fold cross-validation was performed three times for each configuration evaluated, totaling 30 scores per setup.

Considering the type of sample, the trial is the default sample for most setups (setup5 classifies the trial but uses a resampler mechanism to increase the base). In setup4, the classified sample is the one second segment of the signal instead of the trial. The segment does not compose the attribute vector, as in the other configurations, therefore reducing the vector size to 405 (27 channels × 5 components × 3 attributes), but increasing the base sample volume.

Considering the type of decomposition, setups 1–5 apply EMD and select up to five IMFs to compose the feature vector. Setup6 is the only one that doesn't use EMD but breaks the signal down into five frequency band components (delta, theta, alpha, beta, and gamma).

In terms of channel and attribute selection, setup1 is the heuristic approach described in Section 10.2.4. It is the approach with the smallest attribute vector ($=90$) and therefore the least expensive. The remaining setups apply a computational mechanism for attribute selection. The PSO used in setup2 was configured for 30 particles, the k-NN ($k=4$) served as an estimator for the objective function, and we assigned the following values to the parameters: $c_1=0.5$, $c_2=0.5$, $w=0.9$, $k=30$, and $p=2$. RForests, in turn, were used with 100 trees. We can note that RForest was the most frequent method of feature selection used. This is due to its speed compared to PSO and therefore it is less expensive.

The feature vector produced by each setup was then evaluated in three classifiers: MLP, SRC, and SRMLP (Figure 10.2). MLP was trained with 50 neurons in the hidden layer, while OMP was the algorithm used in approaches that included sparse representation of the feature vector.

TABLE 10.1

Groups of Performed Experiments

Experiment ID	Sample Type	Channels	IMF	Feature Selection
setup1	Trial	C3, C4, Cz	3,4	None
setup2	Trial	All	1,2,3,4,5	PSO
setup3	Trial	All	1,2,3,4,5	RForest
setup4	Segment	All	1,2,3,4,5	RForest
setup5	Resampled trial	All	1,2,3,4,5	RForest
setup6	Trial	All	None (frequency bands)	RForest

10.2.7 Metrics

We consider two metrics to evaluate the performance of the experiments: accuracy and the Kappa index. Accuracy is the ratio between the number of correct predictions and the total number of classified samples. In other words, it is the probability of the classifier correctly indicating the class imagined by the patient or user. Its mean and standard deviation were useful in analyzing groups of experiments. The accuracy was calculated using the Eq. (10.4) below:

$$\text{Accuracy} = \frac{\text{TP} + \text{TN}}{\text{TP} + \text{TN} + \text{FP} + \text{FN}} \tag{6.4}$$

where TP indicates true positives, TN indicates true negatives, FP indicates false positives, and FN indicates false negatives.

The Kappa index, in turn, is a metric capable of dealing with multi-class problems, such as the one proposed here. It assesses the level of agreement between datasets, with the maximum value being 1, where values above 0.75 suggest excellent agreement and values between 0.40 and 0.75 indicate a median agreement (De Mast, 2007; Perroca and Gaidzinski, 2003). The Kappa index can be calculated using the Eq. (6.5) below:

$$k = \frac{\rho_o - \rho_e}{1 - \rho_e} \tag{6.5}$$

where ρ_o is the observed agreement or accuracy and ρ_e is the expected agreement, as defined in the Eq. (6.6).

$$\rho_e = \frac{(\text{TP} + \text{FP})(\text{TP} + \text{FN}) + (\text{FN} + \text{TN})(\text{FP} + \text{TN})}{(\text{TP} + \text{FP} + \text{FN} + \text{TN})^2} \tag{6.6}$$

10.3 RESULTS

10.3.1 Database 1

Table 10.2 summarizes the value of the metrics studied for each setup presented in Section 10.2.6. We can observe a pattern of equivalence between the compared classifiers. None of them explicitly excels in any of the metrics.

In Figure 10.5, we can observe the distribution of accuracies presented in Table 10.2. Each boxplot has 30 accuracy values, derived from cross-validation. Some of the configurations have a high interquartile range, having high variance in the results. The smallest variances are observed in the classification of segments (setup4), since there is a greater volume of data in this base, reducing the unpredictability of the classification. The same pattern can be seen in Figure 10.6. However, the results are still far from being of practical use.

The low performance of the metrics suggests that none of the approaches can generalize from the base adopted in this work. However, the averages and deviations

TABLE 10.2

Result of the Mean and Standard Deviation of the Metrics of the Experiments. For Each Setup, 3× Cross-Validation (10-fold) Were Performed, Totaling 30 Scores per Metric

	MLP		SRC		SRMLP	
Exp. ID	Acc	Kappa	Acc	Kappa	Acc	Kappa
setup1	33.37 ± 4.36	0.00 ± 0.07	34.96 ± 4.07	0.02 ± 0.06	33.70 ± 5.08	0.01 ± 0.08
setup2	32.82 ± 4.41	-0.01 ± 0.07	34.13 ± 5.21	0.01 ± 0.08	34.02 ± 5.40	0.01 ± 0.08
setup3	32.58 ± 5.17	-0.01 ± 0.08	33.05 ± 6.60	-0.00 ± 0.10	35.50 ± 5.15	0.03 ± 0.08
setup4	34.01 ± 1.87	0.01 ± 0.03	35.08 ± 2.47	0.03 ± 0.04	34.88 ± 2.26	0.02 ± 0.03
setup5	35.10 ± 4.69	0.03 ± 0.07	34.49 ± 4.89	0.02 ± 0.07	33.33 ± 3.60	0.00 ± 0.05
setup6	33.67 ± 3.87	0.01 ± 0.06	33.37 ± 4.13	0.00 ± 0.06	34.24 ± 4.27	0.01 ± 0.06

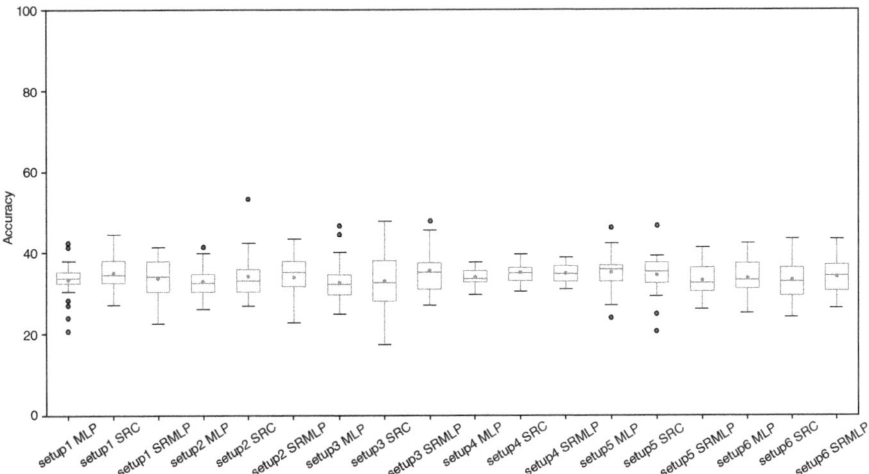

FIGURE 10.5   Accuracies of the MLP, SRC, and hybrid (SRMLP) classifiers, grouped by setup. We observed a similarity in the mean and median across all approaches, around 34%. We also look at similar distributions, making it difficult to determine from these results whether one setting is superior to another.

obtained are very similar, and the high variance suggests a tendency to underfitting. We suspect that the amount of sample in the base is not enough to discriminate well between classes. In this sense, we decided to synthetically increase the base using the SMOTE method (Chawla, Bowyer, Hall, and Kegelmeyer, 2002), which preserves the statistical behavior of the data. Tables 10.3 and 10.4 present the results obtained by increasing the base by 30% and doubling the base size, respectively. Data augmentation was not performed in setup2 due to the high computational complexity of

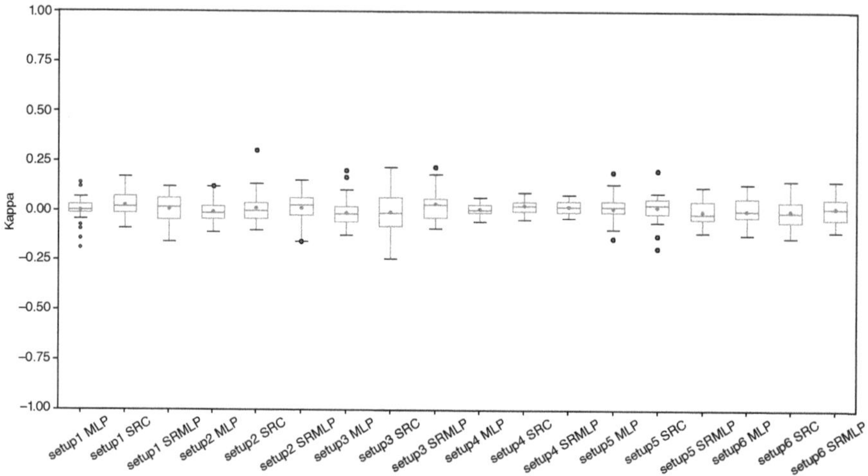

FIGURE 10.6 Kappa coefficients of MLP, SRC, and hybrid (SRMLP) classifiers, grouped by setup. We observe a behavior similar to Figure 10.5 with the coefficient oscillating throughout the value 0.

TABLE 10.3

Result of the Mean and Standard Deviation of the Metrics of the Experiments Increasing the Base by 30%. Setup2 Is Missing, Due to the Computational Complexity of the PSO for Large Volumes of Data. Setup5 Is also Missing, as it Consists of Another Data Augmentation Method, Resampling

	MLP		SRC		SRMLP	
Exp. ID	Acc	Kappa	Acc	Kappa	Acc	Kappa
setup1	48.62 ± 4.01	0.23 ± 0.06	49.35 ± 4.79	0.24 ± 0.07	49.43 ± 4.16	0.24 ± 0.06
setup3	59.89 ± 4.37	0.40 ± 0.07	66.72 ± 3.77	0.50 ± 0.06	66.02 ± 4.55	0.49 ± 0.07
setup4	45.12 ± 2.49	0.18 ± 0.04	63.21 ± 2.14	0.45 ± 0.03	61.41 ± 2.07	0.42 ± 0.03
setup6	60.57 ± 3.78	0.41 ± 0.06	66.86 ± 4.53	0.50 ± 0.07	66.08 ± 4.75	0.49 ± 0.07
Avg	53.55	0.30	61.53	0.42	60.73	0.41
Vs. MLP (%)	–	–	+14.91	+38.52	+13.42	+34.43

the PSO for large volumes of data. SMOTE was not applied in setup5 either, as it already performs another data augmentation method, resampling.

We observe in Table 10.3 that SRC achieved the best average accuracy (61.53%) and a higher percentage increase over MLP (14.91%). The same can be seen with regard to Kappa. SRC gets the highest value (0.42) and the highest percentage increase compared to MLP (38.52%). When we increased the base by 100% (Table 10.4), we noticed the same evolution of the SRC in relation to the average accuracy, obtaining the highest value (83.07%), meaning an increase of 15.84% in relation to MLP. Kappa also represents a high percentage increase (29%). Finally, the SRC method outperformed all others in most setups and second only to the hybrid method (SRMLP) in setup1 (heuristic approach).

When we look at the boxplots of the accuracies (Figures 10.7 and 10.8), we see a proportional increase in intra-setup approaches. It means that all approaches react

TABLE 10.4

Result of the Mean and Standard Deviation of the Experiments Metrics Increasing the Base by 100%. Setup2 Is Missing, Due to the Computational Complexity of the PSO for Large Volumes of Data. Setup5 Is also Missing, as it Consists of Another Data Augmentation Method, Resampling

	MLP		SRC		SRMLP	
Exp. ID	**Acc**	**Kappa**	**Acc**	**Kappa**	**Acc**	**Kappa**
setup1	62.40 ± 3.30	0.44 ± 0.05	62.85 ± 3.77	0.44 ± 0.06	64.52 ± 3.22	0.47 ± 0.05
setup3	84.37 ± 3.23	0.77 ± 0.05	91.43 ± 1.78	0.87 ± 0.03	90.44 ± 2.25	0.86 ± 0.03
setup4	55.94 ± 2.37	0.34 ± 0.04	87.06 ± 1.18	0.81 ± 0.02	85.31 ± 1.17	0.78 ± 0.02
setup6	84.13 ± 2.58	0.76 ± 0.04	90.96 ± 2.03	0.86 ± 0.03	89.93 ± 1.73	0.85 ± 0.03
Avg	71.71	0.58	83.07	0.74	82.55	0.74
Vs. MLP (%)	–	–	+15.84	+29.0	+15.12	+28.14

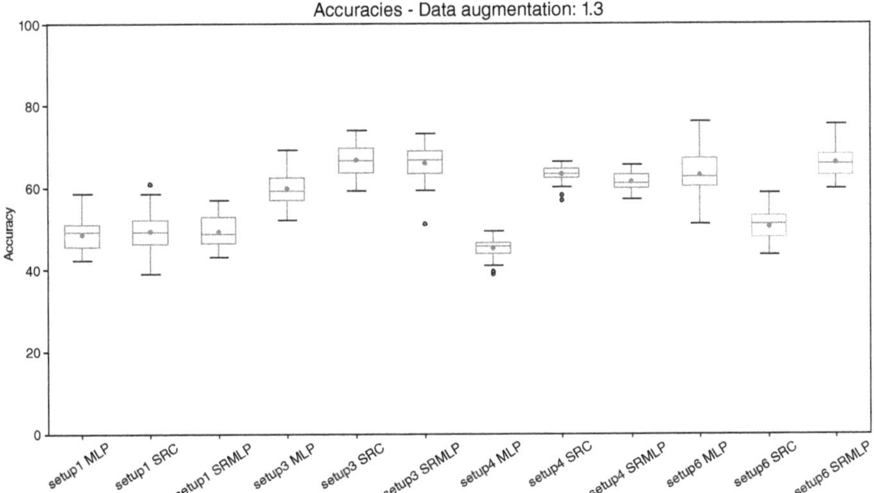

FIGURE 10.7 Distribution of accuracies with a 30% increase in base size, grouped by setup. Setups 3 (IMFs) and 6 (frequency band) appear a little above the rest. It is also possible to observe a small difference between the pure MLP approach and the approaches that use sparse representation. This is most evident in setup4, which has a larger volume of data by sorting segments (1s) rather than trials (8s).

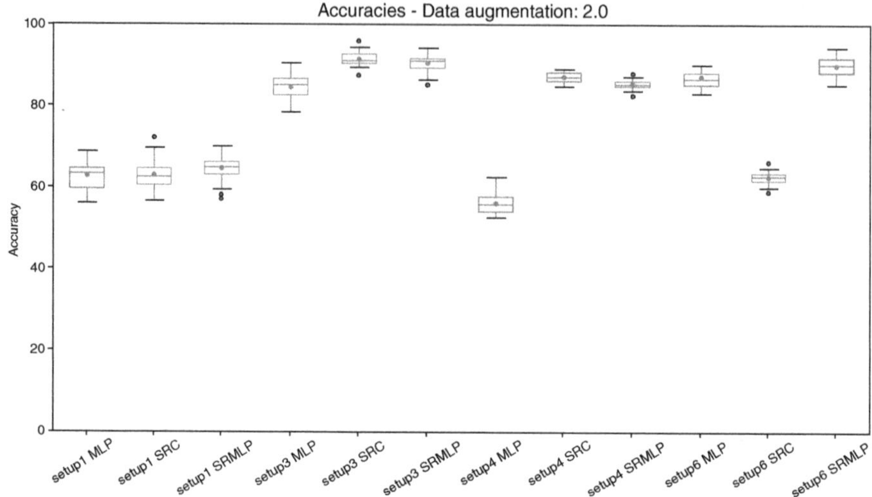

FIGURE 10.8 Distribution of accuracies with a 100% increase in base size, grouped by setup. The differences are most notable. Setup1 (the heuristic approach) is left behind, while the other methods achieve good values. It is also possible to notice the decrease in the accuracy variance in relation to the previous figures. The SRC and SRMLP methods outperform MLP but are very similar to each other.

positively to the increase in the training set, and SMOTE does not seem to privilege a specific method. Setups 3 and 6 appear a little above the others and have in common the selection of attributes through RForest. We also noticed that the more we increased the base size, the smaller the variance of the results, and the better the precision of the methods. There is a similarity in the distribution of results between the methods that use some sparse representation. Both have a certain statistical equivalence. On the other hand, the difference between an MLP and the other approaches is remarkable.

The distributions of the Kappa coefficients, when we increase the base (Figures 10.9 and 10.10), behave similarly to the accuracy distributions. Setups 3 and 5 perform better than the others in almost all classifiers. The variance decreases as the volume of data increases.

We can also observe the results from the perspective of computational complexity. Since the volume of data needs to grow to achieve good results, the more expensive it will be to process. Figures 10.11 and 10.12 show the distribution of the average training time for each model. The experiments were performed on a common computer (a CPU with 2 cores at 2.50 GHz and 4 threads). In general, training times are similar and should have little impact on the choice of algorithm in practice. Except when it comes to the hybrid approach in setup4, which is highly at variance with the others. If we look at the magnitude of the training time, we note that this setup must be chosen with care, as it takes more than 20 minutes (1,200 seconds) to train a model. It is also important to note that the same setup SRC approach has equivalent performance with a much lower computational cost.

Finally, we can assess the computational complexity of classification time. Figures 10.13 and 10.14 present the distribution of the average classification time

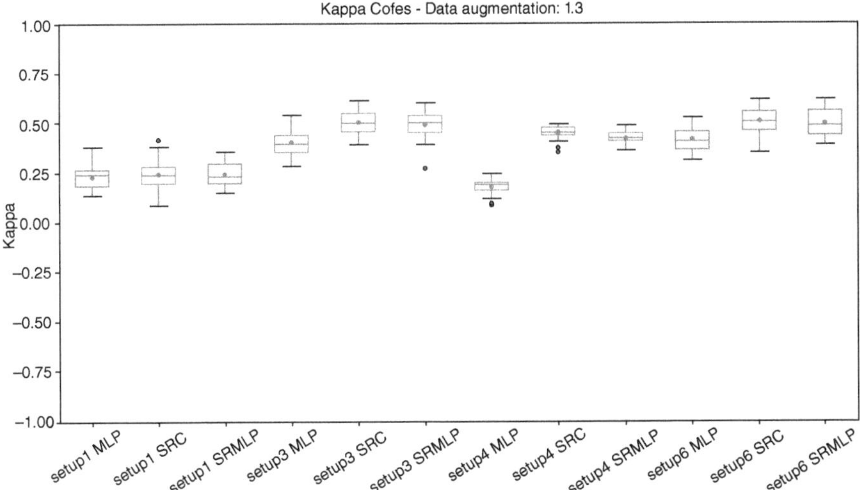

FIGURE 10.9 Distribution of Kappa coefficients with a 30% increase in base size, grouped by setup. The results show the same patterns observed in accuracy for the same base size, signaling an improvement in setups 3 and 6 and a difference between pure MLP and sparse representations.

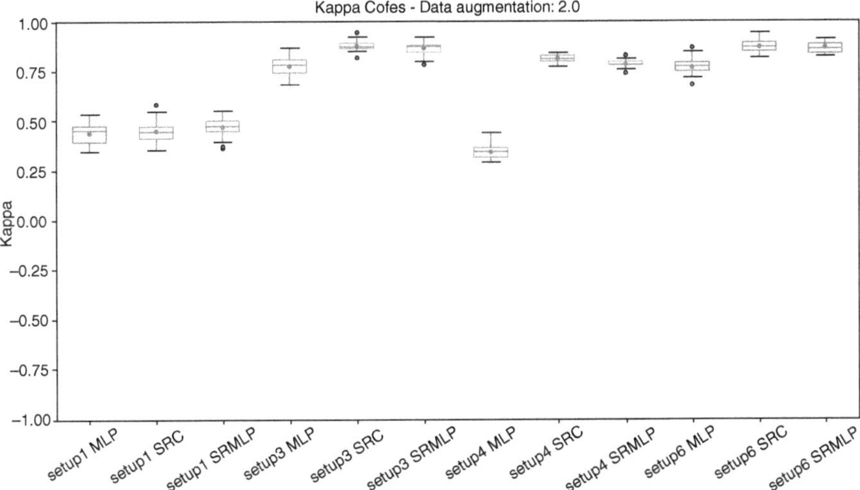

FIGURE 10.10 Distribution of Kappa coefficients with a 100% increase in base size, grouped by setup. The results show the same patterns observed in accuracy for the same base size (Figure 10.8).

of one partition of the cross-validation, that is, it is not about the time to classify a sample, but the test set. In this sense, we also noticed a trend of cost increase for the SRC in the classification of segments (setup4). However, in practice, segment classification should be intended for online applications, whose prediction is given to one sample at a time. This can mitigate the effect of computational costs.

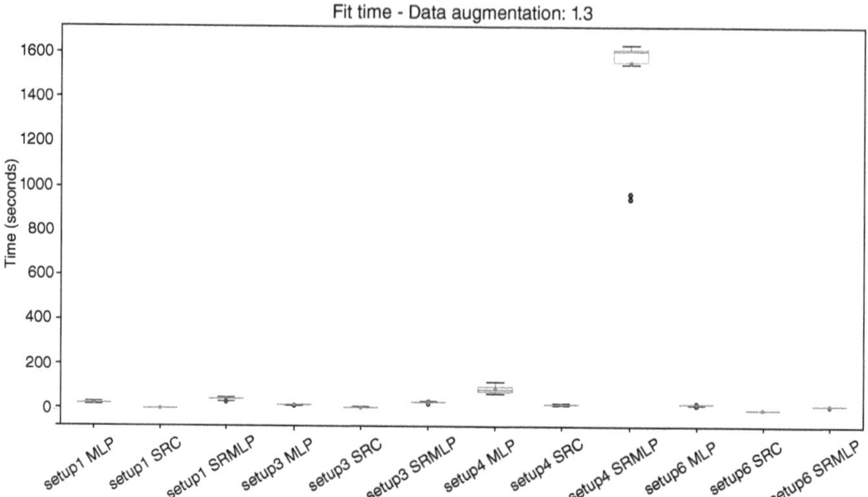

FIGURE 10.11   Distribution of training time with a 30% increase in base size, grouped by setup. The classification of segments using SRMLP (setup4) has a very high cost compared to others. In general, the variance is very small, as the size and characteristics of the base are similar between the cross-validation folds.

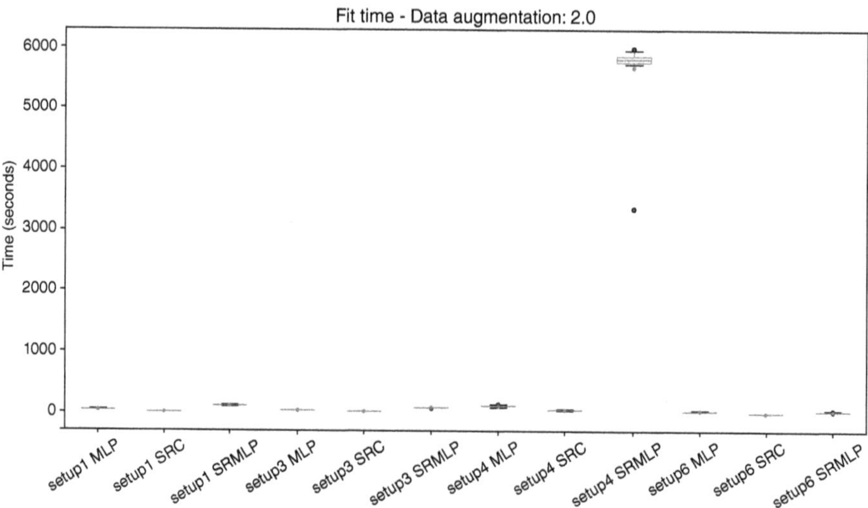

FIGURE 10.12   Distribution of training time with a 100% increase in base size, grouped by setup. Again, the discrepancy between the 4 SRMLP setups and the other configurations is observed.

10.3.2   DATABASE 2: BCI COMPETITION IV 2B

To improve classification accuracy, we generate artificial training data based on real training samples. The data augmentation method is very similar to the one presented by Dai et al. (2020), which shows the effectiveness of the method. Trials

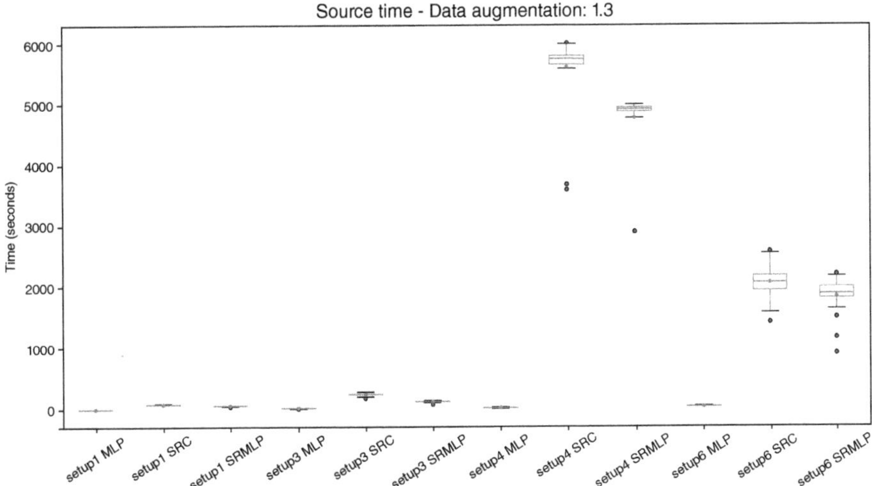

FIGURE 10.13 Distribution of prediction time (test in cross-validation) with a 30% increase in base size, grouped by setup. We observed a high time in setup4 approaches that use sparse representations. However, setup4 consists of segment classification (1s) rather than trials (8s), so it is the base with the most data in your test set.

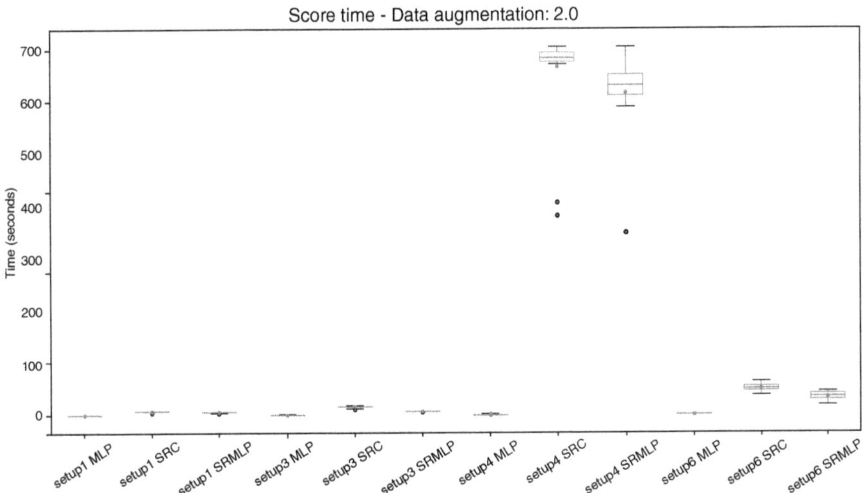

FIGURE 10.14 Distribution of the prediction time (test in cross-validation) with an increase of 100% of the base size, grouped by setup. Shows the same pattern as Figure 10.13.

were segmented into three crops and randomly recombined between trials of the same class and subject, generating new samples. Then the decomposition method is applied (EMD or filtering by frequency bands, according to the experiment setup), and the components are also randomly recombined to generate new samples. This method was applied to triple the size of the training base.

In addition to the classifiers used in the experiments with the previous base (MLP, SRC, and SR+MLP), RForest and SVM were also tested. These algorithms were also used in the classification of the space representation (SRR-Forest and SRSVM). Table 10.5 summarizes the results obtained for each of the 9 subjects in the base (S1–S9) in 3 setups. Setup1 describes the condition in which the experiment does not perform any selection of attributes since the selection of C3, Cz, and C4 is not necessary, since the base already consists of using the same channels. Setups 3 (with EMD) and 6 (with frequency bands) are presented here to allow again the comparative analysis between these techniques. Finally, Figure 10.15 presents the distribution of accuracies for subject 4. The same behavior can be observed in the other subjects and can be deduced from the standard deviation values of Table 10.5.

Table 10.6 considers the most accurate models obtained by the previous experiment and presents the inter-subject average of each setup. The best sparse models achieve an average of 66.7% among the subjects in the base. To obtain this value, we used the average of the SRC of setup3 and the averages of SRMLP, SRR-Forest and SRSVM of setup6. If we consider only the hybrid approaches SRMLP, SRR-Forest and SRSVM, we observe an average accuracy of 69.35%, while non-sparse models reach an average accuracy of 76.05%, that is, the average of MLP, RForest, and SVM models from setup6.

10.4 DISCUSSION

10.4.1 DATABASE 1

The dataset 1, although voluminous, is still not sufficiently representative for the problem of distinguishing three classes of MI. The performance improvement obtained with SMOTE corroborates this thesis. However, the user cannot be expected to have so much time to obtain a significant volume of data. To have an estimate, each collection has 60 trials of eight seconds, which is equivalent to eight minutes per collection. The original base, without data augmentation, has 21 collections, for a total of 168 minutes. However, we only saw a noticeable improvement in the data when we doubled the size of this database (Figures 10.8 and 10.10). It is unfeasible for a person to take that long to provide a massive amount of data. In this sense, the improvement of approaches that use the data augmentation mechanism is essential if we want to reduce the user's reluctance to use BCI. However, the problem is not new. It is possible to observe in the literature the use of data augmentation to increase the size of the training base in EEG signals (Dai et al., 2020).

About the performance obtained in each setup. We can observe that, in addition to adaptive methods (EMD and SRC), the selection of attributes greatly impacts the result. Next, we'll talk about each setup.

The heuristic approach (setup1) is far from being the most promising, as it grew the least as the base increased (Figures 10.7–10.10). This signals that the intentional choice of brain regions (C3, C4, and Cz channels) and frequencies (IMF 3 and 4) is not the best choice. It is possible to affirm that MI information may be better distributed in other regions of the motor cortex and in the frequency spectrum. This reinforces the need to use automatic and adaptive mechanisms for attribute selection.

TABLE 10.5

BCI CIV 2b – Result of the Mean and Standard Deviation of the Accuracies of the Experiments. For Each Setup, 3× Cross Validation (10-fold) Was Performed, Totaling 30 Scores. S1–S9 Identifies the Subjects of the Base

Exp. ID	MLP	R.Forest	SVM	SRC	SRMLP	SRR.Forest	SRSVM
S1 setup1	63.82±2.18	61.37±2.1	66.9±1.03	51.87±2.22	61.54±1.58	58.19±2.05	57.91±2.49
S1 setup3	62.62±2.58	62.22±2.45	66.71±1.06	50.77±2.74	60.75±2.8	60.8±2.2	60.47±2.27
S1 setup6	67.44±3.41	69.56±1.94	67.65±1.45	51.27±2.9	65.51±2.04	59.2±2.56	58.33±2.38
S2 setup1	53.77±2.05	54.24±2.76	50.9±1.05	46.22±2.25	49.41±1.95	50.98±2.58	51.25±1.49
S2 setup3	52.73±2.82	54.07±2.14	51.1±1.37	49.54±2.26	52.59±2.21	51.25±1.87	50.94±2.48
S2 setup6	52.88±1.94	53.1±2.11	55.69±1.16	49.44±1.6	52.05±3.29	53.07±2.6	52.61±2.02
S3 setup1	50.2±2.68	50.68±2.86	49.93±1.75	51.87±3.0	47.26±1.48	49.48±1.77	50.19±2.41
S3 setup3	50.28±2.89	49.93±2.62	50.59±1.71	48.8±2.93	49.65±2.59	48.59±2.43	49.57±1.79
S3 setup6	49.12±2.41	53.57±2.44	50.35±1.6	47.28±2.41	49.2±2.62	48.29±2.67	48.28±2.01
S4 setup1	90.76±0.98	94.95±0.56	90.98±0.83	63.24±1.74	84.1±1.02	81.28±1.49	81.04±1.66
S4 setup3	91.6±0.92	94.86±0.89	90.81±0.53	62.92±1.78	83.02±1.46	81.85±1.55	82.54±1.54
S4 setup6	96.83±0.78	97.2±0.39	94.12±0.35	60.22±1.3	81.68±7.51	79.31±1.7	78.78±2.1
S5 setup1	71.98±1.94	68.77±1.88	69.16±0.81	47.25±1.59	54.47±2.5	52.82±2.05	52.88±1.42
S5 setup3	71.04±2.2	68.41±2.25	69.65±1.09	50.31±2.26	66.01±2.81	52.34±1.78	53.09±2.2

(*Continued*)

TABLE 10.5 (*Continued*)

BCI CIV 2b – Result of the Mean and Standard Deviation of the Accuracies of the Experiments. For Each Setup, 3× Cross Validation (10-fold) Was Performed, Totaling 30 Scores. S1–S9 Identifies the Subjects of the Base

Exp. ID	MLP	R.Forest	SVM	SRC	SRMLP	SRR.Forest	SRSVM
S5 setup6	81.38±2.11	76.91±2.03	81.04±0.79	46.56±1.61	71.48±2.1	65.98±2.16	66.0±2.09
S6 setup1	66.36±1.73	64.08±1.68	68.62±0.88	49.26±2.35	52.36±2.28	54.42±2.25	53.76±2.22
S6 setup3	62.96±2.95	65.22±1.61	68.13±1.27	52.63±2.57	59.32±3.76	54.24±2.48	53.88±2.56
S6 setup6	73.16±2.28	75.31±1.71	73.65±1.17	48.47±2.51	69.65±2.52	63.57±2.15	63.56±2.29
S7 setup1	59.94±1.97	62.69±2.15	62.23±1.2	59.04±2.11	56.31±2.49	56.54±2.91	56.11±3.07
S7 setup3	58.43±2.3	62.44±1.94	61.95±1.23	51.29±2.72	56.06±2.41	56.26±3.01	56.36±2.99
S7 setup6	60.75±2.62	66.02±2.41	64.63±1.48	49.74±3.14	59.01±2.96	55.88±2.27	55.92±2.4
S8 setup1	84.46±2.0	89.17±1.06	87.23±0.81	56.78±1.7	70.25±1.87	71.1±2.02	71.28±2.05
S8 setup3	86.26±2.47	88.91±1.28	86.3±0.93	61.1±3.6	82.04±2.18	70.7±2.8	70.35±2.9
S8 setup6	85.75±2.19	88.99±1.41	85.52±1.01	56.32±2.04	81.72±2.21	69.67±2.52	69.59±2.38
S9 setup1	75.67±1.88	76.67±1.73	79.24±0.84	53.8±1.95	61.16±2.15	60.88±1.81	60.56±1.92
S9 setup3	72.67±2.01	77.33±1.62	79.5±1.11	51.88±3.02	69.88±2.34	60.33±2.76	60.49±1.76
S9 setup6	79.84±2.03	81.93±1.3	79.97±1.0	54.18±2.15	75.77±2.44	67.76±1.68	67.21±2.65

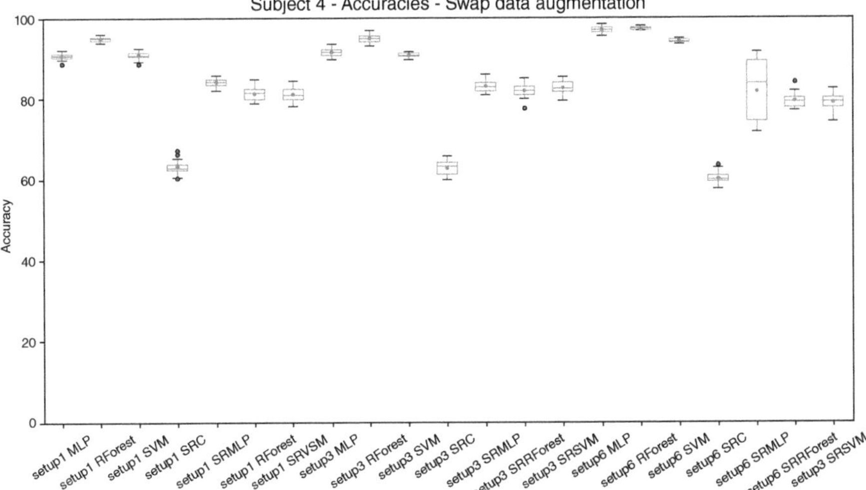

FIGURE 10.15 Distribution of subject 4 accuracies with a 3× increase in base size, grouped by setup. The differences are more notable. The equivalence between the decomposition methods continues to be observed. However, we observed a lower performance of classifiers that use sparse representation. A different result from the first dataset.

Setup2 uses PSO to select attributes among all channels and frequencies. It proved to be very costly for attribute selection, being deprecated in favor of selection by RForest.

Setup3 replaces PSO by selecting RForest. It was one of the settings that grew the most as the base increased (Figures 10.8 and 10.10). It also presented one of the best performances of the SRC and SRMLP, surpassing the conventional technique. We observe with it the first indication of the effectiveness of sparse representations for classifying MI.

Setup4 is similar in setup to setup3, but classifies segments (1s) instead of trials (8s). It is as close to an online rating approach as the user expects real-time feedback (equal to or less than one second). It also corroborates the superiority of the SRC and SRMLP in relation to the MLP, presenting a more notable difference. However, when looking at training and testing time, we must consider it carefully, as the larger the training base, the more costly the SR approaches become. For this case, it is possible to think about optimizing the training dictionary to reduce its size, since the SR dictionary is the set of all training samples in the base. It is also an option to merge the prediction between the pure (faster) MLP model and an SR model. From the degree of certainty that the MLP classifies its samples, we can resort to an SR model to help classify the more difficult samples, as suggested in Betthauser et al. (2017).

Setup5 has a similar setup to setup3, but increases the base by 30% with resampling. It did not stand out in relation to the other methods (Figures 10.5 and 10.6). When it comes to data augmentation, we find it more promising to use SMOTE as it generates new samples close to the group of existing samples.

Setup6 is similar in setup to setup3, but instead of using EMD, it separates the signal into conventional frequency bands (delta, theta, alpha, beta, and gamma). It also

TABLE 10.6

BCI CIV 2b - Accuracy of the Best Models of Each Evaluated Configuration

Exp. ID	MLP	R.Forest	SVM	SRC	SRMLP	SRR.Forest	SRSVM
S1 setup1	67.98	65.79	68.86	55.7	67.11	62.72	62.28
S1 setup3	67.98	67.11	68.86	54.82	66.67	65.35	64.47
S1 setup6	74.56	75.0	69.74	55.26	69.74	64.04	63.16
S2 setup1	57.14	59.18	53.47	50.61	53.06	56.33	53.47
S2 setup3	60.0	57.96	54.29	55.92	57.55	55.1	56.33
S2 setup6	56.73	57.55	57.55	53.47	58.78	59.18	56.33
S3 setup1	55.22	57.83	53.48	58.26	50.0	53.48	54.78
S3 setup3	54.78	56.52	54.35	53.91	54.78	53.48	53.04
S3 setup6	52.17	57.83	53.48	53.48	54.35	53.04	51.74
S4 setup1	92.18	96.09	92.51	67.1	85.67	84.69	84.36
S4 setup3	93.49	96.74	91.53	65.8	85.99	85.02	85.34
S4 setup6	98.37	98.05	94.79	63.52	91.53	84.04	82.41
S5 setup1	76.92	71.79	70.7	50.55	58.24	56.04	55.68
S5 setup3	75.46	73.26	72.16	54.21	71.79	55.68	58.61
S5 setup6	86.08	80.59	82.78	50.18	75.82	71.06	70.33
S6 setup1	70.52	67.33	70.52	52.99	58.17	61.75	57.77
S6 setup3	71.71	69.72	70.92	57.37	65.74	58.17	60.16
S6 setup6	76.89	78.49	76.1	53.39	77.29	68.53	67.33
S7 setup1	62.93	68.1	65.09	63.79	61.64	62.93	62.5
S7 setup3	64.22	65.52	64.22	57.33	63.79	62.93	62.5
S7 setup6	65.09	71.12	67.67	55.17	65.09	62.93	60.78
S8 setup1	88.26	91.3	88.7	61.3	73.04	75.22	75.65
S8 setup3	91.3	90.87	87.83	69.57	85.65	76.52	74.78
S8 setup6	90.87	92.17	88.26	60.43	90.43	76.96	74.78
S9 setup1	78.78	80.41	80.82	57.55	64.9	64.9	64.49
S9 setup3	75.92	80.82	82.04	59.59	75.1	64.9	63.27
S9 setup6	84.08	85.31	82.04	59.59	80.82	70.2	71.84
AVG setup1	72.21	73.09	71.57	57.54	63.54	64.23	63.44
AVG setup3	72.76	73.17	71.8	58.72	69.67	64.13	64.28
AVG setup6	76.09	77.35	74.71	56.05	73.76	67.78	66.52

corroborates the superiority of the SRC and SRMLP over the MLP. However, it has a behavior very similar to that observed in setup3, improving its performance in the same proportion as the database increases (Figures 10.7–10.10). In this sense, the use of EMD does not seem to impact the results. It is possible that the equivalence with processing frequency bands is due to the similarity between the IMFs and the filtered signal in these bands. Figure 10.16 illustrates a comparison between the techniques. It is possible to note the similarity in wave frequency between the two approaches. We can assume that this is so because brain signals do not have very high frequencies and oscillate in a similar way. EMD has little room to generate multi-frequency IMFs.

We observed that the classifiers that use sparse representation have results equivalent to each other, but they outperform the conventional MLP model. The SRC

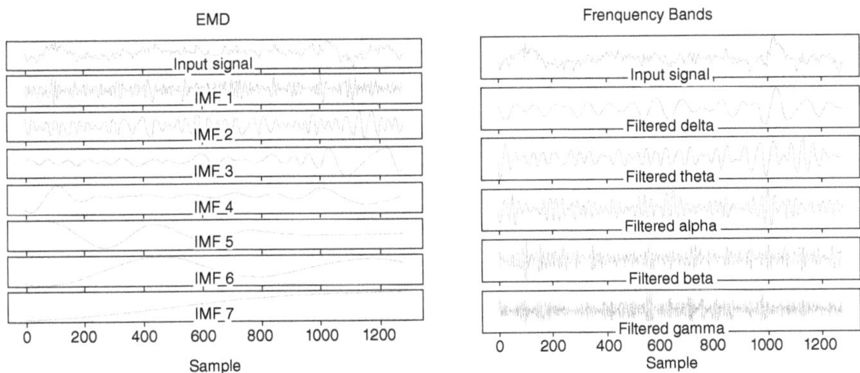

FIGURE 10.16 On the left, we present the EMD decomposition of an EEG signal. The decomposition for the signal in question generated 7 IMF. On the right, we present an EEG signal filtered in 5 frequency bands. It is interesting to note that the 1st IMF has a frequency very similar to the beta filtered signal, while the IMF 2 resembles the signal composition in the alpha and theta bands.

achieves an average accuracy of 83.07%, while the MLP is 71.71%, representing a gain of over 15.84%. The use of EMD in relation to other attribute processing techniques is not superior. However, EMD does not influence negatively; there is room for improvement. Finally, the use of data augmentation proved to be important to obtain relevant results.

10.4.2 DATABASE 2: BCI COMPETITION IV 2B

The results obtained in BCI Competition dataset 2b present a different behavior from the first dataset of this study. When comparing the approaches and observing the attribute processing techniques, it is possible to perceive a small superiority of the filtering by frequency bands in relation to the attributes based on EMD. The average accuracy of the setup6 models generally exceeds the accuracy of setups1 and 3 for most subjects in the base (S1, S5, S6, S7, and S9) (Table 10.5). Regarding the classification algorithm, we can also notice that the models that use sparse representation perform less than the others. Still, among these models, we note that the residual-based algorithm (SRC) is deprecated in relation to models that seek to combine the spatial representation with other algorithms (SRMLP, SRR+Forest, and SRSVM). This is well illustrated in Figure 10.15, referring to subject 4, but which represents the pattern observed in the other subjects. Therefore, the model proposed by Betthauser et al. (2017) in the classification of EMG signals does not seem to be adequate when working with EEG data. However, dictionary optimization techniques can help improve the results by better adapting this approach to the context of MI classification.

When we look at Table 10.6, the previous observations are even more evident; however, this table still allows us to observe which of the tried configurations is the best in the general average. The RForest classification of attributes based on

TABLE 10.7

Comparison between the Accuracies of Different Studies for the BCI Competition IV 2b Base

Subject	Miao et al. SRC	Miao et al. SRC+	Dai et al.	Gaur et al.	Zhu et al.	This Work
S1	69.43	83.83	80.5	62.8	–	75.0
S2	53.00	62.61	70.6	67.1	–	57.55
S3	51.24	61.32	85.6	98.7	–	57.83
S4	93.15	98.11	94.6	88.4	–	98.05
S5	81.23	91.91	98.3	96.3	–	80.59
S6	64.15	85.78	86.6	75.3	–	78.49
S7	76.96	94.39	89.6	72.2	–	71.12
S8	80.03	93.26	95.6	87.8	–	92.17
S9	79.05	91.14	87.4	85.3	–	82.04
AVG	72.03	86.41	87.6	81.6	70.0	77.35

frequency bands (AVG setup6, column 3) is the best configuration among the others, with 77.35% accuracy. It is worth noting that in setup6, the selection of attributes is also carried out by RForest, which explains the reason for the good performance of this combination.

We can then compare it with the cited works that use the same dataset. Table 10.7 presents the performance between the approaches. Miao et al. (2017) use SRC with and without dictionary optimization. However, it only experiences the 3rd collection of each subject, so the training and test data are similar, as they were collected on the same day and time. Therefore, the adaptive factor, where the imagery could vary on different days, cannot be evaluated in these results. The other works, including this one, use the complete base. Zhu et al. (2019) give only the average result of all subjects. Our study thus obtains an average performance in relation to the state of the art. We can attribute this performance to the lack of optimization of the sparse dictionary, considering that its optimization proved to be efficient in increasing accuracy (Miao et al., 2017). The synthetic increase in the training base contributed to increasing the accuracy of our study. It is interesting to note that it is the same data augmentation technique used by the study that had the best performance, but that uses another classification method (Dai et al., 2020).

10.5   CONCLUSION

In this work, we propose to evaluate the combination of two adaptive methods to the subject's context, EMD and SRC, in the classification of three-limb MI. Observing the results, it is possible to affirm that SRC is effective and promising in the detection of MI and can be very useful in BCI applications, generating gains of approximately 15% compared to conventional classifier algorithms. However, the use of EMD does not have a great impact on improving the classification, as the same results can be obtained using other approaches. However, the thesis of the usefulness of the technique still stands when we consider the results obtained by other works (Alam and Samanta, 2017a,b; Alazrai et al., 2017; Bashar and Bhuiyan, 2016; Chen and You, 2017; Davies and James, 2014; Saha and Ali, 2016; Yusoff et al., 2018). In this sense, the evaluation of other databases can also be useful to better understand the impact of the studied techniques. It is noteworthy here that the problem brought up is multiclass, and in the domain of MI it is not a trivial problem, with great variations between databases.

The possibility of combining the methods with other techniques is presented as an option for future work. For example, using wavelet transform decomposition in preprocessing can make the method more noise-resilient (Bajaj, 2020).

Finally, if we want to decrease the cost and effort to use the BCI and still guarantee good performance, we need: (i) to invest efforts in generating new samples to synthetically increase the training base; (ii) to enhance self-adaptive mechanisms that respond efficiently to the user's context and serve as an enhancement for joint use with the SRC.

It is important to realize that, despite the inverse result, we cannot discard the evidence found with the first base experiments. If, on the one hand, the BCI Competition dataset 2b contains more subjects (9 subjects vs 1 subject), on the other hand, the first dataset has a greater amount of subject data (21 collections vs 5). This only suggests that it is necessary to evaluate approaches on a variety of bases in order to observe prevailing behavior and to provide evidence in which contexts one technique may be superior to another.

ACKNOWLEDGEMENTS

The authors are grateful to the Brazilian research agencies FACEPE and CNPq for the partial financial support of this research.

The authors are also grateful to the Research Group on Biomedical Computing at UFPE for the technological support; to the Research Group on Neurodynamics at UFPE for providing the original dataset; and to Neurobots for supporting this study.

CONFLICT OF INTEREST

All authors declare they have no conflicts of interest.

COMPLIANCE WITH ETHICAL STANDARDS

This study was funded by the Brazilian research agencies CAPES and CNPq.

All procedures performed in studies involving human participants were in accordance with the ethical standards of the institutional and/or national research committee and with the 1964 Helsinki Declaration and its later amendments or comparable ethical standards.

REFERENCES

M. M. Ahsan, T. E Alam, T. Trafalis, and P. Huebner. Deep MLP-CNN model using mixed-data to distinguish between covid-19 and non-covid-19 patients. *Symmetry*, 12(9):1526, 2020.

M. E. Alam and B. Samanta. Empirical mode decomposition of EEG signals for brain computer interface. In *SoutheastCon 2017*, Concord, NC, USA, pages 1–6. IEEE, 2017a.

M. E. Alam and B. Samanta. Performance evaluation of empirical mode decomposition for EEG artifact removal. In *ASME International Mechanical Engineering Congress and Exposition*, Tampa, FL, USA, volume 58387, page V04BT05A024. American Society of Mechanical Engineers, 2017b.

R. Alazrai, S. Aburub, F. Fallouh, and M. I. Daoud. EEG-based BCI system for classifying motor imagery tasks of the same hand using empirical mode decomposition. In *2017 10th International Conference on Electrical and Electronics Engineering (ELECO)*, Bursa, Turkey, pages 615–619. IEEE, 2017.

R. Ameri, A. Pouyan, and V. Abolghasemi. Projective dictionary pair learning for EEG signal classification in brain computer interface applications. *Neurocomputing*, 218:382–389, 2016.

S. U. Amin, M. Alsulaiman, G. Muhammad, M. A. Mekhtiche, and M. S. Hossain. Deep learning for EEG motor imagery classification based on multi-layer CNNS feature fusion. *Future Generation Computer Systems*, 101:542–554, 2019.

N. Bajaj. Wavelets for EEG analysis. In *Wavelet Theory*. IntechOpen, London, 2020.

V. A. Barbosa, R. R. Ribeiro, A. R. Feitosa, V. L. Silva, A. D. Rocha, R. C. Freitas, R. E. Souza, and W. P. Santos. Reconstruction of electrical impedance tomography using fish school search, non-blind search, and genetic algorithm. *International Journal of Swarm Intelligence Research (IJSIR)*, 8(2):17–33, 2017.

S. K. Bashar and M. I. H. Bhuiyan. Classification of motor imagery movements using multivariate empirical mode decomposition and short time Fourier transform based hybrid method. *Engineering Science and Technology: An International Journal*, 19(3):1457–1464, 2016.

J. L. Betthauser, C. L. Hunt, L. E. Osborn, M. R. Masters, G. Lévay, R. R. Kaliki, and N. V. Thakor. Limb position tolerant pattern recognition for myoelectric prosthesis control with adaptive sparse representations from extreme learning. *IEEE Transactions on Biomedical Engineering*, 65(4):770–778, 2017.

P. H. Borghi, O. Zakordonets, and J. P. Teixeira. A covid-19 time series forecasting model based on MLP ANN. *Procedia Computer Science*, 181:940–947, 2021.

N. V. Chawla, K. W. Bowyer, L. O. Hall, and W. P. Kegelmeyer. Smote: synthetic minority over-sampling technique. *Journal of Artificial Intelligence Research*, 16:321–357, 2002.

W. Chen and Y. You. Masking empirical mode decomposition-based hybrid features for recognition of motor imagery in EEG. In *2017 3rd IEEE International Conference on Control Science and Systems Engineering (ICCSSE)*, Beijing, China, pages 548–551. IEEE, 2017.

O. Commowick, A. Istace, M. Kain, B. Laurent, F. Leray, M. Simon, S. C. Pop, P. Girard, R. Ameli, J.-C. Ferré, et al. Objective evaluation of multiple sclerosis lesion segmentation using a data management and processing infrastructure. *Scientific Reports*, 8(1):1–17, 2018.

G. Dai, J. Zhou, J. Huang, and N. Wang. HS-CNN: a CNN with hybrid convolution scale for EEG motor imagery classification. *Journal of Neural Engineering*, 17(1):016025, 2020.

S. R. Davies and C. J. James. Using empirical mode decomposition with spatio-temporal dynamics to classify single-trial motor imagery in BCI. In *2014 36th Annual International Conference of the IEEE Engineering in Medicine and Biology Society*, Chicago, IL, USA, pages 4631–4634. IEEE, 2014.

J. De Mast. Agreement and kappa-type indices. *The American Statistician*, 61(2):148–153, 2007.

J. de Vasconcelos, W. dos Santos, and R. de Lima. Analysis of methods of classification of breast thermographic images to determine their viability in the early breast cancer detection. *IEEE Latin America Transactions*, 16(6):1631–1637, 2018.

S. Ding, X. Xu, and R. Nie. Extreme learning machine and its applications. *Neural Computing and Applications*, 25(3):549–556, 2014.

R. C. Eberhart and Y. Shi. Particle swarm optimization: developments, applications and resources. *Proceedings of the 2001 Congress on Evolutionary Computation*, 25:81–86, 2001.

M. Elad. *Sparse and Redundant Representations: From Theory to Applications in Signal and Image Processing*. Springer, Berlin, 2010.

A. R. Feitosa, R. R. Ribeiro, V. A. Barbosa, R. E. de Souza, and W. P. dos Santos. Reconstruction of electrical impedance tomography images using particle swarm optimization, genetic algorithms and non-blind search. In *5th ISSNIP-IEEE Biosignals and Biorobotics Conference (2014): Biosignals and Robotics for Better and Safer Living (BRC)*, Chicago, IL, USA, pages 1–6. IEEE, 2014.

L. Feng, Y. Ong, S. Jiang, and A. Gupta. Autoencoding evolutionary search with learning across heterogeneous problems. *IEEE Transactions on Evolutionary Computation*, 21(5):760–772, 2017.

M. M. Fouad, K. M. Amin, N. El-Bendary, and A. E. Hassanien. Brain computer interface: A review. *Brain-Computer Interfaces*, 74:3–30, 2015.

P. Gaur, R. B. Pachori, H. Wang, and G. Prasad. An empirical mode decomposition based filtering method for classification of motor-imagery EEG signals for enhancing brain-computer interface. In *2015 International Joint Conference on Neural Networks (IJCNN)*, Killarney, Ireland, pages 1–7. IEEE, 2015.

J. C. Gomes, V. A. de Freitas Barbosa, M. A. de Santana, C. L. de Lima, R. B. Calado, C. R. B. Junior, J. E. de Almeida Albuquerque, R. G. de Souza, R. J. E. de Araujo, G. M. M. Moreno, et al. Rapid protocols to support Covid-19 clinical diagnosis based on hematological parameters. *Research On Biomedical Engineering*, 39:509–539, 2021.

M. A. M. Hasan, M. Nasser, S. Ahmad, and K. I. Molla. Feature selection for intrusion detection using random forest. *Journal of Information Security*, 7(3):129–140, 2016.

S. Haykin. Neural networks: principles and practice. *Bookman*, 11:900, 2001.

G.-B. Huang, Q.-Y. Zhu, and C.-K. Siew. Extreme learning machine: theory and applications. *Neuro-Computing*, 70(1–3):489–501, 2006.

G.-B. Huang, D. H. Wang, and Y. Lan. Extreme learning machines: a survey. *International Journal of Machine Learning and Cybernetics*, 2(2):107–122, 2011.

S. Ibrahim, S. A. Kamaruddin, N. N. A. Mangshor, and A. F. A. Fadzil. Performance evaluation of multi-layer perceptron (MLP) and radial basis function (RBF): covid-19 spread and death contributing factors. *International Journal of Advanced Trends in Computer Science and Engineering*, 9(1.4 Special Issue):1 2020.

Y. Jiao, Y. Zhang, X. Chen, E. Yin, J. Jin, X. Wang, and A. Cichocki. Sparse group representation model for motor imagery EEG classification. *IEEE Journal of Biomedical and Health Informatics*, 23(2):631–641, 2018.

G. H. Jóhannesson, T. Bligaard, A. V. Ruban, H. L. Skriver, K. W. Jacobsen, and J. K. Nørskov. Combined electronic structure and evolutionary search approach to materials design. *Physical Review Letters*, 88:255506, 2002.

J. Kennedy and R. Eberhart. Particle swarm optimization. In *Proceedings of ICNN'95-International Conference on Neural Networks*, Killarney, Ireland, volume 4, pages 1942–1948. IEEE, 1995.

K. S. Kumar, V. Sasank, K. R. Praveen, and Y. K. Rao. Multilayer perceptron back propagation algorithm for predicting breast cancer. In *Intelligent System Design*, pages 41–53. Springer, Singapore, 2021.

R. Leeb, C. Brunner, G. Müller-Putz, A. Schlögl, and G. Pfurtscheller. *BCI competition 2008-graz data set B*. Graz University of Technology, Austria, pages 1–6, 2008.

M. Meng, X. Yin, Q. She, Y. Gao, W. Kong, and Z. Luo. Sparse representation-based classification with two-dimensional dictionary optimization for motor imagery EEG pattern recognition. *Journal of Neuroscience Methods*, 361:109274, 2021.

M. Miao, A. Wang, and F. Liu. A spatial-frequency-temporal optimized feature sparse representation-based classification method for motor imagery EEG pattern recognition. *Medical & Biological Engineering & Computing*, 55(9):1589–1603, 2017.

S. Mishra, H. K. Tripathy, P. K. Mallick, A. K. Bhoi, and P. Barsocchi. EAGA-MLP—an enhanced and adaptive hybrid classification model for diabetes diagnosis. *Sensors*, 20(14):4036, 2020.

W. S. Noble. What is a support vector machine? *Nature Biotechnology*, 24(12):1565–1567, 2006.

C. Park, D. Looney, N. Ur Rehman, A. Ahrabian, and D. P. Mandic. Classification of motor imagery BCI using multivariate empirical mode decomposition. *IEEE Transactions on Neural Systems and Rehabilitation Engineering*, 21(1):10–22, 2012.

J. M. S. Pereira, M. A. Santana, R. C. F. Lima, S. M. L. Lima, and W. P. Santos. Method for classification of breast lesions in thermographic images using ELM classifiers. In W. P. dos Santos, M. A. de Santana, and W. W. A. da Silva, editors, *Understanding a Cancer Diagnosis*, 1st edition pages 117–132. Nova Science, New York, 2020a.

J. M. S. Pereira, M. A. Santana, R. C. F. Lima, and W. P. Santos. Lesion detection in breast thermography using machine learning algorithms without previous segmentation. In W. P. dos Santos, M. A. de Santana, and W. W. A. da Silva, editors, *Understanding a Cancer Diagnosis*, 1st edition, pages 81–94. Nova Science, New York, 2020b.

J. M. S. Pereira, M. A. Santana, W. W. A. Silva, R. C. F. Lima, S. M. L. Lima, and W. P. Santos. Dialectical optimization method as a feature selection tool for breast cancer diagnosis using thermographic images. In W. P. dos Santos, M. A. de Santana, and W. W. A. da Silva, editors, *Understanding a Cancer Diagnosis*, 1st edition, pages 95–118. Nova Science, New York, 2020c.

M. G. Perroca and R. R. Gaidzinski. Avaliando a confiabilidade interavaliadores de um instrumento para classificação de pacientes: coeficiente kappa. *Revista da Escola de Enfermagem da USP*, 37: 72–80, 2003.

R. Poli, J. Kennedy, and T. Blackwell. Particle swarm optimization. *Swarm Intelligence*, 1(1):33–57, 2007.

H. Ramchoun, M. A. J. Idrissi, Y. Ghanou, and M. Ettaouil. Multilayer perceptron: Architecture optimization and training. *International Journal of Interactive Multimedia and Artificial Intelligence*, 4(1):26–30, 2016.

R. R. Ribeiro, A. R. Feitosa, R. E. de Souza, and W. P. dos Santos. Reconstruction of electrical impedance tomography images using genetic algorithms and non-blind search. In *2014 IEEE 11th International Symposium on Biomedical Imaging (ISBI)*, Beijing, China, pages 153–156. IEEE, 2014.

A. L. Rodrigues, M. A. de Santana, W. W. Azevedo, R. S. Bezerra, V. A. Barbosa, R. C. de Lima, and W. P. dos Santos. Identification of mammary lesions in thermographic images: feature selection study using genetic algorithms and particle swarm optimization. *Research on Biomedical Engineering*, 35(3):213–222, 2019.

S. K. Saha and M. S. Ali. Data adaptive filtering approach to improve the classification accuracy of motor imagery for BCI. In *2016 9th International Conference on Electrical and Computer Engineering (ICECE)*, Dhaka, Bangladesh, pages 247–250. IEEE, 2016.

S. B. Sakri, N. B. A. Rashid, and Z. M. Zain. Particle swarm optimization feature selection for breast cancer recurrence prediction. *IEEE Access*, 6:29637–29647, 2018.

M. A. Santana, J. M. S. Pereira, R. C. F. Lima, and W. P. Santos. Breast lesions classification in frontal thermographic images using intelligent systems and moments of haralick and zernike. In W. P. dos Santos, M. A. de Santana, and W. W. A. da Silva, editors, *Understanding a Cancer Diagnosis*, 1st edition, pages 65–80. Nova Science, New York, 1 edition, 2020.

M. A. d. Santana, J. M. S. Pereira, F. L. d. Silva, N. M. d. Lima, F. N. d. Sousa, G. M. S. d. Arruda, R. d. C. F. d. Lima, W. W. A. d. Silva, and W. P. d. Santos. Breast cancer diagnosis based on mammary thermography and extreme learning machines. *Research on Biomedical Engineering*, 34:45–53, 01 2018. ISSN 2446–4740.

Y. Shi and R. C. Eberhart. Empirical study of particle swarm optimization. *Proceedings of the 1999 Congress on Evolutionary Computation-CEC99*, 3:1945–1950, 1999.

Y. Shin, S. Lee, J. Lee, and H.-N. Lee. Sparse representation-based classification scheme for motor imagery-based brain–computer interface systems. *Journal of Neural Engineering*, 9(5):056002, 2012.

S. Sreeja, D. Samanta, et al. Distance-based weighted sparse representation to classify motor imagery EEG signals for BCI applications. *Multimedia Tools and Applications*, 79(19):13775–13793, 2020.

S. Suthaharan. Support vector machine. In *Machine Learning Models and Algorithms for Big Data Classification*, pages 207–235. Springer, Berlin, 2016.

E. V. Sylvester, P. Bentzen, I. R. Bradbury, M. Clément, J. Pearce, J. Horne, and R. G. Beiko. Applications of random forest feature selection for fine-scale genetic population assignment. *Evolutionary Applications*, 11(2):153–165, 2018.

F. van den Bergh and A. Engelbrecht. A study of particle swarm optimization particle trajectories. *Information Sciences*, 176(8):937–971, 2006.

X. Wang, J. Yang, X. Teng, W. Xia, and R. Jensen. Feature selection based on rough sets and particle swarm optimization. *Pattern Recognition Letters*, 28(4):459–471, 2007.

D. Wen, P. Jia, Q. Lian, Y. Zhou, and C. Lu. Review of sparse representation-based classification methods on EEG signal processing for epilepsy detection, brain-computer interface and cognitive impairment. *Frontiers in Aging Neuroscience*, 8:172, 2016.

J. R. Wolpaw and E. W. Wolpaw. Brain-computer interfaces: something new under the sun. *Brain- Computer Interfaces: Principles and Practice*, 14, 0001, 2012.

J. Wright, A. Y. Yang, A. Ganesh, S. S. Sastry, and Y. Ma. Robust face recognition via sparse representation. *IEEE Transactions on Pattern Analysis and Machine Intelligence*, 31(2):210–227, 2008.

C. Xu, C. Sun, G. Jiang, X. Chen, Q. He, and P. Xie. Two-level multi-domain feature extraction on sparse representation for motor imagery classification. *Biomedical Signal Processing and Control*, 62:102160, 2020.

M. Z. Yusoff, D. Mahmoud, A. S. Malik, M. R. Bahloul, et al. Discrimination of four class simple limb motor imagery movements for brain–computer interface. *Biomedical Signal Processing and Control*, 44:181–190, 2018.

K. Zhang, N. Robinson, S.-W. Lee, and C. Guan. Adaptive transfer learning for EEG motor imagery classification with deep convolutional neural network. *Neural Networks*, 136: 1–10, 2021.

Y. Zhang, C. S. Nam, G. Zhou, J. Jin, X. Wang, and A. Cichocki. Temporally constrained sparse group spatial patterns for motor imagery BCI. *IEEE Transactions on Cybernetics*, 49(9):3322–3332, 2018.

X. Zhao, H. Zhang, G. Zhu, F. You, S. Kuang, and L. Sun. A multi-branch 3D convolutional neural network for EEG-based motor imagery classification. *IEEE Transactions on Neural Systems and Rehabilitation Engineering*, 27(10):2164–2177, 2019.

Q. Zhu, A. Samanta, B. Li, R. E. Rudd, and T. Frolov. Predicting phase behavior of grain boundaries with evolutionary search and machine learning. *Nature Communications*, 9:467, 2018.

X. Zhu, P. Li, C. Li, D. Yao, R. Zhang, and P. Xu. Separated channel convolutional neural network to realize the training free motor imagery BCI systems. *Biomedical Signal Processing and Control*, 49:396–403, 2019.

11 Prediction of Onset of Seizures from EEG Signals Using ML Techniques

Sumathi A, Priya R Sankpal,
Jyoti R Munavalli, and Anusha A N

11.1 INTRODUCTION

Brain is the most powerful and important part which controls the activities of the human body. The brain is a collection of different neurons which control and decide the behaviour of a human. Understanding and analysing the brain is a critical area for medical researchers. This includes analysing different brain signals and arriving at a solution for different brain-related issues. EEG is a process for recording the electrical activity of the brain. EEG provides data for the analysis of brain signals and issues related to them. The EEG recording process is a painless, non-invasive, and accurate method of recording brain signals. The classification of EEG signals is based on different frequencies due to different states like the movement of the eyeball, opening and closing of the eye, etc.; the range of frequencies associated ranges from 0 to 100 Hz.

The brain is the most critical organ that commands all other organs and coordinates with different muscles and nerves. The brain is basically segmented into two hemispheres: the left and the right. These hemispheres are further split into four regions namely frontal, temporal, parietal, and occipital lobes. The most prominent lobe is the frontal lobe and it is located behind the forehead. The left frontal lobe coordinates with speech and language. It looks after organizing, planning, problem-solving, memory, emotions, etc. Any injury to the frontal lobe leads to personality change, emotional response, difficulties with motivation, decision-making, etc. (Figure 11.1).

The temporal lobes are located just above the brain. It deals with understanding sounds like speech, musical notes, managing emotions, and face recognition. Any injury to the temporal lobe causes difficulty in face recognition, remembering people, reading, etc. The parietal lobes are located above the temporal lobe and behind the frontal lobe. The parietal lobe is responsible to make sense of things touched, such as smooth, sharp, soft, and the body's relation to the object seen as the spatial distance. Any injury to the parietal lobe causes difficulty in naming objects, hand-eye coordination, writing, etc. The occipital lobes are placed at the backside of the brain. The main function of this lobe is visual perception. Any injury to this part affects sight with blurred vision, difficulty identifying colours, recognizing people, words, and things.

DOI: 10.1201/9781003252092-14

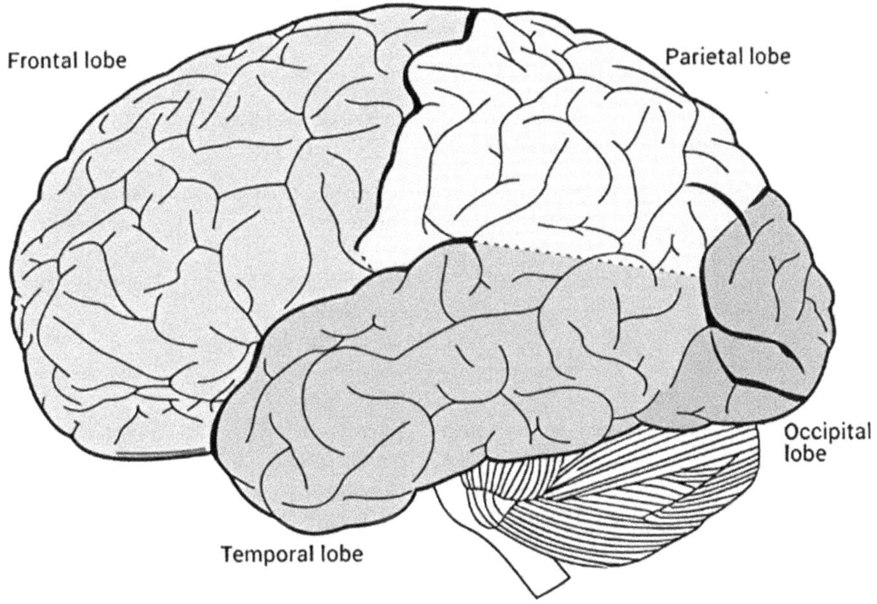

FIGURE 11.1 Lobes of the brain [1].

A technique which reads electrical activity or potential from the brain is called EEG. The measurement of these electrical potentials is called an electroencephalogram (EEG). The device will have electrodes, conductive gel, amplifiers to amplify the weak EEG signals, and analogue-to-digital converters to process the data in the digital domain. Some of the electrodes used can be reusable. Electrodes are placed on the scalp by applying conductive gel to the disc surface. The usual composition of the disc will be gold, silver, and tin, and conductive gel will be made of silver chloride. The cost of the electrode will depend on the metal used for disc. Each electrode will be usually labelled with the letters F, T C, P, O indicating frontal, temporal, central, parietal, and occipital. The middle region is represented by the letter Z and an odd number for the left hemisphere and an even for the right hemisphere. In positioning electrodes, two methods are followed known as referential and bipolar. In the referential electrode method, all the electrodes measure the potential difference with respect to the reference electrode, and in bipolar, the potential difference is measured between paired active electrodes.

EEG signals are classified based on the frequency, amplitude, electrode position, and shape. The most common classification is alpha (8–13 Hz), beta (13–30 Hz), theta (4–8 Hz), delta (0.1–4 Hz), and gamma (3.0–100 Hz) [2]. The table shows different behavioural states and their location of different EEG signals (Table 11.1).

EEG signals are analysed for different brain disorders, such as epilepsy, Alzheimer, learning disability, insomnia, dyslexia, seizure disorder, anxiety disorder, etc.,

TABLE 11.1

Brain Wave Characteristic Table [2]

Type	Frequency (Hz)	Behavioural/ Psychological State	Neurotransmitter/ Hormone	Location
Delta	0–4	Deep rest, dreamless sleep	Human growth hormone, melatonin	Frontally in adults, posteriorly in children
Theta	4–8	Deeply relaxed	Serotonin, acetylcholine, anti-cortisol, endorphins, human growth hormone	Thalamic region
Alpha	8–13	Day dream, calm	Serotonin, endorphins, acetylcholine	Posterior regions
Beta	13–30	Alert, active thinking, anxiety, panic attack, focus, concentration	Adrenaline, cortisol, norepinephrine, dopamine	Frontal and parietal
Gamma	30–100	Combination of two senses	Serotonin, endorphins	Somatosensory cortex

As seizures are unpredictable and uncontrollable, people suffering from epilepsy struggle with their daily lives. Several methods have been investigated to prediction seizures. If seizures are predicted within a reasonable time before their occurrence, patients with epilepsy can take precautions to stay safe during their occurrence or avoid some medications, thereby improving their quality of life.

Epilepsy is a disorder of the central nervous system in which nerve cell activity in the brain becomes disrupted, causing seizures or periods of unusual behaviour, sensations, and sometimes loss of consciousness. An estimated 5% of the world's population has epileptic seizures, but no method exists to cure them. More than 30% of people with epilepsy cannot control seizures. The occurrence of epileptic seizures is unpredictable and predicting seizures is challenging. Seizure prediction can be regarded as the most critical issue in medical science, requiring solutions worldwide. The identification of time for the probable occurrence of a seizure is epileptic seizure prediction. Epilepsy is a disorder of brain activity which is described by many occurrences of seizures. A seizure can be described as a sudden change in behaviour because of an electrical system disorder in the brain. In epilepsy, the electrical signals of the brain are inclined to get imbalanced which causes the patient to have seizures (Figure 11.2).

In patients with epilepsy, the disruption of the normal electric pattern due to bursts of electrical energy causes disturbances in movements, consciousness, and sensation. In most cases, seizures last for a period of 30 seconds to two minutes. If a seizure lasts more than five minutes, it is considered a medical emergency.

Types of seizures: Seizures are broadly classified into two categories.

1. Primary generalised seizures
2. Focal/partial seizures.

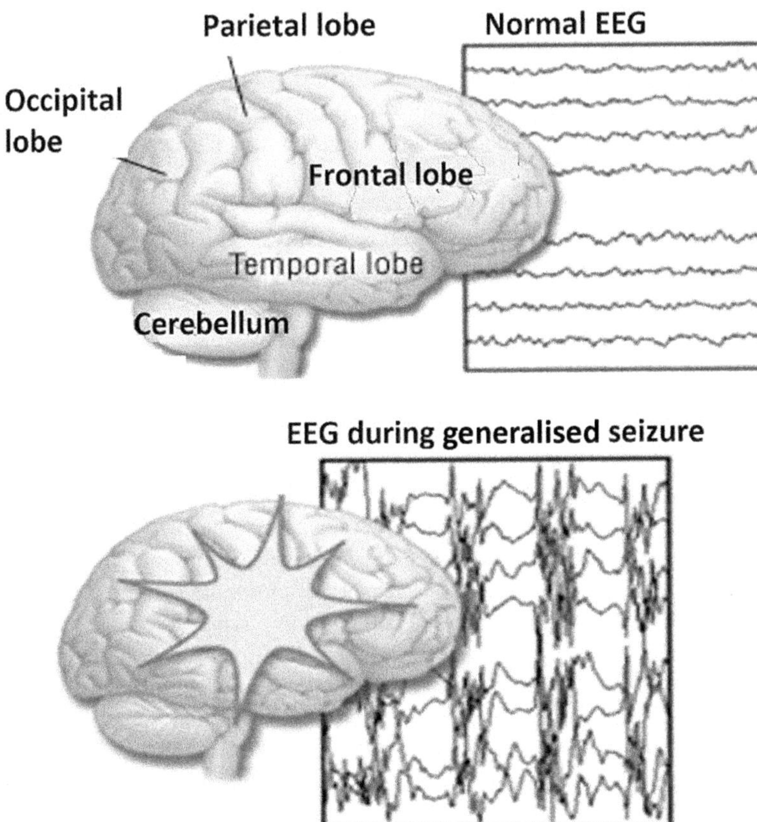

FIGURE 11.2   Brain images with EEG signals [3].

Primary generalised seizures occur due to electrical dysfunction on both sides of the brain. They may have a genetic component and genetic testing can disclose the cause of the seizure.

Generalised seizure can further be classified as:

Absence seizures: Absence seizures most often occur in children. When a child undergoes this type of seizure, it will cause the child to stare at a particular object or make subtle movements like blinking the eyes or smacking the lips. The seizures last for a period of 5 seconds to 10 seconds. It can occur in bunches or a greater number of times in a short period of time and can cause a temporary loss of awareness. In partial seizures, the imbalance of electrical signal is seen only in certain areas of the brain.

Tonic seizures: In this type, muscle stiffness is observed. These seizures more often affect the muscles of the arms, legs, and back. Due to stiffness, people may lose consciousness and fall.

Atonic seizure: This is also called a drop seizure, and it causes the muscle to lose control and hinders muscular movement.

Clonic seizure: This type of seizure causes continuous jerking muscle movements. In this, the muscles of the neck, face, and arms are affected.

Myoclonic seizures: In this type, seizures occur in clusters and involve the arms, neck, and head. Usually, they occur in the morning. If these seizures occur during adolescence along with tonic-clonic seizures, it is called juvenile myoclonic epilepsy.

Tonic-clonic seizure: In this type of seizure, people suffer from stiffness and jerking that cause sudden loss of consciousness. Sometimes it is observed that people lose bladder control and bite their tongue. This may last for a few minutes.

Focal seizure can further be classified as

Focal onset aware seizure: This type of seizure occurs when the person is awake and aware during the seizure. This is also called a simple partial seizure. These also affect the person's behaviour like looking, feeling, smelling, tasting, etc. When a person undergoes this type of seizure, they get angry or feel sad or joyful. Some people even suffer from nausea. Here, the electrical activity affects only one sensory or motor area.

Focal onset impaired awareness seizure: In this type of seizure, the electrical activity affects a larger area of the brain, causing confusion in the person. People experience minor shaking, fumbling, and muscle stiffening. This is also called a complex partial seizure.

11.1.1 CAUSES OF EPILEPSY

The cause of epilepsy is not the same for all people. Different people have different causes, and some people may have no identifiable cause. In contrast, doctors attribute epilepsy directly to genetics, brain infections, autoimmune disorders, metabolic issues, etc.; every case has different symptoms, identification, and treatment. The major cause of the disease can be one of the following:

Genetic influence: Certain types of epilepsy with a part of the brain affected can be hereditary and most likely to have genetic influence. This genetically transmitted disorder might trigger only certain type of environmental conditions causing seizures.

Head trauma: A major accident or other head injury can cause epilepsy.

Brain abnormalities: Due to tumours in the brain or vascular malformations and cavernous malformations, epilepsy can be caused. Stroke is one of the major causes of epilepsy in adults aged 35 and above.

Infections: Certain parasitic infections like meningitis, HIV, etc., are another major cause of epilepsy [4].

Prenatal injury: Brain damage caused before the birth of the child, an infection when the foetus is in the womb, poor nutrition during pregnancy, etc., This damage can cause epilepsy.

Developmental disorder: Developmental disorders, such as autism, can cause epilepsy.

11.1.2 Diagnosis

The diagnosis of epilepsy is initially made with a physical examination and diagnostic tests, such as blood tests, an EEG, magnetic resonance imaging (MRI), a computed tomography scan, or a lumbar puncture.

11.1.3 Treatment

70% of people with epilepsy can become seizure-free with proper treatment. In most low-income countries, more than 75% of people are deprived of treatment. In middle-income countries, around 50% of people with this disease are deprived of treatment. In all other countries, it is diagnosed at the primary health care level without sophisticated medical equipment [5].

Seizures have different phases, namely pre-ictal, ictal, and post-ictal. During the pre-ictal stage, some people will be able to make changes in their body and predict the onset of a seizure. But not all people experience this change. Some of the most common signs during this stage can be anxiety, mood change, feeling lightheaded, sleeplessness. The middle phase, or ictal phase, is the time from the start of the symptom to the end of seizure occurrence. During this phase, an intense change in the brain's electrical activity occurs. Some common signs are loss of awareness, memory loss, difficulty in speaking, confusion, and so on. The final, or post-ictal, stage is seen after the ictal phase of the seizure. This phase is the recovery phase, and the recovery time depends on which part of the brain is affected. Some common signs are tiredness, exhaustion, headache, loss of bladder or bowel function, etc.

11.2 EXISTING METHODOLOGIES

11.2.1 Classification Framework

There are two main approaches to predicting epileptic seizures. The first stream uses a binary classification framework that has been taught to distinguish between pre-ictal and interictal samples. Because of the forecasting valuelessness of the post-ictal and ictal samples, these samples are abandoned during the training method. Researchers who study seizure prediction frequently use this stream. The second stream is predicated on the notion that EEG records contain a certain index that varies with changes in the seizure stage. Some approaches try to monitor this indicator using a threshold and openly describe it. For instance, the indicators have been claimed to be the spike rate zero-crossing intervals and the phase/amplitude-locking value [6].

Research that uses a binary classifier typically combines ML approaches with feature extraction algorithms. Due to the complexity and variety of EEG signals, feature extraction algorithms are frequently used in data preparation. ML techniques then assess the extracted characteristics for providing classifications [6]. ML techniques are used for classification in lung cancer, skin cancer, diabetes, language detection, locust management, and many more [7–10].

11.2.1.1　Pre-processing of Data

Data preparation is one of the most important and necessary phases of ML. When utilising ML algorithms in a data collection, this method is crucial for successful, accurate, and reliable prediction outputs [11]. Data preparation is an approach that entails putting unprocessed, raw data in a manner that will work for classification. Real-world data are frequently incomplete, unreliable, deficient in patterns or behaviours, and/ or contain a variety of errors. A tried-and-true method to address such problems is pre-processing data. To prepare it for further processing, raw data are pre-processed.

11.2.1.2　Feature Extraction

By generating new attributes from the existing ones in the data set, the feature extraction step seeks to reduce the number of attributes. This revised, condensed feature set should summarise most of the data and features in the original data set. The original set can be combined to provide a condensed version of the key features. "Wavelet transform, Q-factor wavelet transform, Fourier neural network, and fractional Fourier transform" are some feature extraction techniques used to learn the high-dimensional representations of samples. To discover the spatial and temporal representations of seizures, ML techniques, including "Support Vector Machines," "Random Forests," "K-Nearest Neighbour," and "Ensemble Learning," are used. Furthermore, deep learning frameworks are now commonly used by researchers to predict seizures. "Convolutional neural networks (CNNs), 3D CNNs, long short-term memory model (LSTM) networks, and cascades of DNNs" are adopted to process the EEG signals.

11.2.2　Classification Algorithms

11.2.2.1　K-Nearest Neighbour

In studies on classification, KNN is one of the supervised learning methods that is often utilised. It is a straightforward, nonparametric algorithm that uses the closest samples to categorise objects in the input space [12]. Although k indicates the number of neighbours, the KNN algorithm refers to the number of neighbours that are closest to the classification-relevant data. Regression and classification issues are both targeted by the KNN classification approach. As the algorithm comes across a new sample of data, it calculates the sample distance across all the samples in the new data. This learning algorithm is called kknn. Class labels are determined by locating the k closest neighbours from the known data samples, comparing them to instances in the new example's education data, and examining their similarities [13]. For instance, if KNNs to the new non-epileptic data sample are all classified as belonging to a non-epileptic class, then the new data sample is assigned to the non-epileptic class and those new epileptic data sample are classified as belonging to epileptic class, a new data sample is assigned to the epileptic class. This assumes that similar data samples tend to belong to the same class. The KNN algorithm is a supervised learning algorithm that can be used to classify data samples.

11.2.2.2　Random Forest (RF)

The recently created RF classifier outperforms the acceleration and bagging approaches in terms of speed and accuracy, despite being two highly recognised collective learning techniques. Compared to other learning strategies, especially the acceleration strategy, the RF classifier trains much more quickly. This classifier is preferred due to its efficiency and accuracy. Even when the meta parameters are left alone, the RF/ML approach typically yields great results and is easy to apply. This technique is one of the most widely deployed ML algorithms for both "classification" and "regression" due to its adaptability and simplicity. This strategy would generate a forest at random. The constructed "forest" is really a "Decision Trees" band. Indeed, this approach is capable of handling large data sets. The data set is sampled randomly, and a decision tree (DT) is built for each sample. Each DT yields a prediction result that is evaluated. Then, vote on the forecast outcome, and the model with the most votes is taken into consideration [14]. If the ensemble is applied to an epileptic seizure data set, each DT will classify the data as either positive or negative, and the model with the most votes will be the final prediction result.

11.2.2.3 Support Vector Machine (SVM)

The SVM searches for a perfect hyperplane capable of isolating examples of any class. Hyperplanes with maximum margins may be used to discover groups that can be separated linearly. Otherwise, if the data cannot be linearly separated, they can be moved to a larger space in order to be linearly separated (i.e., feature space). This conversion is known as the kernel function. This classifier specifies the hyperplane that enlarges the interval of each class to such a hyperplane, separating the spots to place the greatest number of points of a comparable class on the same side. The closest points on the hyperplane make up the support vectors. The smallest distance between them and the points in that class is the distance from a class to a hyperplane. The hyperplane can also be used for regression or grouping. SVM classifies compounds that are not supported by data and divides examples into certain groups. Detachment is completed by playing out the partition on the hyperplane to the nearest training location for any group [13]. The Epileptic Seizure Recognition Data Set was used to evaluate the accuracy of the SVM algorithm. This data set contains 178 instances and 5 classes of epileptic seizures. This data set was divided into a training set with 139 instances and a test set with 39 instances.

11.2.2.4 Artificial Neural Network (ANN)

These are network structures made up of interconnected components called neurons, each of which performs a very straightforward operation and has an input and an output. In general, neural networks develop their capabilities through a learning process. In fact, they determine the rule that supports them by analysing data and sending them to the network. These networks are software applications that can behave like people in the following ways:

- More experienced, gained over time, and via increased exposure to the environment.
- Capable of making logical inferences in addition to doing calculations.
- Provide a workable answer for the brand new circumstances.

Computer architectures called ANNs are designed to resemble the human brain. The input, hidden, and output layers are three examples of the network layers that make up an ANN in general. The input neurons determine all the input attribute values for the data mining model. ANNs, such as voice recognition, picture recognition, and robotics, have enabled a large number of new advances in the field of artificial intelligence [15]. The Epileptic Seizure Recognition Data Set is a well-known example of an ANN used for data mining. This data set includes EEG readings from epileptic patients and is used to classify a seizure from a non-seizure EEG pattern. The data set is used to evaluate the performance of ANNs in detecting epileptic seizures with high accuracy.

11.2.2.5 DT

A DT is a tool for making decisions that use tree modelling. DT is a key method for both classification and regression. DTs are often used in operations and research. The technique for classifying instances based on traits can be defined using a DT model with a tree structure. A DT is used when the result attribute is categorical. The DT graph is made up of the root node, branches, and leaves. The results of each occurrence are stored on the branches, while classification takes place on the leaves. When developing categorisation criteria, the routes from the root node to the child nodes are considered. The DT technique provides both nominal and numerical features. It could put up with noise and erratic values. The DT partitions the nodes from the topmost to the class node in a top-down manner to categorise the entire qualified data set. Each node represents one of the possible values for the test attribute for the instance, which is represented by each node. A DT may easily transform the supplied set of cases into significant patterns going from the top node to the attack class node level by level. The epileptic data set is a good example of a data set that could benefit from the use of DTs. It is a data set with many noisy and erratic values, making it difficult to analyse with traditional methods. By using DTs, it is possible to accurately classify the data and identify patterns that would otherwise be difficult to spot.

11.2.3 PREDICTION METHODS

The common quantitative EEG methods for predicting seizures are "Frequency-Based Approaches, Nonlinear Dynamics (Chaos), and Statistical Analysis" of EEG signals [16]. Most cutting-edge methods for anticipating an epileptic seizure include altering the signal either linearly or non-linearly using one of several mathematical measures and then using the measurement result to attempt to forecast the seizure. These systems can use a class of ML techniques like ANNs or some purely mathematical transformations like the Fourier transform, or they can combine the two. Most of the measures—including observation (inter-ictal), pre-seizure, and seizure periods—are computed from EEG epochs of less than 20 seconds using a moving window technique. Pre-processing and filtering of the EEG epochs are also needed for some metrics. All of these techniques will effectively distinguish between the seizure (ictal) and non-ictal periods [17].

11.2.3.1 Univariate Measures

Time-series analyses, known as univariate analyses, only include a single observation recorded consecutively across equal time intervals. Of course, the time series contains the implicit variable of time. The univariate time series can be graphically represented as a function of time during the entire period of data recording with knowledge of the start time and sampling rate of the data collection. The recorded EEG signal's amplitude value can be stored by the amplitude and phase of a subset of harmonic oscillations that occur at a variety of frequencies, as well as by sampling the signal in the form of a discrete time series. Time-frequency approaches define the map that connects these representations.

A single recording location is used for univariate EEG analysis. Linear univariate metrics characterise the amplitude and phase data of the EEG time series. Non-linear univariate measurements are used to characterise the state and dynamics of the system. The first step in non-linear univariate approaches is to describe the system state at a specific time. A point in m-dimensional space known as the state or phase space, where m is the embedding dimension, describes the so-called system state. The dynamics of the system controls how it changes over time [17].

11.2.3.1.1 Fourier Transform and Short-Term Fourier Transform

One of the most popular methods for anticipating an epileptic seizure is based on calculating the power spectrum of one or more EEG channels. The main theory is that the EEG signal has a signature that differs between the ictal and interictal stages when divided into individual periodic (sine and cosine) waves. The signal's Fourier transform is examined to identify the most prevalent frequencies (in amplitude) in the signal in order to find this signature. In fact, a useful technique to aid in locating the cause of epileptic seizures is the application of time-frequency analysis to seizure EEG activity. The power spectrum is typically not employed as a stand-alone seizure or seizure precursor detector, despite the link between the power spectrum and ictal activity. Usually, it is used in conjunction with another ML or time-series prediction methodology [16].

11.2.3.1.2 Accumulated Energy

This technique uses the EEG time series to calculate a running average of energy. Although this technique has been able to identify EEG seizure precursors under very narrow circumstances, the findings appear to vary among data sets [18,19].

11.2.3.1.3 Autocorrelation and Autoregressive Modelling

A pre-ictal phase may be identified by using autocorrelation techniques for the EEG signal values at various time intervals. The first zero-crossing is used to indicate the decorrelation time. Pre-ictal alterations have been described using techniques from autoregressive modelling. Each time series value is assumed to depend solely on the weighted sum of its previous values and "noise" in linear modelling. The signal's stationarity is the primary presumption in linear modelling. Hence, one must divide non-stationary signals like EEG into stationary components [19].

11.2.3.1.4   Discrete Wavelet Transforms

Like Fourier transforms, wavelet transforms operate on superposition and presume that EEG signals are made up of multiple components drawn from a collection of parameterised basis functions. Fourier transformations can only be used on sine and cosine wave functions, as was previously mentioned. In contrast, the fundamental functions of wavelets must satisfy additional mathematical requirements that make them much more general than simple "sine and cosine" waves. Compared to the Fourier transform, approximating choppy signals with sharp spikes is much simpler when wavelets are used. It is challenging to simulate a spike because "sine and cosine" waves have unlimited support or extend to infinity in the time domain. Adjusting the size of the component basis functions makes it simple to estimate a surge in the EEG signal because wavelets have a finite support. Any time-varying signal, for instance, will be divided into smaller uniform functions, referred to as the basic functions, using discrete wavelets. The fundamental functions are produced by scaling and translating the mother wavelet, a single function of a certain type.

To anticipate seizures, wavelets have been applied to subdural electrocorticogram (ECoG) signals. In one study, the authors used a wavelet-based filter to first separate the ECoG signal into seizure and non-seizure components. The filter did not particularly anticipate seizures. No matter the reason, it signalled a rise in power or a change in frequency. The signal was broken down into its component parts by the filter, and then, it was put through a second filter that attempted to separate the seizures from the other events. Most interictal epileptiform discharges were suppressed by the algorithm's median filter, but power increases in "normal" activity were not "tagged" as seizures. Although not being able to predict electrographic commencement, this technique did identify very brief predictions of clinical seizure onset of 15 seconds or greater [20].

11.2.3.1.5   Statistical Moments

These techniques reveal details about the EEG time series' amplitude and dispersion. Moments and functions of moments can be used to represent an approximation to the distribution of a random variable even when a cumulative distribution function for that variable cannot be found. A particular signal's amplitude distribution can be learned using statistical moments. The statistical moments are typically taken about the mean. The fifth central moment, often known as the distribution's mean, is the first statistical moment.

The variance is the second factor relating to the mean. The level of asymmetry in that distribution is indicated by the skew, which is provided by the third moment about the mean. Kurtosis, which displays the degree to which that distribution is peaked, is the fourth moment about the mean. The ictal and interictal states have been separated using these techniques. Seizure prediction uses the absolute value of skewness. The state transition from interictal to pre-ictal could be detected, but it was unable to be detected, and it could neither detect nor reliably predict a seizure. Yet, in recordings with big-amplitude seizures, statistical moments may be useful for early seizure detection [21].

11.2.3.1.6 Correlation Dimension

The correlation integral is the basis for the measurements known as the correlation dimension, correlation density, and Kolmogorov entropy. These measurements can be computed from the state-space representation of the EEG time series. The progression of a seizure can be traced back to changes in state space throughout time. The EEG time series' state space embedding is used to calculate the correlation dimension. This measurement assumes that there is a chance that any two randomly selected locations in the state space will be close to one another. The correlation dimension can distinguish random signals from deterministic time series. As a result, this measurement can approximate how many dimensions there are in the state space. According to human ECoG time-series investigations, the correlation dimension considerably decreases soon before the commencement of a seizure. The results, however, have not been able to be repeated, as with other non-linear approaches, and statistical validation is needed [19].

11.2.3.1.7 Correlation Density

It is determined by computing the correlation integral for a particular radius and is a closely linked measurement to the correlation dimension. The EEG is processed using both time delays and time spatial embedding. Similar to the correlation dimension, there has been some success in using the correlation density to predict seizures, although the findings have been inconsistent [22].

11.2.3.1.8 Kolmogorov Entropy

The Kolmogorov entropy provides a measurement of the system's future states' level of uncertainty over time. Children receiving ECoG epilepsy evaluations had their EEG time series put through this measurement process. According to results from a limited data set, the Kolmogorov entropy may be beneficial in recognising EEG pre-seizure states. However, a prospective evaluation of these data is lacking [18].

11.2.3.1.9 Dynamical Similarity Index

The dynamic similarity index is said to be able to monitor spatiotemporal changes in brain dynamics minutes before an oncoming seizure. By using the time durations between two positive zero-crossings and the cross-correlation integral to calculate the dynamical similarity between the reference and test windows, respectively, the measure is calculated by reconstructing the EEG time series in phase space. Although one study showed the usefulness of this score in detecting pre-seizure conditions, these preliminary findings have not been replicated in additional trials [17].

11.2.3.1.10 Loss of Recurrence and Local Flow

By estimating the frequency distribution of temporal distances under stationary conditions with respect to each reference point, it is possible to calculate the degree of non-stationarity. Due to a lack of remote time indices in the vicinity of the reference, a non-stationary system exhibits an increase in deviation from this distribution. The loss of recurrence measures how non-stationary a time series is. This decrease in occurrence has been used to predictably forecast when a seizure will occur [17].

11.2.3.1.11   Lyapunov Exponent

EEG signals are intricate and have statistical characteristics that depend on time and space. The presence of limit cycles (alpha activity, ictal activity), instances of bursting behaviour (during light sleep), jump phenomena (hysteresis), amplitude-dependent frequency behaviour (the smaller the amplitude the higher the EEG frequency), and existence of frequency harmonics (for example, under photic driving conditions) are a few non-linear system properties found in EEG signals. The epileptogenic brain may therefore contain components of a non-linear system. The EEG of the epileptic brain has been hypothesised to be a non-linear signal with deterministic and maybe chaotic features by a number of studies [17,18].

The EEG would not demonstrate any observable dynamic changes before the seizure if a sudden and abrupt state transition caused the seizure. This scenario is conceivable for the onset of seizures in primary generalised epilepsy. The second possibility is that this transformation would take place gradually or as a succession of dynamical shifts that could theoretically be recognised and even predicted. Several studies have revealed experimental evidence that changes in the EEG signal's dynamic properties occur before temporal lobe epileptic episodes. Several non-linear time-series analytic techniques have demonstrated promise in their ability to spot pre-ictal dynamic changes required for seizure anticipation. Consequently, it is hypothesised that a seizure represents a change in the dynamic system from a chaotic to an ordered state. According to the idea, individuals may experience a pre-ictal shift minutes to hours prior to having a seizure. The numerous dynamical metrics outlined below can therefore capture this so-called primordial state.

The sensitivity of the initial circumstances affects the Lyapunov exponent, a non-linear measurement of the average rate of divergence or convergence of two nearby paths in a dynamic system. Pre-ictal variations have been identified using this dynamical metric in human EEG recordings collected during ECoG evaluation for epilepsy surgery. The equation of motion defining the temporal evolution of a given dynamic system is used to estimate the Lyapunov exponents, without the equation of motion outlining the dynamic system's course. The Lyapunov exponents have been used in this general way, with varying degrees of success, to find an EEG precursor. Pre-ictal transition was reportedly observed in more than 91% of seizures when the proper sites were picked. By using a paradigmatic chaotic system, these findings have been challenged. These investigations demonstrate that noise and finite-time statistical fluctuations can both seriously impair the ability of Lyapunov exponents calculated from EEG time series to forecast the future. However, a prospective, out-of-sample, class 1 strategy is being used to try and statistically validate this method.

11.2.3.2   Multivariate Measures

EEG signals can be thought of as a multivariate time series, which is a collection of numerical values (voltages) over time and space (gathered from numerous electrodes). Several observations are recorded progressively throughout time in multivariate time-series analysis. Multivariate time series analysis is performed to evaluate how the many parts of the system under investigation interact. We can follow the dynamics of the interactions of various system components by tracking many variables across time, which helps us build a more complete picture of the system. Several EEG channels are evaluated simultaneously using multivariate analysis. Instead of focussing on each channel separately, this strategy considers how they interact and correlate. This is helpful since the brain's many regions frequently interact (for example, synchronise) before a seizure occurs. Bivariate measures that only consider two channels at once and specify how those two channels correlate include the simple synchronisation measure and the lag synchronisation measure. The remaining metrics simultaneously consider every EEG channel. Other multivariate metrics include principal component analysis (PCA), a simple synchronisation measure, correlation structure, phase correlation, autoregressive measures of synchrony, the short-term largest Lyapunov exponent T-index, and phase synchronisation [17].

11.2.3.2.1 PCA

PCA, a dimensionality reduction approach, uses every EEG channel simultaneously. Using the most prominent dimensions from the original data set, PCA takes a multidimensional data set, identifies its most salient dimensions, and then linearly transforms the original data set into a lower-dimensional space. It aims to keep the crucial portions of the data with the highest variance and remove the unimportant portions with the lowest variance. The goal of PCA is to identify a set of input traits that, by reducing the original dimensions of the data, can most effectively describe the distribution of the original data. PCA can do this by increasing variances and minimising reconstruction error through the careful observation of fragmented distances. Each orthogonal axis that is projected onto our primary data is ranked in PCA order of relevance. Unsupervised learning techniques like PCA focus only on diversity and ignore data labels. When PCA is employed, the first few components primarily contain most of the data's variation. As a result, rests are ignored, and only the components with notable changes are kept [15].

11.2.3.2.2 Simple Synchronisation Measure

It is commonly known that different parts of the brain coordinate with one another during specific occurrences. Either focally or in a broader pattern, unusually high levels of extremely synchronised activity are observed during seizures. It has been claimed that this activity can start several hours before a seizure starts. The multichannel EEG model, which describes each point as a linear combination of the prior values from all chosen channels, generates the autoregressive measure of synchrony. The number of events that can synchronise in the signals, expressed as a normalising term, is then divided by the entire count. The result of those synchronisation measures is that they do not detect pre-ictal EEG changes unless information regarding post-ictal changes in closely clustered seizures is provided, even though this metric appears to be very intuitive for seizure prediction.

11.2.3.2.3 Correlation Structure

Another seizure analysis technique is evaluating the correlation across all recorded EEG channels. A correlation is first established over the provided channels. The correlation matrix is determined by analysing an EEG signal segment for a specific window of time. Channels within this time span are then used to normalise the EEG output.

11.2.3.2.4   Phase Correlation

Spectral coherence can be used to measure phase synchrony. These techniques include the detection of maximum values following filtering, as well as amplitude and phase data. The amplitudes of weakly connected non-linear equations change chaotically and are largely uncorrelated, yet they are phase locked. The objective is to uncover this predictive content by transforming the signal using various mathematical techniques.

11.2.3.2.5   Autoregressive Measures of Synchrony

A multichannel EEG model serves as the basis for the autoregressive synchrony measure. Each point in this model is defined as the linear product of the prior values from all chosen channels. This model's EEG fit is best demonstrated by the EEG time series for which it is best fitted. A better match is believed to happen in situations of greater synchronisation between EEG channels. If the post-ictal changes were not also taken into consideration, no significant pre-ictal changes were detected when this measure was used.

11.2.3.2.6   Short-Term Largest Lyapunov Exponent T-Index

Several EEG time-series channels were used to assess STLmax, and a so-called dynamical entrainment was discovered using the T-index, which is obtained from a paired t-test for mean comparison. The authors claim that their model has good predictive capability and a low percentage of incorrect predictions. According to its definition, a measure of "entrainment between important brain recording electrode locations" is the dynamical entrainment. These results, however, have not gone through class 1 validation. Furthermore, as was already indicated, the predictive power of the EEG time-series-derived Lyapunov exponents may be substantially undermined by finite-time statistical fluctuations and noise.

11.2.3.2.7   Phase Synchronisation

Phase synchronisation is the degree of phase lock between two signals over a certain time. This method has proven to be effective at differentiating transient synchronisation in intracranial EEG data. Measures of mean phase coherence reveal a pathologically elevated level of synchronisation during the interictal stage. Several brain synchronisation states have been found before an approaching seizure and in the vicinity of the epileptogenic zone [18].

11.3   PROPOSED METHODOLOGY

In this study, we predict the onset of the start of a seizure through EEG, pulse, and temperature data. These data are taken as input to the Arduino microcontroller. The microcontroller is prestored with the ML models. The ANN model is trained and tested for various data set values. Now, the sensors' new live data values are fed to

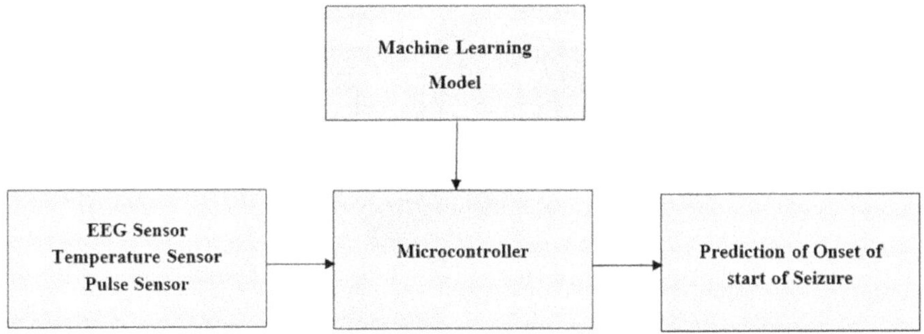

FIGURE 11.3 A diagram illustrating the ML model, showcasing its structure and components.

the ANN model in microcontroller. Based on the learning model, the ANN predicts the onset of seizure (refer Figure 11.3)

To implement the above block diagram of the proposed methodology, we require software as well as hardware. The details of these are as follows:

Prediction models require extensive data to be processed. In order to collect this data, there is a need for hardware components. Once the required data are in proper format, software is used to process this data. The data are input to the ML models based on which prediction is carried out.

11.3.1 Hardware Implementation

11.3.1.1 Sensors

This study used three types of sensors: EEG, pulse, and temperature.

11.3.1.1.1 EEG Sensors

EEG is an electrophysiological monitoring method to record the electrical activity of the brain. There are invasive as well as non-invasive EEG sensors. In the non-invasive, the electrodes are placed on the scalp. The invasive electrodes are used in electrocorticography. An ionic current generated in the neurons of the brain in turn generates voltage fluctuations that EEG measures. EEG records brain's spontaneous electrical activity through multiple electrodes, over a period.

Epilepsy shows changes in EEG signals. So, EEG is the most common method to diagnose epilepsy. It also aids in diagnosing coma, depth of anaesthesia, sleep disorders, encephalopathies, brain dead situations, tumours, strokes, and other brain disorders. Nowadays, other than EEG, imaging techniques like MRI and computed tomography (CT) are used for diagnosis. Yet, EEG remains a valuable tool for research and diagnosis.

EEG sensors are used to capture and record the brain signals (Figure 11.4a). Different kinds of electrodes like dry electrodes, capacitive electrodes, and nanomaterial-based electrodes are used to record EEG signals and each of them has different accuracy, offer comfort, and is practical.

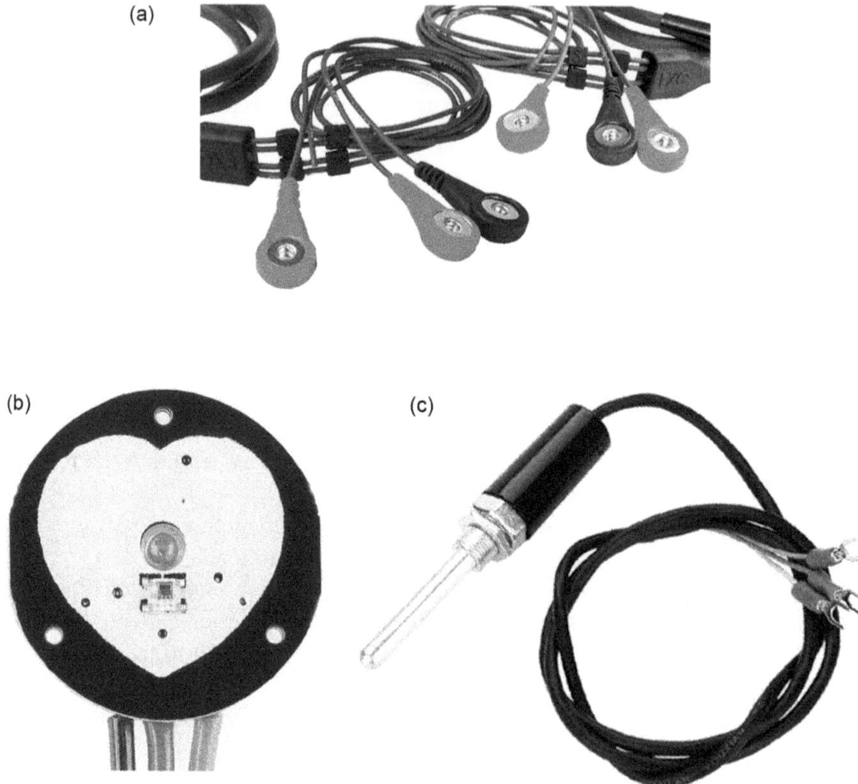

FIGURE 11.4   (a) EEG Sensors, (b) Pulse Sensor, and (c) Temperature sensor [24].

11.3.1.1.2 Pulse Sensors

Pulse sensor monitors volume change in the blood pumped by the heart. The pulse sensor is generally connected from the tip of finger to Arduino/micro controller or from the human ear to micro controller. It has 3 pins: Voltage Common Collector (Vcc), Ground (Gnd), and signal. The working principle is quite simple. The sensor has LED and light sensor connected as first layer. Another layer has the circuitry that takes care of amplification as well as noise cancellation. Pulse sensors are mostly used for sleep tracking, patient monitoring, health bands, and anxiety monitoring.

11.3.1.1.3 Temperature Sensors

Most of the sensors when connected form a part of a larger Internet of Things (IoT) system. One common sensor used these days in automation is temperature sensor. It is a device that detects and measures temperature. There is digital as well as analogue temperature sensors that convert temperature to electrical signals. There are contact and non-contact temperature sensors.

11.3.1.2 Microcontroller

Arduino Mega 2560 is a microcontroller board based on the ATmega2560 micro-controller, which is commonly used for prototyping and educational purposes. It has 54 digital input/output pins, 16 analogue inputs, 4 universal asynchronous receiver/transmitter (UARTs) (hardware serial ports), a 16 MHz crystal oscillator, universal serial bus (USB) connection, power jack, in-circuit serial programming (ICSP) header, and a reset button. The board's 256 KB of flash memory, 8 KB of SRAM, and 4 KB of electrically erasable programmable read-only memory (EEPROM) enable it to handle complex applications and store large amounts of data. It can be used with a variety of sensors and actuators to create interactive projects, including robots, home automation systems, and data-logging devices. The Arduino Mega 2560 is a versatile and powerful platform for electronics enthusiasts and professionals alike (Figure 11.5).

The programming of an Arduino Mega 2560 is done using IDE (Arduino Software). It also supports C-programming language. The board has a memory where the software is dumped, which is needed for interacting with the hardware.

11.3.1.3 Display

LCD is a type of flat panel display technology that uses the properties of liquid crystals to produce images. It features a thin layer of liquid crystals sandwiched between two transparent electrodes activated by an electric current. When the electrical charge is applied to the crystals, they react and change their orientation, which in turn alters the amount of light passing through them. This process causes the pixels on the screen to change colour and brightness, creating a high-quality image. LCDs are widely used in digital watches, calculators, televisions, computer monitors, and many other devices. They offer numerous advantages over traditional cathode ray tube (CRT) displays, including lower power consumption, a longer lifespan, better image quality, and a smaller size. Figure 11.6 shows a typical LCD.

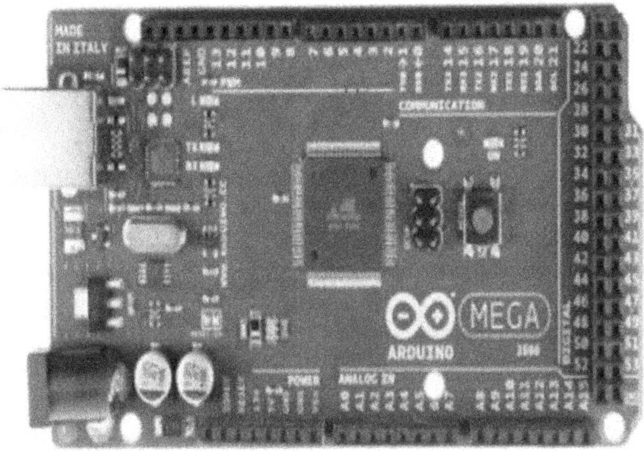

FIGURE 11.5 Arduino Mega 2560.

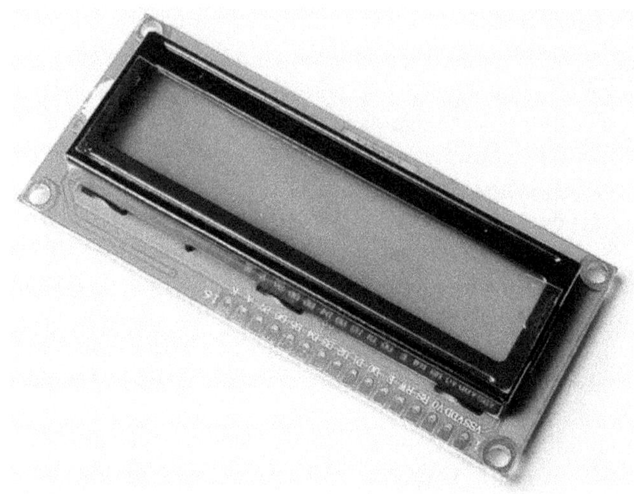

FIGURE 11.6   Display unit.

11.3.2   Software Implementation

Python and R-programming languages are used for scientific computing like data science, ML, large-scale data processing, predictive analytics, etc. Anaconda is a free and open-source distribution that is used by over 15 million users and includes more than 1,500 popular data science packages. It also includes a graphical user interface (GUI), Anaconda Navigator, as a graphical alternative to the command-line interface (CLI). In this study, NumPy, Pandas, Seaborn, Matplotlib, and comma separated values (CSV) were imported.

Data sets:

The data set had a total of 16,100 samples of 3,220 patients where 5 electrodes (0–4) were used to capture the EEG signals in 179 time slots (X1–X179). Table 11.2 shows the data set.

The data set was divided into 70% train data and 30% test data. The data set consisted of 9,200 samples of non-seizure data and 6,900 samples of seizure data (Figure 11.7).

The electrode measurement is in volts, which are further converted to unit variance. Standard Scaler is applied that removes the mean and scales each variable or feature extracted to unit variance (Figure 11.8).

Once trained with the data set, the model gives us 97%–100% accuracy. The prediction from the neural networks is displayed on the LCD screen connected to the Arduino. The LCD screen also displays the EEG values, temperature, and pulse rate per minute of the patient. This helps us in predicting the epileptic seizure beforehand and saving the person from the worst consequences.

Almost 100% accuracy can be reached by maintaining the data set with the proper, required data set. The current data set was designed according to the EEG sensors, using a known, proven data set that was obtained from Kaggle. We implemented

TABLE 11.2

EEG Values for Different Electrodes in Different Timeslots

	X1	X2	X3	X4	X5	X6	X7	X8	X9	X10	...
0	−203	−197	−194	−192	−194	−198	−197	−194	−193	−191	...
1	−563	−429	−294	−117	4	64	−77	−207	−298	−260	...
2	−33	−37	−48	−56	−69	88	−97	−97	−75	−51	...
3	−51	−60	−58	−53	−42	51	−62	−62	−67	−57	...
4	−592	−109	405	822	1095	1192	1149	1015	811	633	...

	X170	X171	X172	X173	X174	X175	X176	X177	X178
0	−110	−119	−125	−136	−141	−147	−150	−153	−154
1	242	247	271	300	−349	402	420	373	255
2	13	3	−12	−19	−15	−1	14	36	47
3	126	142	162	189	203	202	187	181	186
4	−427	−496	−502	−489	−462	−432	−417	−443	−509

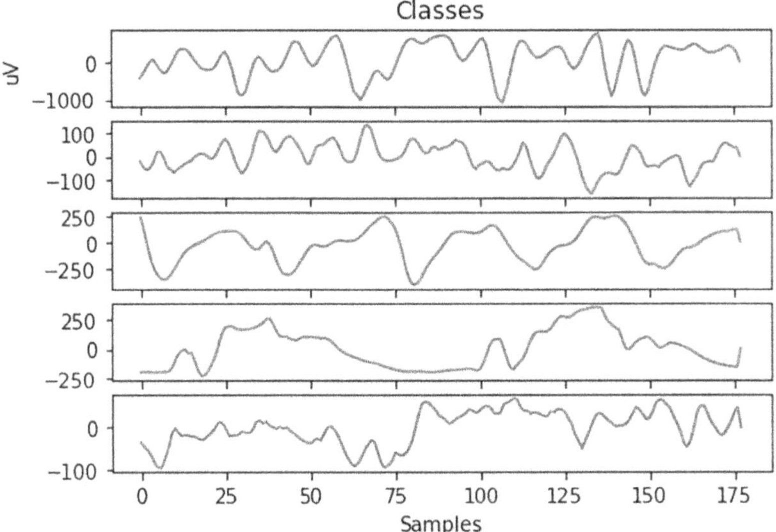

FIGURE 11.7   Split of seizure and non-seizure samples.

different ML algorithms like PCA, logistic regression (LR), SVMs, and KNN to compare the accuracy of prediction (Figure 11.9).

LR was implemented through the sklearn.linear model. The train:test ratio was varied between 80:20 and 70:30. An accuracy of 100% was achieved. Clf.score is the mean accuracy score or accuracy score. The accuracy of LR depends on how balanced the data set is and how much false positives and false negatives are accepted.

SVMs were implemented through sklearn.svm with accuracy of 100%, and KNN was implemented through sklearn.neighbours with accuracy of 97.97%. PCA was

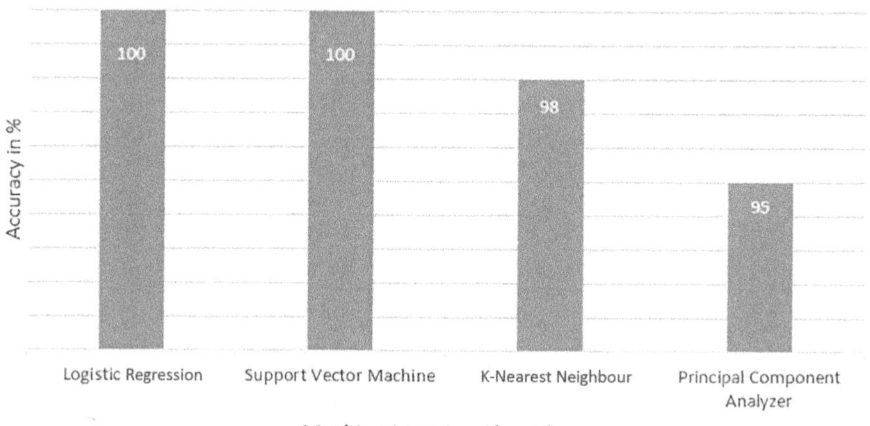

FIGURE 11.8　EEG signals from five electrodes.

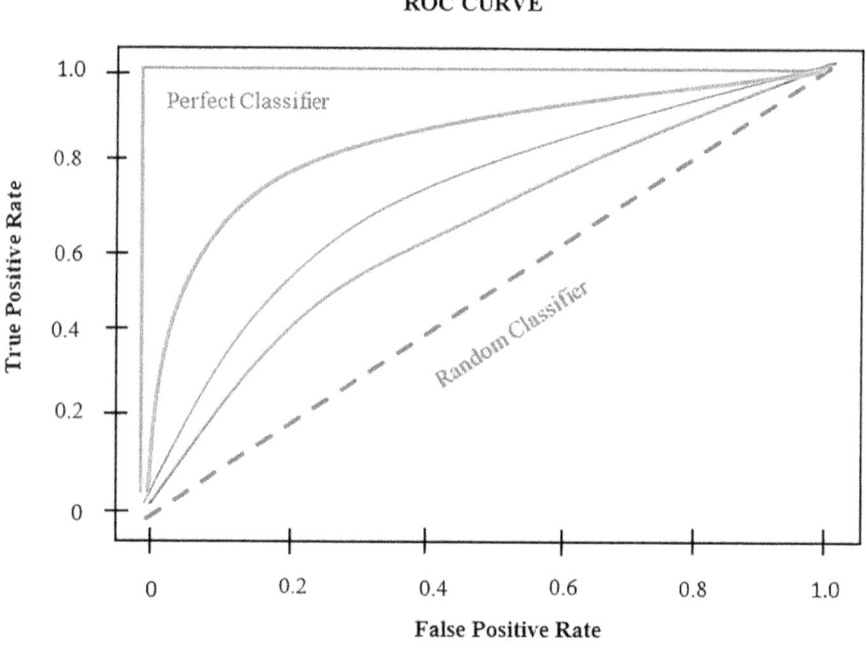

FIGURE 11.9　Comparison of different ML algorithms.

implemented using sklearn.decompose with an accuracy of 95%. It is an unsupervised learning technique for reducing the dimensionality of data. It minimises information loss (Figure 11.10).

The area under the receiving operator characteristic (ROC) curve, which considers both accuracy and sensitivity, is used to calculate correctness scores.

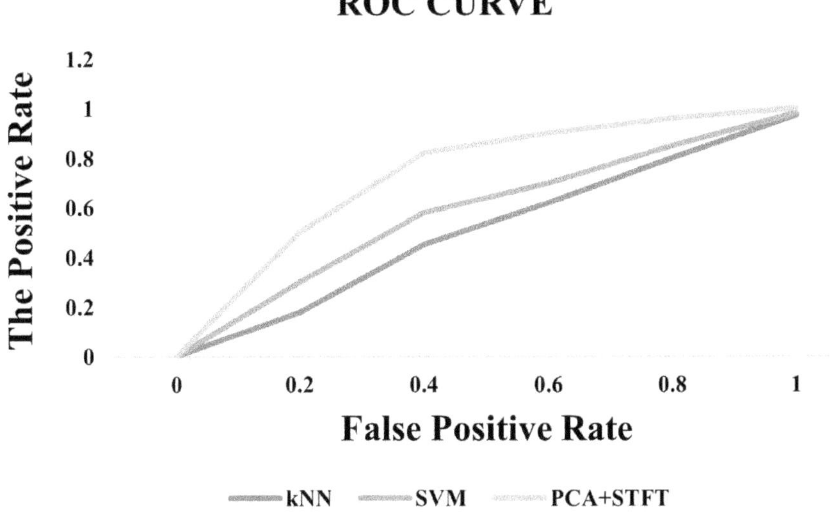

FIGURE 11.10   ROC curve.

In this study, we proposed a new methodology that analyses the Hurst exponent and fractal dimension plots of the EEG data to forecast the beginning of an epileptic seizure. Analysis results for 120 cases revealed that anticipating a seizure's beginning more than 25.76 seconds in advance is achievable. This innovative technology can be useful in the analysis and forecasting of other aberrant brain activity. Additionally, this approach can be utilised to create a portable, handheld device that records EEG signals from the patient's brain using a scalp electrode and then analyses the signal using the approach outlined in this study. Hence, the gadget can inform users prior to the commencement of a seizure, allowing them to take the appropriate prescription to stop the seizure.

The most accurate outcome was obtained using the short-time Fourier transform (STFT) feature extraction, PCA, dimensionality reduction and normalisation, and LR model prediction. Because STFT gave frequency and phase information on each window of each 10-minute EEG film, they were able to deliver robust, domain-specific feature extraction. An even more reliable categorisation feature was supplied by averaging the frequencies from the 30- and 60-second window sizes. Because STFT is a method that is especially used for time-series signal data, the features were domain specific.

Due to PCA's normalisation step, STFT paired with PCA produced findings that were superior to STFT alone. Because it eliminated important latent components of the data, reducing the dimension of the raw signals (carrying out PCA without STFT) decreased classification accuracy to below the baseline. Discrete wavelet transform (DWT) performed less well than STFT because it deleted important latent aspects of the EEG data, like PCA. Although LR outperformed SVM, we reasoned that this was because LR made the fewest previous assumptions about the data set. SVMs classify strictly and frequently fail when there is too much noise in the training data, whereas LR classifies with a probability depending on a data point's distance from the regression line. We want to modify the goal function to support higher variance in order to improve SVM performance and avoid overfitting.

Although KNN was a good starting point method, it was unable to correctly classify test data because it did not offer a sophisticated enough concept of distance between data points.

The first objective is to enhance the SVM model so that it outperforms LR. According to the literature we have studied, SVMs perform at their best, thus the Kaggle data set should not be an anomaly. It hopes to test out more sophisticated categorisation algorithms in the future, like neural networks and RF walks. For this study, neural networks were attempted to be applied, but we encountered severe over-fitting and a classification of non-seizure for almost all data points. To assess neural networks' potential with this data set, it would like to fine-tune them and run them on faster processors. In order to assess the efficacy of the RF model, a recently developed and rapidly gaining technique of categorisation, we will use EEG data to categorise it into two categories: positive and negative.

It is observed that the accuracy improves with various algorithms and it depends on the data set size. This study predicts the onset of the start of seizure so that it will help patients and caretakers to be well prepared during seizure attack. This will minimise the after-effects or impact of seizure-like falls.

REFERENCES

1. Casillo, S. M., D.D. Luy, and E. Goldschmidt. A history of the lobes of the brain. *World Neurosurgery*. 2020. **134**: pp. 353–360.
2. Kumar, J.S. and P. Bhuvaneswari. Analysis of electroencephalography (EEG) signals and its categorization: a study. *Procedia Engineering*. 2012. **38**: pp. 2525–2536.
3. Vezzani, A., R.S. Fujinami, H.S. White, P.M. Preux, I. Blumcke, J.W. Sander, and W. Loscher. Infections, inflammation and epilepsy. *Acta Neuropathologica*. 2016. **131**(2): pp. 211–234.
4. Lehnertz, K. Seizures/Seizure prediction. In *Encyclopedia of Basic Epilepsy Research*, ed. P.A. Schwartzkroin. Academic Press, Oxford, pp. 1314–1320, 2009.
5. Peng Peizhen, S.Y., Y. Lu, and W. Haikun. Seizure prediction in EEG signals using STFT and domain adaptation. *Frontiers in Neuroscience*. 2022. **15**: pp. 825434.
6. Koundinya, T.S., S.C. Gowda, and J.R. Munavalli. Dhanvantari: An intelligent diagnosis tool to classify malignant skin disease and lung conditions using deep learning. In *2022 6th International Conference on Computation System and Information Technology for Sustainable Solutions (CSITSS)*, Bangalore, India, 2022.
7. Koundinya, T.S., S. Brinda, S. Nikhil, M.A. Thelapurath, R. Chinmayee, and J.R. Munavalli. A comparative study of joint and bolt structures with and without edge detection using CNN. In *2023 International Conference for Advancement in Technology (ICONAT)*, Goa, India, 2023.
8. Neha, H. and J.R. Munavalli. Automated real-time locust management using artificial intelligence. *International Journal of Engineering Applied Sciences and Technology*, 2020. **5**(4): pp. 133–138.
9. Shashank Simha, B.K., M. Rahul, J.R. Munavalli, and P. Anand. Dual-language detection using machine learning. In *International Conference on VLSI, Communications and Computer Communication, Advances in Intelligent Systems and Technologies*. AnaPub Publications, Kenya, 2022.

10. Rachana R., A.N. Vaidya, B. Shreyas, and J.R. Munavalli. Predictive and comparative analysis for diabetes using machine learning algorithms. *International Journal of Advanced Science and Technology*. 2020. **29**(3): pp. 14407–14416.
11. Yağanoğlu, M. and C. Köse. Real-time detection of important sounds with a wearable vibration based device for hearing-impaired people. *Electronics*. 2018. **7**(4): p. 50.
12. Li, H. and L. Wu. EEG classification of normal and alcoholic by deep learning. *Brain Science*. 2022. **12**(6): p. 778.
13. Fawagreh, K., M.M. Gaber, and E. Elyan. Random forests: from early developments to recent advancements. *Systems Science & Control Engineering*. 2014. **2**(1): pp. 602–609.
14. Nahzat, S.Y. and M. Yağanoğlu. Classification of epileptic seizure dataset using different machine learning algorithms and PCA feature reduction technique. *Journal of Investigations on Engineering and Technology*. 2021. **4**(2): pp. 47–60.
15. Blanco, S., S. Kochen, O.A. Rosso, and P. Salgado. Applying time-frequency analysis to seizure EEG activity. *IEEE Engineering in Medicine and Biology Magazine*. 1997. **16**(1): pp. 64–71.
16. Carney, P.R., S. Myers, and J. D. Geyer. Seizure prediction: methods. *Epilepsy & Behavior*, 2011. **22**(Suppl 1): ppp. S94–101.
17. Esteller, R., J. Echauz, M. D'Alessandro, G. Worrell, S. Cranstoun, G. Vachtsevanos, and B. Litt. Continuous energy variation during the seizure cycle: towards an on-line accumulated energy. *Clinical Neurophysiology*. 2005. **116**(3): pp. 517–526.
18. Mormann, F., R.G. Andrzejak, C.E. Elger, and K. Lehnertz. Seizure prediction: the long and winding road. *Brain*. 2007. **130**(Pt 2): pp. 314–333.
19. Osorio, I., M.G. Frei, and S.B. Wilkinson. Real-time automated detection and quantitative analysis of seizures and short-term prediction of clinical onset. *Epilepsia*. 1998. **39**(6): pp. 615–627.
20. McSharry, P.E., L.A. Smith, and L. Tarassenko. Prediction of epileptic seizures: are nonlinear methods relevant? *Nature Medicine*. 2003. **9**(3): pp. 241–242.
21. Hajare, R. and S. Kadam. Comparative study analysis of practical EEG sensors in medical diagnoses. *Global Transitions Proceedings*. 2021. **2**(2): pp. 467–475.
22. Eickenscheidt, M., P. Schäfer, Y. Baslan, C. Schwarz, and T. Stieglitz. Highly porous platinum electrodes for dry ear-EEG measurements. *Sensors*. 2020. **20**(11): pp. 3176.

Index

O

ocular artifacts 150, 151
onset 6, 12, 245–247, 252, 254, 256, 257

P

Parkinson's disease 128
power spectral density 39, 63, 81, 192
pre-processing 98
principal component analysis 81, 103, 106, 152, 255

Q

quality 33, 34, 94, 130, 133, 143, 160, 167, 214,
    244, 259

R

radial basis function 136
recurrent neural networks 7, 9
root mean square 12, 134

S

schizophrenia 11–13
segmentation 161, 215
short time Fourier transform 63, 81, 106
signal processing 3, 19, 25, 61, 80, 89, 93,
    105, 221

sleep disorders 33–35
sleep stages 46
smote 222, 223, 230, 233
software 21, 22, 24, 36, 63, 132, 249, 257, 259
spatial filtering 48, 51
spectral EEG 5
spindle pattern 5
steady state visually evoked potential 60–63
support vector machine 39, 81, 106, 114, 136, 168

T

tonic 6, 244

U

unsupervised 7, 8, 11, 41, 255, 262

V

valence 19, 95, 97, 99, 101
validation 25, 79, 100, 138, 160, 194,
    253, 256

W

wavelet transformation 37, 39
windowing 63, 104, 113, 191

For Product Safety Concerns and Information please contact our EU
representative GPSR@taylorandfrancis.com
Taylor & Francis Verlag GmbH, Kaufingerstraße 24, 80331 München, Germany

www.ingramcontent.com/pod-product-compliance
Ingram Content Group UK Ltd.
Pitfield, Milton Keynes, MK11 3LW, UK
UKHW022316100726
473146UK00009B/504